E 26- 50

Preventing Dance Injuries:
An Interdisciplinary Perspective

Edited by:
RUTH SOLOMON
SANDRA C. MINTON
JOHN SOLOMON

Copyright © 1990

American Alliance for Health,
Physical Education, Recreation and Dance
1900 Association Drive
Reston, VA 22091

ISBN 0-88314-425-5

Preventing Dance Injuries:

An Interdisciplinary Perspective

Dedication

To Jean Erdman, who taught me
to teach so that the individual
artist in each of us could emerge
without damage to the body or psyche.

R.S.

Contents

About The Editors

Ruth Solomon has been a distinguished performer and choreographer in the modern dance idiom for many years. She is also a dance educator of note, having directed the dance program at the University of California, Santa Cruz since 1970. Her highly successful teaching technique has been documented in an hour-long video, "Anatomy as a Master Image in Training Dancers" (1988). Other aspects of Ms. Solomon's multi-faceted career are represented by her publications. Her articles on dance have appeared in all major periodicals in the field, and more recently her research in dance medicine has produced articles in such medical journals as *The Physician and Sportsmedicine* and *The Journal of Bone and Joint Surgery*, and in the ground-breaking book, *Dance Medicine: A Comprehensive Guide (1987)*.

Sandra Cerny Minton, Ph.D., is coordinator of the Dance Program at the University of Northern Colorado. From 1985-87 she was publications director for the National Dance Association. Books she has authored include *Modern Dance: Body and Mind; Choreography: A Basic Approach Using Improvisation;* and *Body and Self: Partners in Movement*. Dr. Minton pursued kinesiology as an area of emphasis in her doctoral work, and she currently does workshops which develop understanding of body and self.

John Solomon, Ph.D., is a freelance editor.

Contributors

Stephen P. Baitch, P.T., is coordinator of the foot and biomechanics program, Sports Medicine Center, Union Memorial Hospital, Baltimore, MD, and has a private physical therapy practice in Lutherville, MD, specializing in treatment of foot-related problems. He is a frequent presenter on lower extremity biomechanics and foot related abnormalities at various meetings at both national and local levels.

Robin Chmelar, M.S., is a former dancer with Repertory Dance Theatre, has her Master's in Sports Medicine/Exercise Physiology, and is presently clinical, medico-legal, and insurance Research Specialist for Cybex, which designs and manufactures musculoskeletal rehabilitation equipment. She also serves as program consultant for Sports Medicine & Rehabilitation Therapy in Huntington, NY. Her research on dancers has appeared in *The Physician and Sportsmedicine, Journal of Orthopaedic and Sports Physical Therapy, Dance Research Journal,* and *Medical Problems of Performing Artists.*

Karen Clippinger-Robertson, M.S.P.E., is kinesiologist at Seattle Sports Medicine and a consultant to Pacific Northwest Ballet. She has presented over 300 lectures/workshops throughout the United States and in Canada and Japan at such events as the 1984 Olympic Scientific Congress, 1986 Congress on Research in Dance, American College of Sports Medicine, and American College Dance Festival. Her dance publications include chapters and articles on principles of dance training, increasing range of motion, patellofemoral pain, and injury prevention.

Sally Sevey Fitt, Ed.D., is a professor of Modern Dance at the University of Utah, where she has taught since 1976. She is the author of *Dance Kinesiology* (Schirmer Books, 1988), and co-author with Robin Chmelar of a soon to be released book, *Dancing at Your Peak: Diet.*

James G. Garrick, M.D., is an orthopedic surgeon and currently the director of the Center for Sports Medicine at Saint Francis Memorial Hospital in San Francisco. He has long had a special interest in dance and, with Patrice Whiteside, founded a DanceMedicine division in

1983, designed especially for the treatment and rehabilitation of dance-related injuries. He is the orthopedic consultant for the San Francisco Ballet, Oakland Ballet, many modern and jazz companies, and physician for visiting ballet companies such as the Bolshoi, the Joffrey, and the American Ballet Theatre. Dr. Garrick has written a number of books, the latest of which is *Be Your Own Personal Trainer*.

Steven R. Kravitz, D.P.M., is assistant professor in the Department of Orthopedics, Pennsylvania College of Podiatric Medicine. He is associated with numerous podiatric societies, and serves as consultant to the Pennsylvania Ballet Company and the School of Dance at Philadelphia University of the Performing Arts. His most recent publications are, "The Mechanics of Dance and Dance-Related Injuries" (*Sports Medicine of the Lower Extremity*, 1989) and "The Dancer's Foot" (*Current Therapy in Podiatric Surgery*, 1989).

Sandra Kay Lauffenburger, B.Ed., M.Sc., C.M.A., is a certified movement analyst based in Houston, TX. She specializes in sports, dance, public fitness, athletics, and rehabilitation. Her work focuses on the efficient use of the body for improved performance, a prolonged and active movement career, and increased mental, physical, and spiritual well-being. She presents workshops throughout the United States, Asia, and Australia, and has authored numerous articles on the application of Laban Movement Analysis to movement issues.

Lyle J. Micheli, M.D., is assistant clinical professor of Orthopaedic Surgery, Harvard Medical School, and director of the Division of Sports Medicine at Children's Hospital, Boston, MA. He is an associate editor of *Medicine and Science in Sports and Exercise*, and serves on the Editorial Board of *Kinesiology and Medicine for Dance*. For the last 12 years he has been attending physician to the Boston Ballet and the School of the Boston Ballet, and he is the current president of the American College of Sports Medicine.

Richard N. Norris, M.D., is a specialist in Physical Medicine and Rehabilitation. He is director of the Performing Arts Medicine Clinic in Braintree, MA, and clinical assistant professor at Boston University School of Medicine. He also serves on the Board of Directors of the Performing Arts Medicine Association, and has studied various forms of dance for 14 years.

Raymond Novaco, Ph.D., is associate professor, Program in Social Ecology, at the University of California, Irvine. His research has focused on the correlations of mind, environment, and stress, and especially on the therapeutic regulation of anger. He serves on the editorial boards of *Cognitive Therapy and Research* and the *American Journal of Community Psychology*.

Janice Gudde Plastino, Ph.D., is a professional performer and choreographer of ballet, opera, musicals, and modern dance. She co-directed Penrod Plastino Movement Theater, a modern dance company, for 12 years. Her publications include numerous articles and the book (with James Penrod), *The Dancer Prepares*. She is professor of Dance at the University of California, Irvine, and heads the Dance Medicine/Science program on that campus.

Ralph K. Requa, M.S.P.H., is an epidemiologist and currently the research director of the Center for Sports Medicine at Saint Francis Memorial Hospital in San Francisco. He has co-authored numerous articles concerning the epidemiology of injuries in sports ranging from aerobic dance to wrestling.

Allan J. Ryan, M.D., practiced general surgery at the Meriden Hospital, Connecticut, and served as chairman of the Department of Rehabilitation and athletic teams physician at the University of Wisconsin-Madison. Former editor-in-chief of *The Physician and Sportsmedicine*, he is now director of Sports Medicine Enterprises in Minneapolis, Minnesota. His recent publications include *Dance Medicine: A Comprehensive Guide* (1987), and *The Dancer's Complete Guide to Health Care and a Long Career* (1988).

Marie Schafle, M.D., is a primary care sports physician at the Center for Sports Medicine at Saint Francis Memorial Hospital in San Francisco. In 1986, after practicing emergency medicine for almost 10 years, Dr. Schafle elected to follow a long-time interest in sports medicine by accepting a fellowship at Michigan State University, where she had the opportunity to start a dance medicine program. She is currently a physician for the San Francisco Ballet.

Ruth Solomon is professor of Theater Arts and director of the Dance Theater Program at the University of California, Santa Cruz. Her approach to teaching has recently been documented in an hour-long video, "Anatomy as a Master Image in Training Dancers" (1988). She is widely published in the field of dance medicine.

Robert E. Stephens, Ph.D., is the director of Sports Medicine and associate professor of Anatomy at the University of Health Sciences Medical School in Kansas City, MO. He is also the Dance Medicine

Advisor for *Shape* magazine and the co-author of *Dance Medicine: A Comprehensive Guide* (1987) and *The Dancer's Complete Guide to Health Care and a Long Career* (1988).

Carol C. Teitz, M.D., is an orthopedic surgeon who chairs the Division of Sports Medicine at the University of Washington. She studied dance for 11 years prior to entering the School of Medicine at Yale University. She has served as a faculty member of Scientific Aspects of the Art of Dance, Northwest University Dance Conference, Congress on Research in Dance, International Dance Exercise Association, and the dance program of the 1984 Olympic Scientific Congress. Her work related to dancers' musculoskeletal problems has been published in *Foot and Ankle, JOPERD, Pediatric Clinics of North America,* and *The Dancer as Athlete.*

Elly Trepman, M.D., is a clinical fellow in Orthopaedic Surgery, Harvard Medical School, and Fellow in Sports Medicine, Children's Hospital, Boston.

Arleen Walaszek, P.T., is staff physical therapist, Children's Hospital, Boston, and physical therapist to the Boston Ballet Company.

Cover Design: Mary Cosenza, University of California, Santa Cruz
Cover Photography: Don Fukuda, University of California, Santa Cruz

Introduction

Dance medicine is in some respects an outgrowth, or sub-set, of sports medicine. Many of the same doctors and other professionals in the health sciences who have studied and ministered to the needs of athletes for decades have more recently included dancers in their purview. Prestigious medical journals now find room in their pages for research in dance as well as sports. The national convention of the American College of Sports Medicine has begun to include dance-oriented presentations in its agenda. Like professional sports teams, some larger dance companies have formed affiliations with their own physicians. Dance medicine will in all likelihood never rival its better established and more attractive sister in terms of either social or financial allure, yet it has undeniably become a presence in its own right.

The common element is, of course, that both sports and dance require endless physical training in order to achieve peak performance, and culminate in concentrated, often risk-involving expenditures of physical energy. Thus, the bodies of dancers and athletes tend to be exposed to far greater stress than are those of the population at large. This unfortunately produces injury with greater frequency than the norm, calling for an unusual amount of medical attention. Similarly, those who study the workings of the body from a scientific point of view—exercise physiologists, biomechanists, kinesiologists, etc.—find in the dancer, like the athlete, a condensed subject for their investigations. The dancer is also of special interest to those involved through our schools in sports psychology and physical education.

For their part, today's dancers have clearly benefited in many ways from this new attention. More readily than ever before they find sympathetic, appropriate care for their medical needs; they are training by means that are both safer and more efficient; they have available to them a greater body of knowledge, and are therefore better able to take care of themselves. Further, they have begun to return the favor: having absorbed and made use of information for promoting healthy practice of the art form, they are utilizing their unique perspectives as performers and teachers to make their own contributions. Increasingly, dancers are assuming a symbiotic relationship with those in the medical and research sciences who supervise their well-being.

This book illustrates the richly interdisciplinary nature of dance medicine as an emerging field of inquiry. While focusing on the specific issue of how to prevent injuries in dance, it draws upon the expertise of authors in various branches of medicine, exercise physiology, kinesiology, psychology, physical education, dance education, and the body therapies. Thus, in addition to tapping into a tremendous wealth of specific information, it also provides a general overview of the multiple perspectives from which its subject might be considered.

A microcosmic example of how this interdisciplinary approach works can be seen in the chapters of this book which deal with the dancer's foot and ankle. Podiatrist, Steven Kravitz takes a biomechanical look at the anatomy of the region to explain how its most common malalignment, pronation, can cause problems when subjected to the wear and tear imposed by dance training. Professor Sally Fitt, a university-based kinesiologist, discusses, with the use of illustrated exercises, how to strengthen the unit to ward off injury. Dr. Richard Norris, a specialist in rehabilitative medicine, explains in some clinical detail how the most common foot and ankle injuries happen, what they entail, and how they are dealt with. Accumulatively, these chapters provide both an excellent anatomical and theoretical orientation to the region, and various indications of how this knowledge can be put to use.

Precisely because it is interdisciplinary, the material presented here raises questions of audience that have been central to the editorial process: To whom, exactly, is this book addressed? How much knowledge of medicine/science can they be expected to have? What are their main concerns likely to be? Our solution to these vexing questions has been essentially to invite in as contributors authors who are known to be in the forefront of their respective fields, and to publish without major emendation what they have provided. Happily, the result is far more than a something-for-everyone potpourri. In one chapter after another ideas, observations and images recur, each author making use of what is clearly becoming a shared body of knowledge to further his/her ends. What this felicitous continuity serves to do, we feel, is establish baselines for the current state of the art. It also proves (as is being demonstrated at the national conventions of various organizations these days) that medical people and dancers *do* share in common enough information and language to be able to interest one another. Nonetheless, we have included glossaries of medical and dance terms at the end of this volume to aid in the communication process.

The book is divided into four parts. Part One is given over entirely to a huge survey of injury patterns in three different dance forms. Hence, it provides an overview for all that follows. The second section deals with anatomy. The foot, knee, hip, and spine are discussed in detail, as they represent the areas most vunerable to injury in all dance forms. Part Three looks at injury prevention through the use of a variety of approaches, including strengthening, stretching, stress reduction, and dance technique classes based on anatomical imaging. Finally, the book concludes with two chapters on practical matters: how to find a physician who is sympathetic to dancers' needs, and dealing with insurance liability and worker's compensation in injuries related to dance.

Dance medicine is a new field, and its importance should not be exaggerated. For most doctors it will always represent a marginal aspect of their practice. Many dancers would, frankly, prefer to ignore it; the risk of injury is simply something one lives with in the pursuit of an aesthetic goal. Those concerned with the science of body mechanics are likely to find greater inducements for the study of sports. Nevertheless, as this book demonstrates, dance medicine has captured the attention of first rate minds in all these fields (and more), so its future appears bright.

The Editors

Acknowledgments

The editors wish to thank the following individuals for their help in preparing this manuscript for publication: T.E. Baldwin, M.D., Family Physicians, and Keith Thompson, M.D., Surgeon, Greeley, Colorado; George Sage, Ed.D., Department of Kinesiology, Dan Libera, M.S., Head Athletic Trainer, Dave Stotlar, Ed.D., Department of Physical Education and Dance, and William Hudspeth, Ph.D., Department of Psychology, University of Northern Colorado. Additional thanks go to Lynne Fox, M.L.S., and Kathy Earle, M.L.S., both of the Michener Library, the University of Northern Colorado, and to Margaret McCray and Rebecca Fuson of the University of California, Santa Cruz.

PART I:

Survey

1

A Comparison of Patterns of Injury in Ballet, Modern, and Aerobic Dance

Marie Schafle, M.D.
Ralph K. Requa, M.S.P.H.
James G. Garrick, M.D.

Introduction

Although ballet, modern, and aerobic dance forms are distinctly different with regard to the actual tasks performed, they have much in common, and their similarities tend to distinguish them from other athletic-type activities. For example, the fact that these activities are "choreographed" sets them apart from team sports, which abound with unexpected, and perhaps injurious situations. Also, unlike many athletic endeavors, dance is commonly a year-round activity, with no "off season" to provide rest and rehabilitation. It is quite natural, then, to look for injury patterns that are unique to dance.

1

Several studies have addressed injury patterns within a single dance form.[1, 2, 3] Solomon and Micheli related injury patterns to variations in different modern dance techniques.[4] It is useful to compare injury patterns among dance forms, but large numbers of dance patients are required for the comparisons to be reliable.

Almost 3,500 dance injuries were examined and treated at the Center for Sports Medicine during the first eight and one-half years of its operation (through April 1988). The population of dancers utilizing the Center includes ballet, modern, and aerobic dancers, as well as a potpourri of other dance styles from ethnic and jazz to square and ballroom dancing. Participants range in skill and intensity from professionals of the very highest caliber to those engaging in dance more as an athletic or recreational activity. Dance medicine alone has become such a large part of the practice that a separate section was established in 1984 for the diagnosis and rehabilitation of injured dancers. Although there is a substantial variety of dance activities represented, here we review only the dance injuries falling into ballet, modern, or aerobic dance categories (93 percent of all our dance injuries).

As with other areas of sports medicine, it seems likely that increasingly more dancers are seeking sports-oriented medical care. This may appear true in our case in part because of our interest in dance and our involvement with several professional dance companies. As important, however, is what we see as an increasing willingness on the part of athletes of all persuasions to seek specialized care for their athletic-related concerns.

While most of the actual injuries associated with dance are not unlike those seen in other athletic activities, the frequency with which certain problems occur does indeed appear to reflect the tasks performed in each of these dance forms. This descriptive analysis of the injuries seen emanating from ballet, modern, and aerobic dance styles is an attempt to compare and characterize the patterns of musculoskeletal problems of each of these activities.

Method

The computerized records of all dance injuries that presented to a sports and dance medicine facility over the eight and one-half year period from January 1979 through April 1988 were reviewed. All patients were examined by at least one of the nine physicians practicing full-time in the facility. Diagnostic codes, uniform among the physicians, were assigned to each injury. These consisted of two parts: the pathology, or type of injury, and the anatomy, or location of injury. During the last six years of data collection, the injuries were additionally coded as being either the result of a single specific incident or rather having a more gradual—and less well defined—onset. The "overuse" designation was employed as a category of pathology for these latter injuries, such as plantar fasciitis, tendinitis, or "chondromalacia" of the patella.

An injury was defined as a medical condition resulting from dance activity that prompted the patient to seek formal medical care. Due to the retrospective nature of the study no control group was available, nor was it feasible to estimate the population at risk in any of these activities. Hence, *rates* of injury are unavailable from these data. Without rates it is not possible to estimate what the risk of sustaining a particular injury might be, nor can we say that an injury occurs more often in one dance form than another. What *can* be compared is how common an injury type or category is within the injuries presenting from that dance form compared to another. This not only reflects to a significant extent the clinical reality that patients from the various dance forms present, but also suggests something of the nature and intensity of the activities involved.

Results

During the period of study, 3,251 dance related injuries were evaluated. Fifty-five percent occurred in ballet, 15% in modern, and 30% in aerobic dance. Seventy-nine percent of the injuries occurred to females. Seventy-six percent of the ballet, 80% of the modern, and 86% of the aerobic injuries were to females.

Figure 1.1 shows the percent of injuries within each dance form by age group. The greatest proportion of ballet injuries was reported in the 13 to 18 year-old group, whereas modern and aerobic dance injuries were most often seen in the 26 to 39 year-old group. There were few in the 12 and under age group with the exception of ballet. Altogether, 43% of the ballet injuries occurred in the 18 and younger group. In contrast, less than 1% of the aerobic injuries were seen in that age group. Aerobic dance tended to have much more representation in the older groups compared to ballet.

Figure 1.2 illustrates the relationship of dance form to anatomic location of injury. In all groups, the knee was the most often affected area, with about one-third of the modern and aerobic injuries and a little more than one-fifth of the ballet injuries (21%). In all groups, the foot/toe area was the next most frequent site of injury. For the ballet dancers, foot and toe injuries were virtually as common as knee injuries. Ankle injuries were third for ballet and modern with 16 and 13%, but were less common among aerobic dancers (7%). The spine, hip/

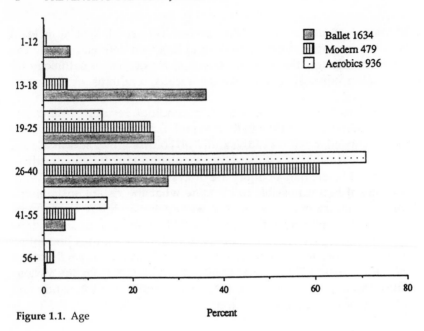

Figure 1.1. Age

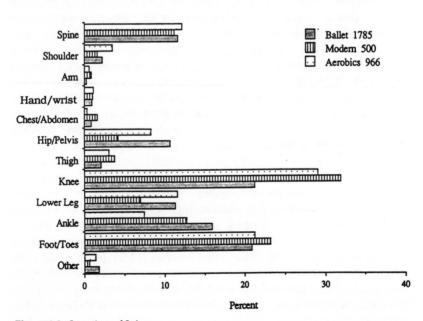

Figure 1.2. Location of Injury

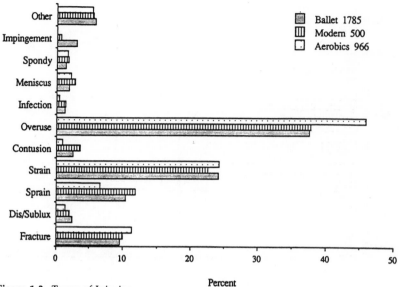

Figure 1.3. Types of Injuries

Percent

pelvis and lower leg seemed to fall generally in the 8-12% range for all three forms (although modern is lower at the hip/pelvis).

Figure 1.3 shows the distribution of types of injuries reported for each dance form. Fractures, the majority of which were stress fractures, were reported by about 10% of each form. Strains were very common and were reported to make up approximately one-quarter (23%-24%) for all three dance forms. Overuse injury was the most common category for all groups; of the three, aerobic dance had the highest proportion of injury in this category. Strains were of both the acute and overuse varieties, with the latter predominating.

Comparing types of injury at specific anatomic locations showed some variation among forms, as illustrated by Figures 1.4-1.9.

We found that most of the spine injuries (70-76%) occurred to the lumbar area. As seen in Figure 1.4, strains were very common; they made up 67, 60, and 64% of the spine injuries for ballet, modern, and aerobic dance, respectively. Spondylolistheses ("Spondy") constituted 12 to 17% of the spine injuries.

Overuse problems made up 42% of the ballet and about one-third of the modern and aerobic hip injuries (Figure 1.5). Strains were the most common type of injury at the hip and formed almost equal proportions in all groups, between 54 and 58%.

Among knee injuries, overuse problems were by far the most common: about two-thirds of the ballet and modern, and 80% of the

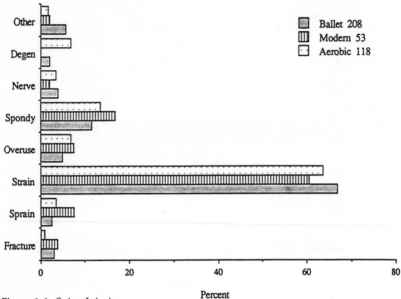

Figure 1.4. Spine Injuries

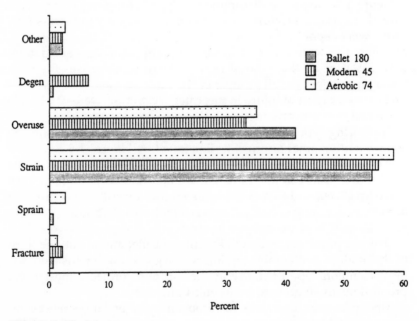

Figure 1.5. Hip Injuries

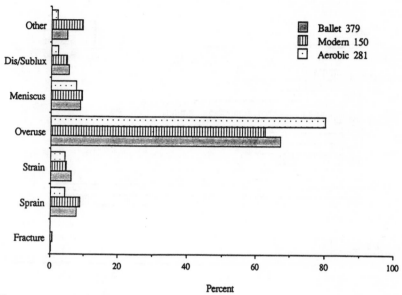

Figure 1.6. Knee Injuries

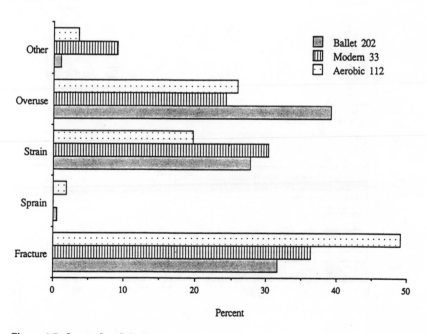

Figure 1.7. Lower Leg Injuries

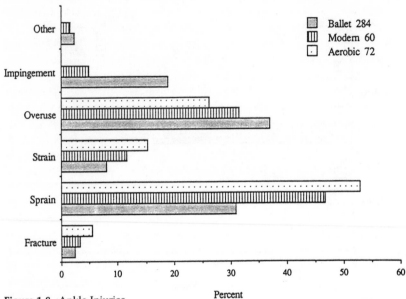

Figure 1.8. Ankle Injuries

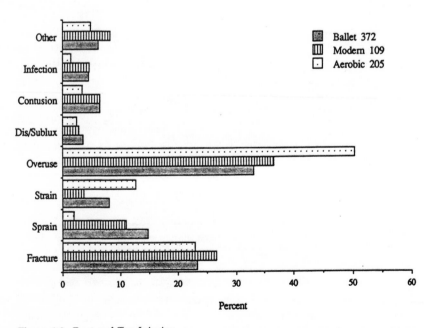

Figure 1.9. Foot and Toe Injuries

aerobic dance injuries were of the overuse variety (Figure 1.6). The remaining categories of injury were relatively uncommon.

Almost one-half of the aerobic dancers' injuries to the lower leg were fractures, compared to about one-third each for ballet and modern dance (Figure 1.7). Strains were about 30% of the injuries for ballet and modern dance and about 20% of the aerobic dancers' injuries. Overuse injuries were about one-quarter of the modern and aerobic and almost 40% for the ballet dance injuries.

About half of the ankle injuries were sprains for aerobics and modern dance; for ballet, overuse injuries outnumbered sprains (Figure 1.8). Overuse injuries were also common with between 26-37% of the injuries at the ankle. Ballet dancers had the highest percent of ankle impingement; almost one in five ankle injuries were so classified, compared to 5% of the modern and none of the aerobic dancers' ankle injuries. Overuse injuries were common among foot and toe injuries (Figure 1.9). Aerobic dancers had the highest proportion, one-half; the other forms had between 33% and 37%. Fractures were also common and accounted for similar proportions in each form, 23% to 27%. Ballet and modern dancers had the higher percentages of sprains (15% and 13%), aerobic dancers the highest percentage of strains (13%).

Discussion

There are obvious differences between these three dance categories, and even within a single form, where great uniformity might be expected, variations between schools or approaches create differences in the patterns of injury.[4] The choreography practiced in aerobics is clearly different from that of ballet and modern dance. Further, aerobic dance is largely a recreational or fitness activity, as opposed to the discipline and precision of the more traditional dance forms. For these reasons, one might anticipate that aerobic dance would have an injury pattern that differed markedly from the others. Yet this did not seem to occur. One is struck by the overall similarity among categories, rather than by the differences between them.

Age

The distribution of injury by age within dance form did vary; a much higher proportion of ballet injuries were in the adolescent and pediatric age groups, while most injuries in modern and aerobic dance involved mature dancers. Quite likely this reflects the age distribution of participants in the three dance forms.

Thirty-seven percent of the ballet injuries occurred in the 13 to 18 year-old group. These are young dancers who are beginning to participate seriously, to take more classes per week, and to make concerted efforts to increase turnout and perfect technique. This is also the age when *pointe* classes begin, with all the demands for strength and balance which are characteristic of work *en pointe*. Twenty-five percent of the ballet injuries occurred in the 19 to 25 year-old group, which included the professional dance population. The professional dancer is not only subject to long hours of dancing (often 6-8 hours a day, 6 days a week), but also to varying demands of choreographers, from highly classical to ultra-modern techniques. Frequent changes from one choreographic style to another can be problematic, and in our experience are as likely to produce injury as is an abrupt change in training regimen in any sport.

In modern and aerobic dance most injuries occurred in the 26 to 39 year-old group, where in all likelihood most participation also occurs. Modern dancers tend either to begin dancing later in life than ballet dancers or to change from ballet to modern in their mid-20s. Participants in aerobic dance include many women who, for one reason or another, have not previously been involved in other forms of dance and exercise. These women, in their 20s and 30s, have embraced aerobic dance as a satisfying form of exercise and perhaps as an outlet for the desire to dance.

Overuse Injuries

These dance forms have in common several factors that tend to contribute to overuse injuries. First, there is a requirement—or predilection—for repetitive movement in ballet and modern dance as a means of perfecting a certain skill, and in aerobic dance as a method of working a particular muscle group to exhaustion. Second, delays of weeks or months between onset of symptoms and medical treatment were common, and may have converted acute problems into overuse injuries. In some instances the delay was caused by an inability to pay for care, but often the insidious onset of symptoms resulted in the dancer ignoring the problem until there was finally a perceptible loss of function. Not surprisingly, injuries occurred almost exclusively to the lower extremity, with overuse problems predominating. The differences in the patterns observed by anatomic area should be considered primarily useful for generating discussion, since most comments about possible reasons for the differences are *post hoc* and therefore speculative.

Overuse injuries were present in every anatomic location. Those regions with higher proportions of acute injuries (sprains, fractures) included the ankle, spine, lower leg, and foot/toes, although in the case of both the leg and the foot/toes many injuries in the fracture category were gradual and stress-related, and therefore more overuse than acute. About one-third of the hip injuries were from overuse, as compared to knees with about two-thirds overuse injuries.

Within specific anatomic areas a few differences in overuse injuries between dance forms were seen. Aerobic dancers' knee injuries had the highest proportion of overuse problems, and they also had the highest percent of leg injuries classified as fractures. The repetitive calisthenic-style jumping that is a part of most aerobic programs may play a role here. Ballet dancers had proportionally fewer fractures and the largest proportion of overuse problems of the leg.

Anatomic Area

The anatomic areas injured provided the most obvious associations with the involved dance forms. In all forms, the knee was most often injured. This is probably the result of several factors. First, most active people regard an injured knee as serious, perhaps because of media attention devoted to many professional athletes' knee injuries. Thus the relatively high proportions of knee injuries seen in these dancers may be, in part, a reflection of heightened concern for this anatomic region. However, biomechanical nuances common to other athletic activities appear to exist in the dance world as well. In all three dance forms vigorous maneuvers are performed from a "turned out" position. In ballet, many dancers will attempt to "force" turnout. Forcing turnout often involves external rotation from the knee distally. The resulting lateral displacement of the patellar tendon insertion increases compression of the lateral patellar facet, leading to what is sometimes referred to as "chondromalacia" of the patella. This is especially likely to occur in dancers who do not have a great degree of natural turnout (external rotation) at the hips.

Modern dancers may also increase the possibility of injury by performing maneuvers in which the dancer is kneeling or dropping onto the knees, although the extent may vary according to the modern style.[4] If, as is the case for a surprising number of dancers, the quadriceps muscles lack flexibility, the probability of knee injury might be expected to increase.

Aerobic classes are often taught by instructors who have had some ballet training, who may inadvertently teach in a *turned out* position. In an effort to emulate their instructors, students may place their feet in a turned out position as well, but fail to externally rotate their thigh/ knees. Even if the students are instructed to avoid this practice, the custom of leading from the front of the class combined with the reality of often large classes makes it almost impossible for even the sophisticated instructor to check students individually. Repeating these movements incorrectly would place the adult aerobic dancer at risk for injuries identical to those incurred by adolescent ballet dancers who force turnout.

Leg injuries, common in ballet and aerobic dancers, were usually of the overuse variety; even the fractures were most often not acute. Although the term *overuse* would encourage one to assume that the rate of occurrence of these injuries would increase dramatically with increasing exposure time, at least one study of aerobics has found this to be untrue.[1] Garrick found that injuries per hour of exposure (exercise) decreased with increasing participation. Even though this meant additional risk for an average individual as his or her exposure increased, the rate of increase was not linear, making the additional hours less hazardous on a per hour basis. This phenomenon may have been due to the "training effect" of regular, consistent participation. Experience with technique may also provide a degree of protection from injury in those exercising more often.

Modern dancers had the lowest percent of lower leg injuries. If this difference reflects something real, perhaps it is the slightly less repetitive and routinized nature of the movements in modern dance. If instead this represents underreporting of the injury, perhaps the background of university training that many modern dancers have may in some part predispose them to manage this type of injury themselves, more so than they would an injury to the knee or ankle. Modern dancers may also feel somewhat unappreciated and misunderstood by the traditional medical community due to the relative lack of acquaintance that most physicians have with modern dance as compared to ballet. This is speculation, of course; still, even "dance medicine" is unfortunately less sophisticated and experienced in dealing with modern dancers than with ballet and aerobic dancers.

Ankle, foot, and toe injuries were common among the ballet and modern dancers. Together, they are in the neighborhood of the knee in frequency of injury. Aerobic dancers had similar proportions of foot and toe injuries, but fewer to the ankle. Ballet and modern dance require a far more strenuous use of the foot than does aerobic dance. *Pointe* in ballet, and *demi-pointe* and aerial movements with landings on one foot in both ballet and modern dance, are ubiquitous. In aerobic dance, of course, no such use of the foot is required. Although, because of their training, ballet and modern dancers' feet are quite strong and flexible, the demands made on those same feet are often more than the dancers can tolerate. Impingements at the ankle, and inflammations, strains, and sprains at both the ankle and foot/toe area, result.

Another major difference between aerobics, ballet, and modern dance is the footwear worn in each. The design of aerobic dance shoes is heavily influenced by the perceived need to protect and cushion the foot.[5] Not so in ballet and modern dance, where footwear serves little protective function and in many instances is not even worn. Whether the absence of any protective footwear is responsible in part for the injury patterns seen in modern dance and ballet is difficult to determine.

While there are major differences in how the feet are used in the various dance forms, except for the impingement problems seen in ballet, the proportions of pathologies within each dance form are not dramatically dissimilar. One tends to think of ballet and modern dance movement as composed of repetitive, rehearsed elements, likely to be more precise and controlled than those in the less structured, recreational setting of the aerobic dance studio. While this may well be so, aerobic dance led in both the percentages of overuse (50%) and strain (13%) injuries to the feet, and trailed in percent of sprains, 2 percent vs 15 percent and 11 percent for ballet and modern, respectively.

Comments

Dancers are a unique group among the athletic population, combining as they do elements of both art and exercise. The physician, trainer, therapist, or instructor who cares for the injured dancer requires a thorough knowledge of the demands of the dance form both to fully appreciate the problem and to communicate effectively with the dancer. Understanding the exact nature of the injury, while critical, is only the initial step in its proper management. Because so many problems in dance are either partly or wholly related to overuse, analyzing the techniques responsible and altering them where feasible are essential steps in preventing recurrence of injury. Needless to say, any suggested alterations involving a dancer's program, particularly to the advanced dancer, should be discussed thoroughly with his or her teacher or company artistic director.

Tailoring the dance class to allow the injured dancer to continue to dance "around the injury" can provide enormous psychological support as well as effective maintenance conditioning. Ballet dancers can often be allowed to do *barre*, even when injured (e.g., with stress fractures). If weight-bearing is impossible, a floor *barre* or water *barre* can be utilized. Modern dancers can amend their classes to include only the warm-up and stretch portions, or they may do a ballet type *barre*. Aerobic dancers may omit inappropriate portions of their routine and instead substitute exercise cycling, swimming, or arm ergometer work.

Dancers' injuries often require a good deal of time from the physician, dance instructor, or any practitioner trying to aid the dancer. Time spent gaining insight into the origins of the problem coupled with informed and practical treatment can, however, result in real benefits to the patient. The goal, of course, is to keep the dancer dancing, while bringing about a return to full function. The most effective way to accomplish this is through a coordinated effort that includes all members of the health care team.

References

1. Garrick, J.G., Gillien, D.M., Whiteside, P. (1986, Jan/Feb.). The epidemiology of aerobic dance injuries. *American Journal of Sports Medicine, 14*, 67-72.
2. Francis, L.L., Francis, P.R., Welshons-Smith, K. (1985, Feb.). Aerobic dance injuries: a survey of instructors. *The Physician and Sportsmedicine, 13*, 105-111.
3. Richie, D.H., Kelso, S.F., Bellucci, P.A. (1985, Feb.). Aerobic dance injuries: a retrospective study of instructors and participants. *The Physician and Sportsmedicine, 13*, 130-140.
4. Solomon, R.L., Micheli, L.J. (1986, Aug.). Technique as a consideration in modern dance injuries. *The Physician and Sportsmedicine, 14*, 83-92.
5. Garrick, J.G. (1987). Aerobic dance injuries and their prevention. In: Ryan, A.J., Stephens, R.E., eds. *Dance medicine: a comprehensive guide*. Chicago and Minneapolis: Pluribus Press/The Physician and Sportsmedicine.

PART II:

Anatomy

2

Pronation as a Predisposing Factor in Overuse Injuries

Steven R. Kravitz, D.P.M.

From the earliest examples onward, one of the major themes of the literature devoted to dance medicine has been that injuries to dancers result most often from overuse. By this we mean simply that the constant repetition of prescribed movements required by the practice of dance can wear body parts down to the point that they give way. Research in the field of biomechanics has been particularly useful in explaining how this happens. Using everything from the common tools of measurement to state-of-the-art computer and laser technology, the biomechanists have demonstrated how the body's natural configurations—especially its malalignments—interact with the stresses applied to them by dance training to produce injuries.

Perhaps the anatomical region at which these stresses are most intense in all forms of dance is the foot and ankle. Many common malalignments result in excessive pronation; hence, from an injury-prevention point of view, pronation is a subject of particular concern to dancers. This chapter looks briefly at the mechanisms by which pronation predisposes the dancer to injury, and some of the things that might be done to counteract them.

Anatomically, the ankle joint consists of the articular aspects of the distal tibia and fibula surrounding the articulating joint surface of the talus (Figure 2.1). This joint primarily allows dorsiflexion and plantarflexion of the foot on the leg. The joint just below the talus, the "subtalar joint," allows for articulation between the talus and the calcaneus. This joint has three facets, or joint surfaces, where the two bones lie in direct contact with one another. These three areas, as with all movable joints, have a smooth surface of hyaline cartilage over bony areas at the corresponding facets which decreases friction and allows the opposing bones to move with respect to one another. The structure of the anterior, middle, and posterior facets of the subtalar joint classify it as a "saddle joint"; that is, it allows the talus to rotate and slide as well as plantarflex or dorsiflex relative to the calcaneus.

Thus, articulations at the ankle and subtalar joints allow for motion in all three cardinal body planes—frontal for eversion/inversion, sagital for dorsiflexion/plantarflexion, and transverse plane for inward

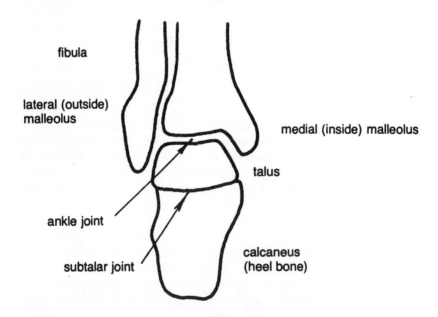

Figure 2.1. Ankle and subtalar joints: frontal plane view from the back (posterior) aspect of lower leg and foot.
Illustration: Barry La Point

rotation (adduction)/outward rotation (abduction). This range of available motion is made possible by the fact that the axis around which it occurs is oblique to all three cardinal body planes and thus not parallel to any one plane (Figure 2.2).

A full description of the mechanics relative to these anatomical structures will not be covered within the space of this chapter. However, the athlete and dancer should remember that, due to the structural and dynamic factors briefly described above, the various mechanical aspects of the subtalar joint complex allow the foot to pronate and supinate, and thereby affect the stability of the foot. This mechanical action causes the foot to function as both a mobile shock absorber (when pronated) and as a rigid lever (when supinated) which can be used to propel one forward from step to step, or off the ground to perform a jump, or in the case of a ballerina on to her *pointe* stance.

Simply stated, pronation describes a foot which collapses medially as one bears weight upon it. Pronation at the subtalar joint allows the calcaneus to evert, and thus leads to the foot rolling in upon itself (Figure 2.3). Small amounts of calcaneal eversion during heel contact may occur normally, but the calcaneus should reduce to perpendicular during the middle of the stance phase of the walking cycle. Calcaneal

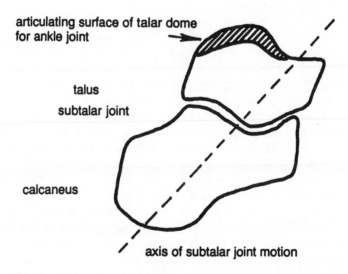

Figure 2.2. Sagittal plane view of the talus and calcaneus. The axis of the subtalar joint is near 45 degrees to the frontal and transverse planes, producing equal motion in both planes.

Illustration: Barry La Point

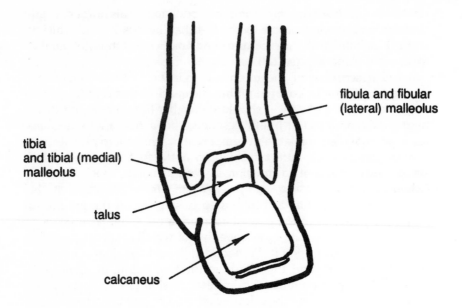

fibula and fibular
(lateral) malleolus

tibia
and tibial (medial)
malleolus

talus

calcaneus

Figure 2.3. Excessive pronation as viewed from the rearfoot, with marked calcaneal eversion.
Illustration: Barry La Point

eversion in this period of the walking or running cycle is often indicative of excessive pronatory motion and should be evaluated for biomechanical instability.

As the calcaneus everts, the talus is forced to rotate internally and plantarflex. As already mentioned, motion at the subtalar joint occurs in all three body planes; thus, as the heel everts relative to the calcaneus, the talus is forced to perform the other two motions described. Heel eversion cannot occur by itself; the other two movements must simultaneously develop in a weight bearing attitude.

The internal rotational force of the talus transfers through the ankle joint to the lower tibia and fibula, forcing the leg to rotate internally. The leg rotates at a faster rate than the thigh (when not extended and locked), leading to a significant shearing force at the knee and a tendency to pull the patellar tendon internally, directing the knee cap off its normal track. The resultant effect to this joint often produces chondromalacia, or "dancer's knee," as the under surface and the surrounding tissues around the knee cap become inflamed.

Furthermore, plantarflexion of the talus can lead to anterior movement of the upper tibia, thus increasing strain to the foot as well as the knee. As the talus plantarflexes, the inside column of the arch unlocks, enhancing the collapsing effect on the foot. This produces the typical "rolled in foot" appearance, and can encourage the development of many overuse injuries, such as heel pain, shin splints, and stress fractures.

The mechanism for heel pain is easily demonstrated. Make an arch out of your hand and picture a rubber band attached around the end of the thumb and forefinger. As you open this arch, you can easily imagine the rubber band being stretched. Similar mechanisms occur on the plantar aspect of the foot, where a traction or stretch is placed upon the multiple tissues located there, especially the fascia. The plantar fascia is a thick piece of tissue which is attached as a narrow band to the calcaneus, and then broadens as it runs distally toward the metatarsal heads one through five. Collapse of the arch structure places considerable strain on this tissue, and is a common cause of arch and heel pain.

Shin splints may also be associated with these mechanisms. This is especially true of strain involving the tibialis posterior muscle, which will often overwork in an attempt to maintain the arch in an appropriate functioning position. Muscles are generally necessary to provide motion to bones respective to one another at joint interfaces, and are not designed to support unstable structures. One function of the tibialis posterior muscle is to provide foot supination; thus, the collapsing foot places excessive strain on this muscle and can initiate a posterior shin splint.

Excessive pronation can also contribute to stress fractures. The internally rotating leg establishes torque forces relative to the internally rotating talus, and may develop a type of stress fracture which often presents as pinpoint pain over bone 3.0-5.0 cm. proximal to the fibular malleolus found at the outside of the ankle joint. Second metatarsal stress fractures are also commonly associated with this pathology. The mechanisms here relate to the only way the foot can truly "roll in": Calcaneal eversion with excessive subtalar joint pronation causes the first metatarsal to become hyper-mobile, and ultimately to dorsiflex; as this occurs, the first metatarsal moves toward the top surface of the foot and one "loses the inside pillar of support" to the foot; the rolled in appearance with associated calcaneal eversion is the result. As the first metatarsal dorsiflexes, it loses its ability to maintain weight bearing function. The weight which normally would have been absorbed by the first metatarsal is transferred to the much thinner second metatarsal. During aggressive propulsive activity, too much force may be received on the second metatarsal bone, causing it to develop a small hairline fracture known commonly as "stress fracture" or "march fracture."

A small amount of pronation is normal and indeed needed to absorb shock; however, excessive pronatory motion can lead to many overuse injuries of the type commonly seen in dancers. These syndromes may occur anatomically from the lower lumbar spine distally through the bottom plantar aspect of the foot.

The overly pronated foot can be treated with support to decrease injury potential. The athlete, dancer, and athletic trainer should bear in mind that all means of foot support may be helpful in decreasing symptomatology associated with the mechanisms herein addressed. Thus, foot strapping and padding applied to stabilize the arch is often an effective means of adjunctive therapy. Shoes with strong heel counters and longitudinal arch pads can be helpful. Shoe inserts, orthotics, can be made by professionals in the field from a cast impression of the foot, and are the best device for providing needed support. Orthotics can help to decrease multiple overuse injuries and the rate of deformity development—e.g., bunions, hammertoes, and heel spur syndrome—to which the pronated foot is especially susceptible. This holds true for the pediatric patient as well as the individual with a more developed foot. That is not to say that all children need orthotic support; indeed, most do not. However, professional opinion must be sought when the need is questioned.

One last point: appropriate muscle balance with well-toned leg musculature is an excellent shock absorber and may be adjunctively helpful in decreasing shock transmittal between foot and leg, thus decreasing potential injury associated with excessive pronatory mechanisms. Hence, a well developed dance regimen should serve this preventative function.

In summary, foot pronation is a very important shock absorbing mechanism. The subtalar joint, just below the ankle, is a primary factor in transmitting various forces from the foot to the leg, and it defines how the foot pronates in reaction to these forces. Excessive pronation is commonly associated with "malalignment," as well as with many overuse injuries and developmental foot deformity. Controlling the pronatory factors may decrease the rate of deformity, and is definitely advantageous in reducing the overuse injury potential. Supporting the foot with appropriate footwear and, when necessary, orthotics, can be very helpful.

3

Some Common Foot and Ankle Injuries in Dancers

Richard N. Norris, M.D.

This chapter discusses four of the most common foot and ankle injuries seen in dancers: ankle sprains, flexor hallucis longus tendinitis, sesamoid injuries, and achilles tendinitis. In each case it describes the basic anatomy involved, the typical mechanisms of injury, the treatment modalities and prognosis, and the rehabilitation procedures to be considered. It is hoped that this information will help dancers to understand more fully what is involved in diagnosing and dealing effectively with injuries to this most vulnerable anatomical unit.

Ankle Sprains

Ankle sprains are very prevalent in dancers.[1] Too often treated as insignificant, these injuries can have a major impact on a dancer's life and ability to perform. Before discussing treatment of ankle sprains, it is important to understand just how the ankle joint is constructed and how these injuries can occur.

The talus is the part of the ankle on which the tibia, or shin bone, rests. It is relatively wide in the front and narrow in the back.[2] The talus fits into what is called the ankle mortise, which is a niche formed by the end of the fibula and tibia. The medial aspect of the ankle has three very strong ligaments, the deltoid ligaments. These are rarely sprained. There are also three major ligaments on the lateral side of the ankle. The anterior talofibular ligament (ATF) runs from the fibula to the talus in a horizontal fashion. When a dancer is in the *demi-pointe* position the ATF becomes vertical instead of horizontal.[3] This provides some mechanical stability and prevents the foot from supinating. The ATF also gives rotational stability,[3] preventing the talus from rotating out of its mortise, especially on outside turns. Despite its stabilizing

21

role, or perhaps because of it, the ATF ligament is most commonly involved in minor ankle sprain.

Muscles also play a role in stabilizing the ankle joint. Among these the most important are the peroneal muscles. They run from the top of the fibula down the outside of the lower leg. The peroneus longus then runs along the side of the ankle and inserts under the ball of the great toe, or hallux. The peroneus brevis inserts into the base of the fifth metatarsal. On the medial side of the leg the tibialis posterior muscle originates from underneath the calf muscle and sends its tendon around the medial malleolus, inserting on the inner aspect of the mid-foot. When the foot is on *demi-pointe* the narrow rear part of the talus is in the mortise, and thus there is very little or no mechanical (bony) stability in this position.[4] In high *demi-pointe* there is some stability gained from the locking of the calcaneus against the posterior aspect of the tibia. When the ankle is dropped even a few degrees out of a very high *demi-pointe* the responsibility for stabilizing the ankle falls predominantly on the ATF ligament and the peroneal and posterior tibial muscles, which form a yoke around the ankle.

There are many causes of ankle sprains. Perhaps the most important one is inadequate rehabilitation of previous ankle sprains, since these injuries are often taken too lightly. Another is poor technique in landing from jumps, particularly with the foot supinated.[5] Certain dance steps also seem to carry a higher risk for ankle sprains, such as the *entrechat six*.[6] At the end of a long day, when fatigue is a factor, rehearsing new, unfamiliar, or advanced steps can be a very real threat. It is essential that dancers stay attuned enough to the workings of their bodies to know what their limits are, and when those limits are reached. Other disorders, such as arthritis of the great toe joint (hallux rigidus) can cause a sickling in of the foot when attempting *relevé*, which then may predispose to ankle sprains. Dance surfaces that are hard or uneven or steeply raked may also be a factor.[7]

Ankle sprains are usually classified into three grades, grade 1 being the mildest and grade 3 the most severe (and fortunately the least common). It should be remembered that the amount of pain experienced is not a reliable indicator in diagnosing the degree or severity of an ankle sprain. A grade 1 sprain means there has been partial tearing of the fibers in the ligaments of the muscles, while a grade 2 involves a more severe tear. A grade 3 is a complete disruption or tearing of one or more of the ligaments. The ankle develops what is called a "talar tilt sign"; that is, when the ankle is placed under a lateral stress the talus tilts and opens up, creating a gap laterally. This can be measured and diagnosed by taking a stress x-ray in which the ankle is manipulated to simulate stress under normal movement conditions.[6] A "talar tilt sign" during this test indicates a complete rupture of the calcaneofibular ligament, which normally assists with lateral stability of the ankle. Clinically, a grade 3 sprain of the ATF ligament is confirmed when there is a positive "draw sign"; when the tibia is stabilized and the heel is pulled forward, there is an anterior shifting of the talus out of the mortise joint.

The first aid treatment for ankle sprains is the acronym RICE, standing for rest, ice, compression, and elevation. This minimizes the bleeding and swelling that occurs in and about the ankle joint following the sprain. Controlling the swelling significantly reduces recovery time. For first and second degree sprains an air cast or gel cast ankle brace is very useful. This consists of two plastic shells containing air- or gel-filled bladders, which are arranged on either side of the ankle and held in place by a flat stirrup which fits inside the shoe, and by straps wrapped around the ankle. With each step and release the bladders cause a change of pressure, which helps force out some of the swelling. The construction of the brace prevents painful pronation and supination while still allowing for nearly full flexion and extension. The dancer wearing this device is able to bear weight earlier, walk more naturally, and return to activities in less time.[6]

Rehabilitation aims at restoring full range of motion, the normal levels of strength and endurance, and position sense, or proprioception. In many cases exercises are addressed to a number of these rehabilitative principles or goals simultaneously. An attempt should always be made to rehabilitate the dancer in as functional a manner as possible[8]; it is very important to maintain overall body flexibility and strength while the dancer is injured and recuperating. Allowing the entire body to become deconditioned because of an injury to a specific part is a common problem in any sport, and one that is easily avoidable. In the case of ankle injuries, swimming is often an excellent solution, or a ballet *barre* may be done in the water.[5]

The flexibility of the achilles tendon must be restored through stretching, as the achilles often becomes tight following an ankle sprain. Strengthening the peroneal muscles can be done most effectively by using a theraband, which is a broad elastic or rubber band that comes in different degrees of resistance, each color coded. The band can be wrapped around the balls of both feet so that when the feet are opened up to a V shape, keeping the heels together, the band applies the desired resistance. This should be done with the feet pointed as well as flexed, because the peroneal muscles come into play primarily when the foot is up on *demi-pointe*, and therefore must be rehabilitated in that position. The yoke muscles, that is, the peroneal and the posterior tibialis muscles, can also be strengthened very effectively using manual resistance. Holding the foot, the therapist (or the dancer him/herself) will resist movement in two different diagonals, referred to by physical therapists as "close pack" and "loose pack."[8] The diagonals are from dorsiflexion with supination to plantarflexion and pronation—that is up and in, down and out—and the opposite, dorsiflexion and eversion or pronation (up and out) to plantarflexion and supination (down and in). Resisting these movements in a smooth but progressively intense fashion has an advantage over the theraband in that it rehabilitates the muscles in more directional planes.

Within the substance of the ankle ligaments and joint capsule lie sensory nerve endings called proprioceptive endings. These nerve endings transmit position information to the brain, so that it can direct muscle control about the ankle and thereby maintain stability. When the ankle is sprained these pathways are often disrupted, and must be restored through functional rehabilitation. The wobble-type board is an excellent means of doing this. Such a board can be constructed by simply fixing a half-round dowel or half of a hard wooden ball to the underside of a piece of plywood about a foot and a half square. It can be used initially in a seated position with no weight bearing, and then with progressive weight bearing. A more sophisticated version of this device is called the BAPS, or biomechanical ankle platform system, manufactured by Camp International, Jackson, Michigan. The BAPS has five different sized hemispheres that can screw to the underside of the board. The board is designed to accommodate the difference in range of motion between pronation and supination. There are mechanisms for adding weights in different positions around the foot and ankle to provide progressive resistive exercises in addition to proprioceptive rehabilitation.[8] The BAPS board is also useful for rehabilitation of knee injuries.

Molnar, in her article, "Rehabilitation of the Injured Ankle," outlines quite a number of ankle rehabilitation exercises (with photographs), and the reader is referred to this article for more detailed information.[8]

A sensible plan for rehabilitation is essential to a full recovery. The following 7-10 day program is designed primarily for mild ankle sprains. More serious grades would use a similar progression but with greater length between the stages.

Day 1: ice with elevation and compression; no weight bearing; air cast or gel cast.

Day 2: active exercises for ankle and foot two to three times a day; ice after each period; conditioning exercises for entire body, and walking when necessary with air cast.

Day 3: massage elevated lower leg, stroking upward towards heart; swimming and pool exercises; resistive exercises for ankle two to three times a day; walking with air cast.

Day 4: stretch to normal range of motion; increase resistance exercises; use balance board; continue using ice after exercise.

Day 5: warm-up foot and ankle; contrast baths; *barre* work, slowly with foot in tape; strength and flexibility exercises, then ice.

Day 6: continue body conditioning exercises; resistance exercises for ankle; full *barre* all speeds; walk in *pointe* shoes, but don't work on *pointe.*

Days 7-10: begin small jumps and turns; resisted balance positions; rehearsals and slow *pointe* work.[9]

One further comment about third degree (complete) sprains: There is some controversy among dance orthopedists as to how these injuries are to be managed. Some feel that conservative or "closed" management is adequate,[10, 11] whereas others favor "open" or surgical repair.[6] It is, however, agreed that if a reconstructive procedure does become necessary to stabilize a joint, the peroneal tendons should not be sacrificed to serve as a reinforcement. The peroneal tendons are too important for stability *en pointe* to be sacrificed.[3]

Flexor Hallucis Longus Tendinitis

The flexor hallucis longus tendon (FHL) runs behind the medial malleolus of the ankle, along with the tendons of the posterior tibialis and flexor digitorum longus. This muscle and tendon can be thought of as the achilles tendon of the great toe, since it does for the toe what the achilles does for the foot—i.e., completes push-off during striding or jumping. When a dancer is experiencing tendinitis about the inner side of the ankle, this is the tendon that is usually involved (rather than the posterior tibialis tendon).

The FHL tendon is unique among the three tendons behind the medial malleolus in that it passes through a fibro-osseous tunnel just behind the malleolus (Figure 3.1). This is one of the anatomical reasons why this tendon is so often involved in tendinitis. In the dancer who has an abnormally low insertion of the muscle belly on the tendon, the muscle belly tends to be jammed down into the mouth of the fibro-osseous tunnel when the foot and great toe are both dorsiflexed, as in doing *grand pliés* in fifth position (Figure 3.2). This causes irritation, often resulting in inflammation and adhesions in this area. Interestingly, the condition seems to arise more often in the left foot than the right, perhaps due to the predominance of right turns *(pirouettes, fouettés)* in ballet choreography.[12] If adhesions *do* occur, they can mimic

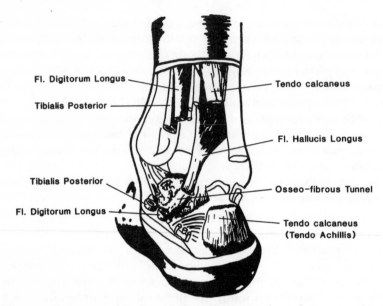

Fl. Digitorum Longus

Tibialis Posterior

Tibialis Posterior

Fl. Digitorum Longus

Tendo calcaneus

Fl. Hallucis Longus

Osseo-fibrous Tunnel

Tendo calcaneus
(Tendo Achillis)

Figure 3.1. The tendon of the flexor hallucis longus muscle can be seen entering the fibro-osseous tunnel behind the medial malleolus.

Illustration: Barry La Point

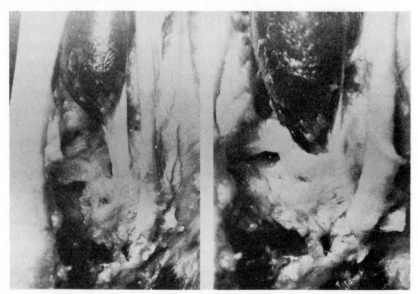

Figure 3.2. As the ankle and great toe dorsiflex, the belly of the flexor hallucis longus is pulled down into the mouth of the tunnel. This can be a source of irritation, especially in those individuals with a low insertion of the muscle belly.

From Thomasen, E. (1982). *Diseases and Injuries of Ballet Dancers.* Denmark: Universitetsforlaget I. Arhus, 35. Reprinted by permission.

an arthritic condition of the metatarsophalangeal joint of the great toe (pseudo hallux rigidus), in that it will not allow for dorsiflexion of the great toe. Even without adhesions, dorsiflexion of the great toe and ankle may be limited, but when the ankle is plantarflexed the great toe can then be dorsiflexed, as plantarflexion of the ankle releases the tension on the FHL tendon.[13]

Another common cause of FHL tendinitis is pronation, as a result of either a natural malalignment or of faulty technique (dancers with inadequate turnout at the hips will often "cheat" by turning out from the knee down, thus encouraging a pronated alignment of foot and ankle, especially in fifth position). Pronation, in *relevé* (sickling out) also predisposes to FHL tendinitis in combination with a short first toe, the so-called Morton's foot, or lack of strength about the ankle.

Occasionally nodules may form in this region, resulting in triggering and snapping of the great toe.[6, 13]

Treatment primarily consists of anti-inflammatory medications, thermotherapy in the form of ultrasound, and ice massage. Electrical stimulation may be useful to decrease inflammation and swelling. Stretching and strengthening the FHL tendon with physical therapy techniques is also required. Orthotics used in street footwear may be of benefit in the dancer who has a naturally pronated foot. Injection of steroid solution is favored by some, but is difficult in this area as to be effective the steroid solution must enter the fibro-osseous tunnel. Additionally, steroid injections can weaken tendons and, in the worst-case scenario, predispose to rupture. Rupture is rare, but should it occur the treatment is surgical repair with six weeks in a cast and extensive rehabilitation. Full recovery may take up to one year.[4]

Sesamoid Injuries

The sesamoid bones are small isolated bones found in multiple locations in the foot and ankle. This discussion will be limited to the sesamoids on the undersurface of the first metatarsophalangeal (MTP) joint. These bones lie within the tendon of the flexor hallucis brevis, and their articular surfaces are covered with hyaline cartilage (Figure 3.3).[14] There are generally two sesamoids. The medial or tibial sesamoid tends to be larger and longer compared to the sesamoid on the fibular or lateral side. In addition to the flexor hallucis brevis muscle, the adductor hallucis and abductor hallucis tendons also contribute tendons to the sesamoids. The sesamoids may also be bipartite—that is, in two parts—or multipartite. These variations are said to occur in approximately 10-33 percent of all feet.[15, 16] It has been estimated that forces equal to three times the body weight occur beneath the

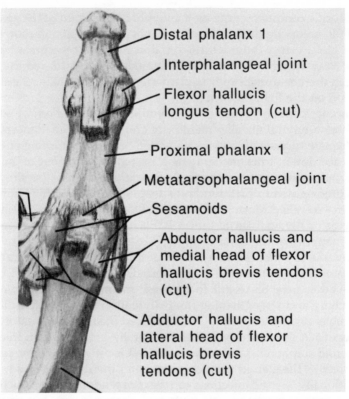

Distal phalanx 1

Interphalangeal joint

Flexor hallucis
longus tendon (cut)

Proximal phalanx 1

Metatarsophalangeal joint

Sesamoids

Abductor hallucis and
medial head of flexor
hallucis brevis tendons
(cut)

Adductor hallucis and
lateral head of flexor
hallucis brevis
tendons (cut)

Figure 3.3. A view of the plantar aspect of the first metatarsal head with the two heads of the flexor hallucis brevis muscle cut revealing the sesamoids embedded in their tendons.

From Hamilton, W.G. (1985). Surgical anatomy of the foot and ankle. *CIBA Clinical Symposia Annual, 28.* Adapted by permission.

sesamoids during the normal gait cycle, particularly at push-off.[17] These studies also show that the sesamoids aid push-off during gait by accentuating the flexor strength of the flexor hallucis longus. During weight bearing, particularly in *relevé,* the tibial or medial sesamoid bears most of the weight, thus accounting for the higher incidence of injury in this bone. Certain ethnic dances (e.g., Japanese) may be particularly irritating to the sesamoids because they employ slapping forefoot steps.[18]

The sesamoids are subject to numerous pathological processes, including fracture, stress fracture, chondromalacia and osteoarthritis, tendinitis of the flexor hallucis brevis, osteochondritis of the sesamoids, and ganglion cysts between the sesamoids.[19] Sesamoid problems may be localized clinically by forcibly dorsiflexing the great toe with one hand while palpating the undersurface of the head of the first metatarsal with the opposite thumb. Fracture and stress fracture must be ruled out through radiographs or bone scan, and bipartite sesamoids should be differentiated from fractures by the same means (Figures 3.4, 3.5). Stress fractures often do not show up for several weeks, but the bone scan will confirm their presence or absence.

Sesamoid problems must be treated vigorously, not only to relieve chronic pain and disability in the dancer, but to avoid consequential injury. The dancer with pain under the head of the first metatarsal will often compensate by supinating the forefoot during *relevé*. This may then lead to ankle sprains, fifth metatarsal fractures, etc. The dancer should be examined in the *relevé* position, as pain in this region that was not apparent when palpated by the examiner's thumb may become evident upon weight bearing.[19]

Treatment should include physical therapy modalities such as ultrasound, deep friction massage, ice massage, and electrical stimulation. However, the cornerstone of therapy is relief of weight bearing on the sesamoids. There are several considerations to address here. Sesamoiditis is typically treated with a sesamoid "pad" which lifts up the first metatarsal and extends far enough distally to lift up the second through fifth metatarsals when the dancer is in *relevé* (Figure 3.6). I have found this to be not entirely satisfactory. While it is necessary to relieve weight bearing on the sesamoids, it is also important to prevent the MTP joint from flexing during normal gait, as this places increased stress on the sesamoids. The best way to accomplish this is by use of a rigid or wooden-soled shoe with a rocker bottom, which causes the foot to roll through the push-off phase of the gait cycle. A router can then be used to grind away the wood from underneath the first metatarsal head, all the way out to beyond the end of the great toe. This space is then filled in with a very soft foam (Figure 3.7). Such a device not only relieves weight bearing on the sesamoids and prevents MTP joint flexion during push-off, but also inhibits or discourages contraction of the flexor hallucis brevis during push-off, as there is nothing substantive for the pad of the distal phalanx of the great toe to push down against. This prevents strain on the sesamoids from contraction of the flexor hallucis brevis muscle, within whose tendons the sesamoids are located.

The dancers should be told that they may be in for a long course of treatment with sesamoiditis, particularly if there is a stress fracture or frank fracture of the sesamoids. I have, however, successfully treated several fractured sesamoids with the above protocol.

If at all possible, sesamoid problems should be treated nonsurgically, as sesamoidectomy can create imbalance, particularly with the

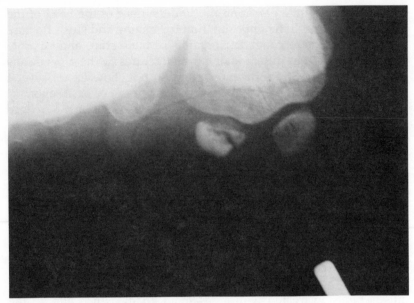

Figure 3.4. Fracture of the lateral sesamoid in a 24 year old dancer.

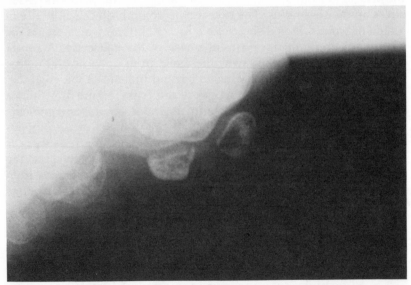

Figure 3.5. After 3 months of treatment with a modified shoe (Figure 3.7) the fracture is nearly healed as shown by x-ray, and the patient is asymptomatic.

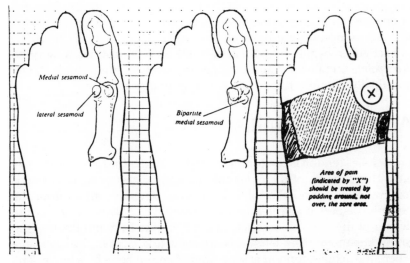

Figure 3.6. Standard padding of the sole of the foot for sesamoiditis. This is often ineffective for reasons explained in the text.

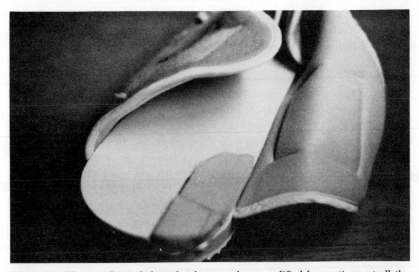

Figure 3.7. The wooden soled, rocker-bottom shoe, modified by routing out all the wood from behind the first metatarsal head to beyond the toe and filling the space with soft foam (plastazote). This not only relieves weight bearing on the injured sesamoid, but prevents additional irritation by eliminating metatarsophalangeal flexion on push-off and inhibiting isometric contraction of the flexor hallucis brevis, the tendons of which contain the sesamoids.

exaggerated forces generated in the *relevé* position in dance. Removal of one sesamoid also places excessive force on its mate.[20]

When symptoms are resolved the dancer may gradually return to full activities, beginning with *demi-pointe* on both feet, working up to *demi-pointe* on one foot, and then progressively to jumps on both feet and finally one foot jumps, such as *jetés* or *assemblés*.

Achilles Tendinitis

The achilles tendon is the common tendon for the triceps surae (Figure 3.8). This consists of the outer calf muscle, or gastrocnemius, which has two bellies, and the soleus. The gastrocnemius arises from the posterior aspect of the femoral condyles. The soleus, which is the deeper of the two calf muscles, arises from the tibia and fibula distal to the knee joint. The tendon is attached to a facet in the calcaneus where the achilles tendon is separated from the bone by a bursa. The tendon is shaped somewhat like an hourglass, with the narrow part 4-7 cm above the calcaneal insertion. There is no true synovial tendon sheath around the achilles tendon. Rather, it is covered by fascia, and a sheath, or paratenon, is formed by the fascia. The two muscle groups of the triceps surae have a different but similar function. The gastrocnemius flexes both the knee and the ankle in an open kinetic chain, whereas the soleus only plantarflexes the ankle. It has been observed that the gastrocnemius is used primarily in jumps, whereas the soleus has a more static function. In *relevé* both of these muscles act together, and due to the physics involved, the pull on the achilles tendon is less in high *relevé* or full *pointe* than in low *relevé*.[13]

There are numerous factors which contribute to achilles tendinitis in the dancer: 1. Tightness of the heel cords, which is quite common in dancers, as they do most of their work in plantarflexion; 2. Anatomic variation of the achilles, with persons having smaller and thinner achilles tendons being more susceptible to strain; 3. Supination or pronation of the foot; and 4. A low *relevé* which, as mentioned previously, places more stress on the achilles than a high *relevé* because of the physics involved. Additionally, a prominence of the posterior superior portion of the calcaneus may cause mechanical irritation and tendinitis of the achilles and/or the retrocalcaneal bursa in *plié*.[21] A personal observation is that the neoclassical *en pointe* position, with its exaggerated plantarflexion, may cause toe shoe ribbons to bite tightly into the back of the achilles right in the vulnerable area.

Achilles tendinitis occurs in various degrees, from mild irritation or fraying of the fibers to intratendonal tears or fusiform swellings.

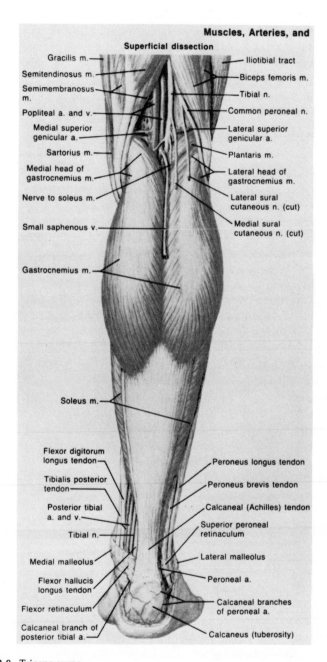

Figure 3.8. Triceps surae.

From Hamilton, W.G. (1985). Surgical anatomy of the foot and ankle. *CIBA Clinical Symposia Annual*, 20-21. Reprinted by permission.

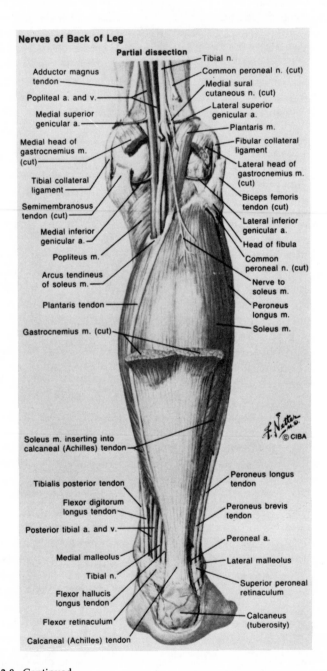

Nerves of Back of Leg

Partial dissection

Tibial n.

Adductor magnus tendon

Common peroneal n. (cut)

Popliteal a. and v.

Medial sural cutaneous n. (cut)

Medial superior genicular a.

Lateral superior genicular a.

Plantaris m.

Medial head of gastrocnemius m. (cut)

Fibular collateral ligament

Tibial collateral ligament

Lateral head of gastrocnemius m. (cut)

Semimembranosus tendon (cut)

Biceps femoris tendon (cut)

Medial inferior genicular a.

Lateral inferior genicular a.

Popliteus m.

Head of fibula

Arcus tendineus of soleus m.

Common peroneal n. (cut)

Plantaris tendon

Nerve to soleus m.

Gastrocnemius m. (cut)

Peroneus longus m.

Soleus m.

Soleus m. inserting into calcaneal (Achilles) tendon

Tibialis posterior tendon

Peroneus longus tendon

Flexor digitorum longus tendon

Peroneus brevis tendon

Posterior tibial a. and v.

Medial malleolus

Peroneal a.

Tibial n.

Lateral malleolus

Flexor hallucis longus tendon

Superior peroneal retinaculum

Flexor retinaculum

Calcaneus (tuberosity)

Calcaneal (Achilles) tendon

Figure 3.8. Continued

Chronic tendinitis may result in nodule formation or adhesions between the tendon and paratenon.[21]

Recently, magnetic resonance imaging has been used increasingly in the diagnosis of achilles tendinitis. This can be most useful in differentiating a simple tendinitis from intratendonal tears. These latter must be treated more aggressively, as they may herald impending achilles rupture.

Nonsurgical management includes anti-inflammatory medications, ice massage, ultrasound with electrical stimulation to reduce edema, contrast baths, and range of motion only up to the point of mild discomfort, not pain. There is no place in the conservative management of achilles tendinitis for steroid injections, as this runs the risk of weakening the tendon and predisposing towards rupture. A heel lift in the shoe is of benefit in taking some of the tension off the achilles, and the dancer with mild achilles tendinitis may use a character shoe or jazz shoe with a small heel to reduce strain on the achilles during *plié*. For more severe cases of achilles tendinitis this author uses an air cast walking brace with an added heel lift (Figure 3.9). This immobilizes the ankle, and the rocker-type sole prevents stretching of the achilles just before push-off. The walking brace should be removed every 3-4 hours, and active, *pain-free* range of motion exercises performed to prevent stiffness of the ankle joint.

Once pain has diminished, full range of motion and then strength and endurance must be gradually restored. Pilates equipment, which allows for horizontal jumps on a spring-loaded board, or else doing jumps in a swimming pool, can both be used for this purpose. Dancers should be encouraged to do adequate heel cord stretching both in and out of class in an effort to prevent this injury.

Foot and ankle injuries, being so common and potentially disabling, are of the utmost importance to those concerned with dance medicine. Understanding the role of certain muscles should encourage preventative strengthening programs. Early and aggressive rehabilitation, stressing functional activities, *full* restoration of strength, range of motion, proprioception and endurance, and gradual return to dance activities, will serve to minimize disability. The importance of maintaining good general physical condition during the rehabilitation process cannot be overemphasized. Finally, appreciating that inadequate treatment often leads to recurrence of injury should cause us to look at these injuries as seriously as they deserve.

References

1. Liebler, W.A. (1976). Injuries of the foot in dancers. In: Bateman, J.E., ed. *Foot Science*. Philadelphia: W.B. Saunders, 284-287.

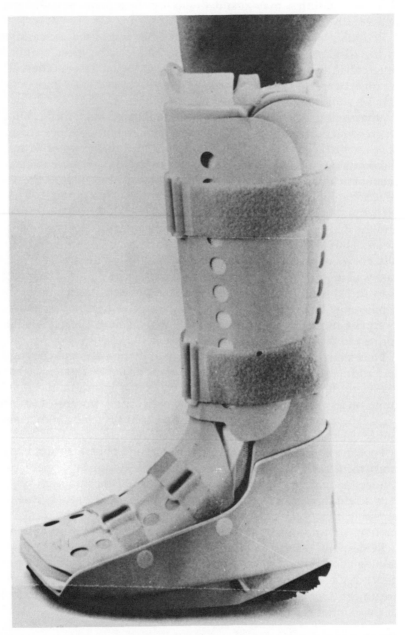

Figure 3.9. The aircast walking cast provides protection of the inflamed achilles tendon by eliminating ankle motion during ambulation and by placing the foot-ankle complex in slight plantarflexion. The advantage over a traditional cast is easy removal for gentle range-of-motion exercises to prevent joint stiffness and muscle atrophy.

2. Inman, V.T. (1976). *The joints of the ankle*. Baltimore: Williams and Wilkins.
3. Gould, N., Seligson, D., Gassman, J. (1980). Early and late repair of the lateral ligament of the ankle. *Foot and Ankle, 1*(2), 84-89.
4. Sammarco, G.J. (1982). The foot and ankle in classical ballet and modern dance. In: Jahss, M.H., ed. *Disorders of the Foot*. Philadelphia: W.B. Saunders, 1626-1659.
5. Hardaker, W.T., Angelo, J.C., Malone, T.R., Myers, M. (1988). Ankle sprains in theatrical dancers. *Medical Problems of Performing Artists, 3*(4), 146-150.
6. Hamilton, W.G. (1982). Sprained ankles in ballet dancers. *Foot and Ankle, 3*(2), 99-102.
7. Seals, J.G. (1983). A study of dance surfaces. *Clinics in Sports Medicine, 2*(3), 557-561.
8. Molnar, M.E. (1988). Rehabilitation of the injured ankle. *Clinics in Sports Medicine, 7*(1), 193-204.
9. Hamilton, W.G., Molnar, M. (1983, April). Back to dancing after injury. *Dance Magazine, 57*, 88-90.
10. Norris, R. (1988). [Personal communication with Lyle Micheli, Director, Division of Sports Medicine, Children's Hospital, Boston, Massachusetts].
11. Norris, R. (1988). [Personal communication with John Bergfeld, Orthopaedic Surgeon, Cleveland Clinic].
12. Hamilton, W.G. (1977). Tendinitis about the ankle joint in classical ballet dancers. *American Journal of Sports Medicine, 5*(2), 84-88.
13. Thomasen, E. (1982). *Diseases and injuries of ballet dancers*. Denmark: Universitetsforlaget I. Arhus.
14. Richardson, E.G. (1987). Injuries to the hallucal sesamoids in the athlete. *Foot and Ankle, 7*(4), 229-244.
15. Hamilton, W.G. (1985). Surgical anatomy of the foot and ankle. *CIBA Clinical Symposia Annual, 37*(3).
16. Jahss, M.H. (1981). The sesamoids of the hallux. *Clinical Orthopaedics and Related Research, 157*, 88-97.
17. Drez, D. (1982). Forefoot problems in runners. In: Mack, R.P., ed. Symposium on the foot and leg in running sports. St. Louis: C.V. Mosby, 73-75.
18. Sammarco, G.J. (1988). The dancer's foot and ankle. In: Postgraduate advances in sports medicine, University of Pennsylvania School of Medicine. Forum Medicum.
19. Novella, T.M. (1987). Dancers' shoes and foot care. In: Ryan, A., Stephens, R.E., eds. *Dance medicine: a comprehensive guide*. Chicago and Minneapolis: Pluribus Press/The Physician and Sportsmedicine, 139-176.
20. McBryde, A.M., Anderson, R.B. (1988, Jan.). Sesamoid foot problems in the athlete. *Clinics in Sports Medicine, 7*, 51-60.
21. Hamilton, W.G. (1988, Jan.). Foot and ankle injuries in dancers. *Clinics in Sports Medicine, 7*, 143-173.

4

Knee Problems in Dancers

Carol C. Teitz, M.D.

Introduction

In dancers, the vast majority of injuries occur in the lower extremity. Lower extremity injuries in various studies have accounted for from 58 percent to 88 percent of all dancers' injuries.[1,2,3] The rate of knee injuries ranges from 14 percent to 17 percent (Table 4.1). Quirk studied professional ballet dancers and found that patellofemoral problems and patellar tendinitis accounted for approximately 16 percent of knee injuries seen.[4] Patellar subluxation accounted for 0.3 percent, and meniscal problems for 16 percent of knee injuries in this group of dancers. Patellar tendinitis is also seen commonly in aerobic dancers. Torn menisci are more common in male than in female dancers, particularly in folk dancers, in whom percussive squatting activities put the meniscus at risk during rapid flexion and extension of the knee.[3,5] The following discussion describes the anatomy and pertinent biomechanics of the knee, followed by typical causes, clinical presentations, and recommended treatment for common knee problems.

TABLE 4.1

Percent of Dancers' Injuries By Anatomic Location as Reported in Previous Studies

Location	Theatrical Dance (Washington, 1978)	Ballet & Modern (Rovere et al., 1983)	Ballet (Quirk, 1983)	Aerobic Dance (Garrick et al., 1986)
Knee	14	15	17	14
Foot & Ankle	23	37	42	37
Other Lower Extremity	21	19	21	31
Back & Other	42	29	20	18

Anatomy

The knee is a complex joint with no inherent bony stability. It is made up of articulations between the femur and tibia, and the patella and femur, and is surrounded by both a layer of synovial tissue that produces fluid and by a tough, fibrous capsule. Within the synovial tissue are folds called plicae. A plica is a synovial band that is a remnant of an embryologic partition in the knee. The medial plica is present in approximately 60 percent of adults and rarely produces any symptoms. However, when knee irritation results in synovial thickening, this band can harden to the point where it rubs back and forth on the undersurface of the patella, producing wear and pain.[6,7]

Ligaments lend support to the connective tissue capsule around the knee. There are four major ligaments supporting the knee joint, two collateral ligaments, medial and lateral, and two cruciate ligaments, anterior and posterior. The collateral ligaments are located on either side of the knee, whereas the cruciate ligaments cross each other in the center of the knee. They form an axis about which the knee rotates. The medial collateral ligament has two components, a superficial and a deep component, both running from the medial femoral condyle onto the proximal portion of the tibia. The deep portion of the medial collateral ligament is attached to the capsule of the knee joint and the medial meniscus; hence injuries that tear both the medial collateral ligament and the medial meniscus can occur. The lateral collateral ligament is outside the capsule of the knee. The anterior cruciate ligament originates on the lateral femoral condyle and inserts on the anterior aspect of the tibia. The posterior cruciate ligament originates on the medial femoral condyle and inserts on the posterior-most margin of the tibia. The designation of these ligaments as anterior or posterior is derived from the site of insertion on the tibia (Figure 4.1).

The patella is a triangular-shaped bone with the apex pointing toward the foot. On its posterior surface (the surface making contact with the femur), the patella has facets which are designed to articulate with the trochlear groove in the femur. The patella lies within the quadriceps tendon and is held in position by connective tissue bands from the quadriceps muscle, the iliotibial tendon, and the patellar tendon. These attachments compose the patellar retinaculum. The mobility of the patella as well as its position in the trochlea is determined by the relative flexibility or tightness of these retinacular attachments, as well as by the length of the patellar tendon (Figure 4.2).[8] The stability of the patella in turn is determined by its position in the

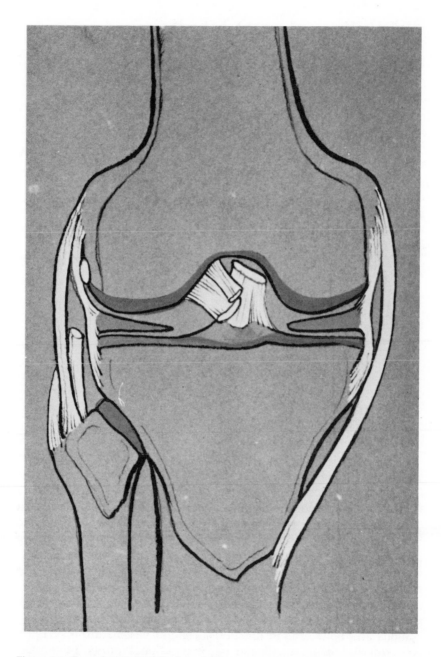

Figure 4.1. Frontal section of the knee joint

From Teitz, C.C. (1983). Office management of common knee problems. *Current concepts in pain, 1*(4), 12. Reprinted by permission.

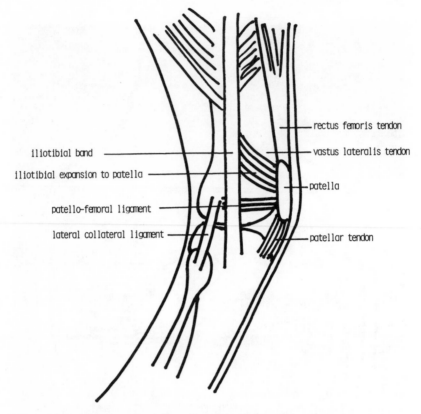

rectus femoris tendon

iliotibial band

vastus lateralis tendon

iliotibial expansion to patella

patella

patello-femoral ligament

lateral collateral ligament

patellar tendon

Figure 4.2. Lateral view of patellar retinacular attachments

trochlear groove, the depth of the groove, and the tightness of the retinacular attachments (Figure 4.3).

The patellar tendon is made up of dense, regularly arranged collagen fibers, that function to transmit force from the quadriceps muscle to the tibia, causing the knee to straighten. Similarly, the hamstring tendons transmit forces from their respective muscles (semimembranosus, semitendinosus, biceps femoris) to the tibia, causing the knee to bend. At their insertions into bone, tendon fibers become incorporated into relatively avascular fibrocartilage. The blood supply to a tendon is variable. Blood supply may originate both at the musculotendinous and bone tendon junctions. Tendon vasculature is compromised at sites of friction, torsion, or compression. Proprioceptive information is obtained through nerve endings near the musculotendinous junction.

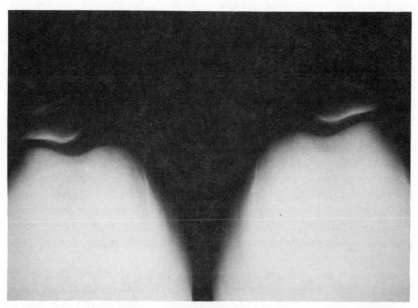

Figure 4.3. The "sunset" view reveals an abnormal lateral position of the patella
From Teitz, C.C. (1983). Office management of common knee problems. *Current concepts in pain,* 1(3),5. Reprinted by permission.

In addition to collagen, which accounts for 30 percent of the wet weight of tendon, tendon contains 2 percent elastin, and 58 percent to 70 percent water. Where collagen is predominantly responsible for the structural integrity of tendon and for resisting deformation, elastin contributes to the flexibility of tendon. Scar contains almost no elastin, resulting in its relatively stiff behavior.

The menisci are small, wedge-shaped semilunar cartilages in the knee, with their thickest portion at the periphery and a paper-thin portion at their innermost margin. The menisci function in a number of ways. They increase the congruity between the femur and tibia, thereby distributing weight evenly and preventing excessive wear in any one area. By pushing synovial fluid around, they contribute to the lubrication of the knee and to the nourishment of the articular cartilage. They also act as shock absorbers, and provide some stability to the knee joint by acting as spacers (Figure 4.1). The medial meniscus is attached to the capsule all along its peripheral margin, and is also attached to the medial collateral ligament. The capsular attachment of the lateral meniscus, on the other hand, is interrupted in its mid to posterior third by the passage of the popliteus tendon from the tibia up to the lateral femoral condyle. The inner margins of the menisci are free (Figure 4.4). Their peripheral attachments provide the outer 20-30 percent of the meniscus with a blood supply.[9] When a tear occurs in the periphery, i.e., the vascular area, the meniscus is capable of healing. However, the vast majority of tears occur in the nonvascular area, and therefore have no potential for healing.

Biomechanics

Knee joint motion is quite complex; it includes flexion and extension, rotation, rolling, and gliding. Because the lateral femoral condyle has a smaller radius of curvature than does the medial femoral condyle, the condyles move at different rates across the tibia during knee flexion and extension. During the first 10° to 15° of flexion, the femur rolls posteriorly farther on the lateral tibial plateau than on the medial tibial plateau. This creates a passive internal rotation of the tibia with respect to the femur during flexion.

Ligaments are collagenous connective tissue structures that act to restrain joints. Fibers in the ligaments run in the direction necessary to control loading. The collateral ligaments resist medial and lateral angulatory forces. The cruciate ligaments resist both anterior and posterior translation of the tibia on the femur, as well as rotational stresses. Due to the differences in radius of curvature between the medial and lateral femoral condyles, tension in the cruciate ligaments

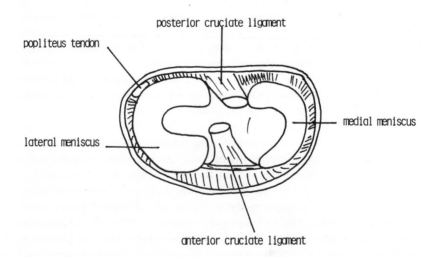

Figure 4.4. Section through the knee joint looking down from above

changes during flexion and extension. The anterior cruciate ligament tightens around the posterior cruciate ligament during internal rotation of the knee. Both the anterior and posterior cruciate ligaments are tight when the knee is in full extension and when it is flexed to 90°. Both are lax when the knee is flexed between 30° and 60°. These changes in tension are due to the twisting of the ligaments around each other, and to the twist of the fibers within the ligaments themselves.[10] Because collagen is viscoelastic, rate of stretch is an important factor in ligament failure. Other factors include age, ligament strength, and axis of loading. Ligament strength increases with exercise and decreases following immobilization.[11] During kinematic studies of the knee, it becomes apparent that there is a fine line between stability brought about by ligaments and the freedom of movement necessary as the knee moves through a range of motion. In order to totally appreciate the functional stability of the knee, one must also consider the dynamic stability brought about by muscle use.[12] Stabilization provided by the muscles is important not only in the normal knee, but also in the previously injured knee.[13] However, when a sudden deforming force is applied, muscle contraction usually does not occur rapidly enough to prevent damage. When forces are applied more slowly, proprioceptive input from the ligaments and capsule is relayed to the neighboring muscles, which then contract to resist the force.

The articulation of the patella with the femur varies as a function of knee flexion. When the knee is in full extension, the patella rests on a fat pad just above the trochlear groove. As the knee begins to flex, the patella moves downward and engages the trochlear groove.[14] The compressive forces between the patella and the femur are generated predominantly by the pull of the quadriceps muscle and the patellar tendon. (Although the patellar tendon is the anatomic termination of the quadriceps muscle, for purposes of biomechanical analysis they are considered as separate structures.) These forces can be considered in two planes. When looking at the knee from the front, one can draw a line along the axis of the quadriceps muscle and tendon, and a second line along the axis of the patellar tendon. The acute angle formed between these two lines makes up what is known as the Q (quadriceps) angle. The larger this Q-angle, the larger will be the "lateral vector" tending to pull the patella laterally in the trochlear groove (Figure 4.5). Looking at the knee from the side, the forces generated by the quadriceps muscle also can be analyzed using vectors. The resultant of the quadriceps vector and the patellar tendon vector produces compressive forces between the patella and the femur (Figure 4.6). As knee flexion increases, this force also increases.[15] The magnitude of quadriceps force has been found to increase 6% per

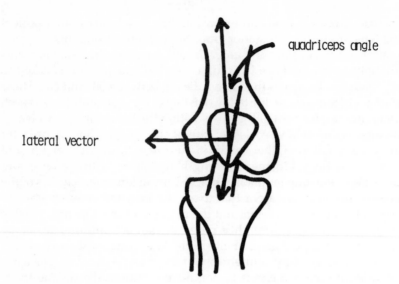

quadriceps angle

lateral vector

Figure 4.5. Quadriceps angle

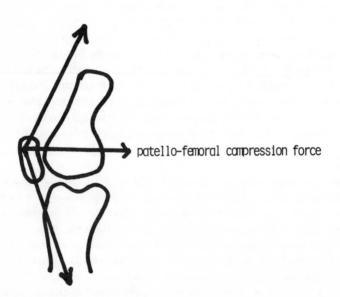

patello-femoral compression force

Figure 4.6. Patellofemoral compression force

degree of flexion. Reilly and Martens found that the patellofemoral force was half body weight during level walking, three times body weight going up and down stairs, and 7.6 times body weight during a deep knee bend.[16] Perry, Antonelli, and Ford found that the amount of quadriceps force required to stabilize the knee when the knee was flexed to 30° equalled 50 percent of maximum quadriceps strength.[17]

The behavior of tendon under load is a function of the structural orientation of the fibers, the properties of collagen and elastin, and the proportions of collagen and elastin. Both the range of motion of a musculotendinous unit and the force applied to the tendon are in part a function of the orientation of the muscle fibers relative to the axis of the tendon. The greater the longitudinal array of muscle fibers, the greater is the range of motion of the muscle and tendon. The greater the obliquity of the muscle fibers, the more force is dissipated laterally relative to the axis of the tendon. A fusiform muscle (spindle-shaped, tapering at both ends) exerts greater tensile force on its tendon than does a pennate (feather-shaped) muscle because all of the force in a fusiform muscle is applied in series with the longitudinal axis of the tendon.

The ability of tendon to deform without suffering structural damage is due in part to its viscoelastic properties. A viscoelastic material exhibits both solid and fluid properties, and the rate at which forces are applied determines the amount of force that the tendon can withstand prior to rupture. Tendon is most vulnerable to injury when tension is applied quickly or obliquely, when the tendon is tense before the trauma, or when the attached muscle is maximally innervated.[18] Eccentric muscle contraction is associated with a higher incidence of tendinitis than is concentric contraction.[19] During an eccentric contraction the muscle fibers lengthen (i.e., are stretched) while the sarcomeres (contractile units) contract to produce force. This occurs, for example, when the quadriceps muscle is used to decelerate the descent of the body when landing from a jump. Concentric contraction occurs when the muscle shortens while producing force. This occurs in the quadriceps muscle during final straightening of the knee in *développé*, for example. The force production during eccentric contraction appears to be greater than during concentric contraction.

Exercise improves both the mechanical and structural properties of tendon. These improvements appear to occur through changes in the synthesis of the collagen and proteoglycan matrix, changes in the collagen cross-links, and changes in the deposition and arrangement of collagen fibers.[20]

The collagen within the meniscus is aligned much like barrel hoops to withstand centrifugal stress. In the most superficial layer of the meniscus, the fibers are predominantly radially oriented. In the deeper layers, the collagen is circumferentially oriented, with random branching fibers that may link the circumferentially oriented bundles. Loading of the meniscus causes radial displacement that must be resisted by the radially oriented collagen fibers (Figure 4.7). This knowledge of collagen alignment becomes important during consideration of partial meniscal excision following tears. The lateral meniscus absorbs most of the weight applied to the lateral aspect of the knee, whereas the weight applied on the medial side is shared equally between the medial meniscus and the articular surface. Obviously, when menisci are removed there is a considerable loss of energy absorbing function, and increased load is transmitted to the articular cartilage.[21,22] Meniscal tears usually result from compression and/or shear forces. Due to the differences in collagen orientation between the superficial and deeper layers, the biomechanical behavior of the meniscus is not homogeneous in its response to various stresses (Figure 4.8).[23]

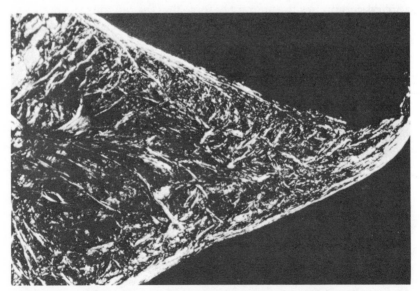

Figure 4.7. Collagen fiber orientation in a cross section of a medial meniscus
Ackeson, W., Woo, S.L.-Y., Amiel, D., Frank, C. (1984). From: The chemical basis of tissue repair. In: Hunter, L.Y., Funk, F.J., eds. *Rehabilitation of the injured knee*. St. Louis: C.V. Mosby, 189. Reprinted by permission.

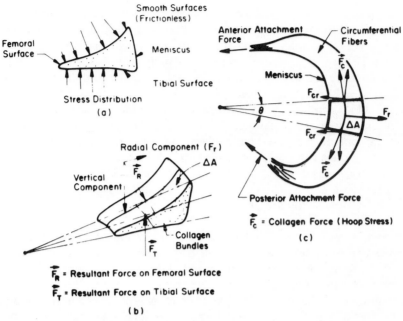

Figure 4.8. Forces acting on the meniscus

From Arnoczky, S., Adams, M., DeHaven, K., Eyre, D., Mow, V. (1988). Meniscus. In: Woo, S.L.-Y., Buckwalter, J.A., eds. *Injury and repair of the musculoskeletal soft tissue.* Parkridge, Illinois: American Academy of Orthopaedic Surgeons, 509. Reprinted by permission.

Problems

Medial Knee Strain

The word strain, by standard definition, refers to a change in length, and often is used to describe a microscopic tear in connective tissue. In dancers medial knee strain is seen predominantly in those who are poorly trained, either children or adult beginners. It is rare in the accomplished dancer. The strain occurs in the capsule on the medial aspect of the knee.[24]

Etiology: During *plié* an imaginary plumbline dropped from the knee should land over the second toe. When the plumbline falls medial to the foot during *plié,* the medial capsule and collateral ligament are stretched and strain occurs. In ballet in particular, emphasis is placed on turnout, or external rotation of the lower extremities. In the ideal turned out position, the weight should fall from the body to the thigh and directly through the center of the knee and ankle (Figure 4.9). This distribution of weight can be achieved if the external rotation of the lower extremities occurs at the hip. When external rotation of the hip is lacking, or as a result of poor instruction, a dancer may attempt to gain more rotation by doing a *demi-plié*, "turning out" the feet, and then straightening the knees. Weight will then fall medial to the knee and ankle, producing tensile stresses on the medial side of the knee and first metatarsophalangeal joint (Figure 4.10), as well as pronation of the foot. In the usual ballet class, approximately one-half to two-thirds of class time is spent at *barre* exercises, many of which include *pliés* in various positions. In addition, *pliés* are fundamental to initiating and landing jumps. Hence, if one's *plié* technique is incorrect, musculoskeletal problems are likely to occur.

Symptoms and Signs: Medial knee strain presents as pain along the medial side of the knee, with no history of specific injury. Pain is usually worse after class, and gradually decreases if there is a day or two hiatus between ballet classes. There is no history of knee swelling or locking. Physical examination often reveals some tenderness along the medial aspect of the knee, but not specifically over the joint line. No effusion (excessive fluid in the joint) is present. Ligamentous laxity, meniscal signs, and patellar tenderness are lacking. Radiographs are not usually required in this situation. One can confirm the suspicion of medial knee strain by asking the dancer to do a *plié*. If the positioning is inappropriate (as in Figure 4.10) rather than appropriate (as in Figure 4.9), technique is quite likely the culprit causing this minor problem.

Treatment: This problem requires no specific medical care, but rather technical training. The best way for finding a dancer's proper position using external rotation of the hip is to have the dancer stand with his or her legs and feet together (Figure 4.11). Instruct the dancer to move his or her legs from parallel to a position of comfortable external rotation, keeping the back straight and head up (Figure 4.12). (Keeping the back straight is important because students may increase their lumbar lordosis to achieve increased external rotation of the lower extremity. Increasing lordosis decreases the tension on the iliofemoral ligament, allowing increased external rotation of the hip. However, it will strain the lumbar spine.) The "turnout" achieved by starting in parallel and then turning out while the knees are kept straight will be a function of the dancer's femoral neck-shaft angle (Figure 4.13). Keeping the knees straight ensures that the rotation will occur at the hips. Once in this position, the dancer can be instructed to keep his or her feet at this angle when assuming the various ballet positions.

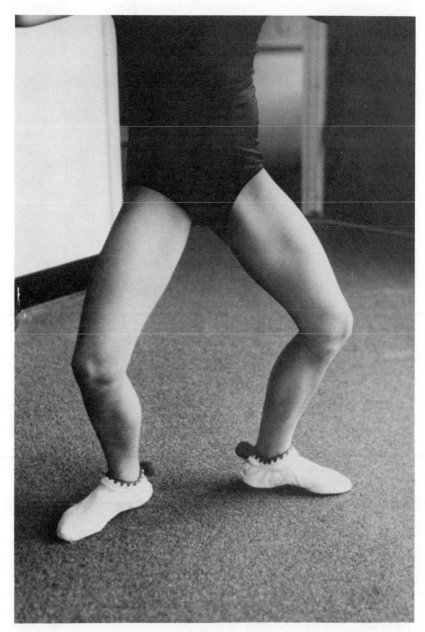

Figure 4.9. Ideally, weight should fall through the center of the knee and ankle
From Teitz, C.C. (1982). Sports medicine concerns in dance and gymnastics. *Pediatric Clinics of North America, 29*(6), 1402. Reprinted by permission.

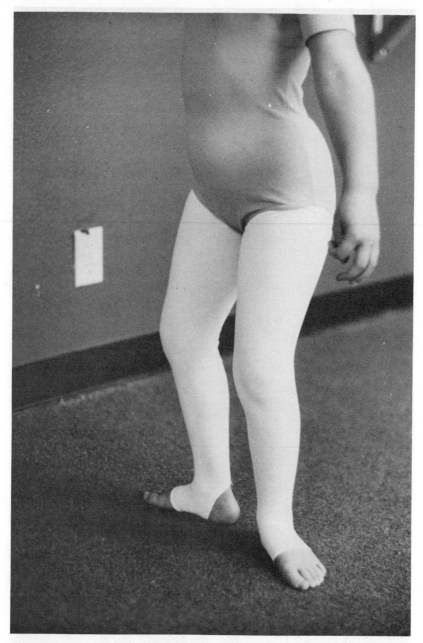

Figure 4.10. Turnout attained from the floor upward places abnormal stresses on the medial knee, ankle, and foot structures

From Teitz, C.C. (1982). Sports medicine concerns in dance and gymnastics. *Pediatric Clinics of North America, 29*(6), 1405. Reprinted by permission.

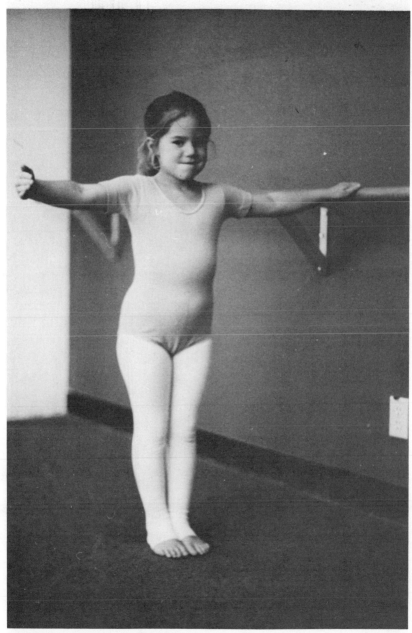

Figure 4.11. Begin with legs parallel
  From Teitz, C.C. (1982). Sports medicine concerns in dance and gymnastics. *Pediatric Clinics of North America, 29*(6), 1409. Reprinted by permission.

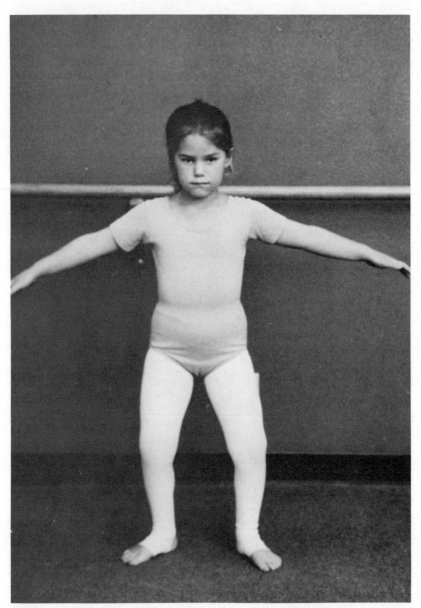

Figure 4.12. This child's "natural" turnout allows second position with the feet at a 145° angle

From Teitz, C.C. (1982). Sports medicine concerns in dance and gymnastics. *Pediatric Clinics of North America, 29*(6), 1410. Reprinted by permission.

Often fifth position will resemble third, and the feet will not be parallel in fourth position. While performing *pliés* in these positions, the knees should fall directly over the feet (Figures 4.9 and 4.12). Most good ballet instructors will accept this variation in positioning of their students, realizing that not all students can achieve a 180° angle with their feet. In addition, good instructors will teach their students to obtain more external rotation by using the short external rotators of the hip, rather than "cheating" through excessive lordosis of the lumbar spine or twisting the knee (see under Torn Cartilage).

Patellofemoral Pain

Patellofemoral pain is responsible for a large percentage of knee complaints in dancers. When one has a good grasp of the basic biomechanics of the patellofemoral joint (described above), it is not difficult to understand why abnormalities in lower extremity alignment, overuse, and faulty dance technique can lead to pain originating in the patellofemoral joint.

Etiology: Small variations in anatomic alignment of the lower extremities can produce patellar problems in dancers due to the requirements for frequent knee flexion and for turnout. The most common form of lower extremity malalignment seen is a triad of excessive femoral anteversion, external tibial torsion, and pronated feet. Femoral anteversion describes the angle of the femoral neck at the hip relative to the plane of the femoral condyles at the knee. In most individuals this angle is 10°. In individuals with excessive femoral anteversion, the angle between the neck of the femur and its shaft may equal as much as 20° (Figure 4.13). This is reflected clinically by an excessive amount of internal rotation of the hip. The tibia compensates for this excessive

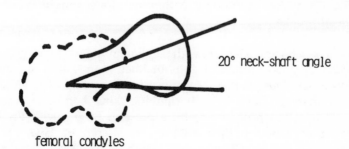

20° neck-shaft angle

femoral condyles

Figure 4.13. Looking down from above, the angle of the femoral neck in relation to the shaft of the femur

internal rotation at the hip by rotating externally with relation to the femur. Finally, in order to get the foot flat on the ground, it must pronate at the subtalar joint. As femoral anteversion and tibial torsion increase, so do the Q-angle and the lateral vector, tending to pull the patella laterally. Subsequent abnormal patellar tracking with wear of the articular surfaces, patellar subluxation, or excessive pressure on the lateral facet of the patella results. The first has been called chondromalacia of the patella, whereas the last is known as excessive lateral pressure syndrome. Both produce similar symptoms.

Overuse and poor technique also create abnormal pressure in the patellofemoral joint. Excessive compressive loading of the patella occurs due to the frequency of knee flexion, and to improper use of the quadriceps muscle. Many students contract their quadriceps muscles tightly during an entire *plié*, producing constantly high patellofemoral compression forces that theoretically will wear patellar and femoral surfaces. In addition, quadriceps strains will result from chronic eccentric use.

Additional minor aberrations in *plié* technique, repeated over time, may produce clinical problems. In the dancer with excessive femoral anteversion, particularly the dancer attempting ballet, knee pain is frequently produced due to the lack of turnout at the hips, and compensatory faulty technique. The dancer who attempts to achieve turnout from the floor upward uses the iliotibial band to gain further external rotation of the tibia. This is called "screwing the knee" because of the torque applied. Simultaneously, the patellar attachments of the iliotibial band pull the patella into an abnormal lateral position while it is being subjected to the large compressive forces generated during a *plié*.

Determining the exact source of anterior knee pain in a dancer— e.g., malalignment, thickened plica, or faulty technique—demands a thorough history and physical exam by someone versed in dance technique as well as in anatomy, pathophysiology, and clinical musculoskeletal problems.

Symptoms and Signs: Dancers with patellofemoral problems generally complain of poorly localized anterior knee pain that is aggravated by dance activities, particularly those incorporating *plié*. This pain is generally aggravated by stair climbing, knee bends, or running, particularly when pronated feet are present. Sitting with the knee flexed for any length of time will produce discomfort. Giving way is common and due to reflex quadriceps inhibition. A crackling sound is described commonly, but is also present in many people without patellofemoral problems.[25]

Treatment: For most dancers with a patellofemoral problem, improving the position of the patella with regard to the femur and correcting faulty technique and training schedules will solve the problem and prevent recurrence. In some cases assistive bracing, and rarely surgery, are required to relieve the pain and return the dancer to full activity. In order to try to gain optimal position of the patella in the trochlear groove, overstrengthening the vastus medialis obliquus component of the quadriceps muscle is recommended.[26] Vastus medialis strengthening should include isometric contractions and straight leg raises with the leg externally rotated, as well as isotonic short arc exercises. We recommend that the student keep a finger on the vastus medialis to obtain "biofeedback" on correct muscle usage during straight leg raises. It is easy to cheat and to raise the leg using hip flexors, or to rotate the leg inward and use the vastus lateralis. Full arc isotonic exercises are generally discouraged due to the high patellofemoral compression forces produced. In dancers who have difficulty contracting the vastus medialis muscle, or who have pain during isometric exercise, electrogalvanic muscle stimulation will produce a vastus medialis contraction with less force across the knee joint than a voluntary quadriceps contraction.[27]

Close assessment of technique and correction thereof is often necessary. Dancers should be taught to position their feet to correspond to their hip rotation. Additional turnout can be achieved by working the short external rotators at the hip and stretching the iliofemoral ligaments anteriorly.[24] Hamstring strengthening and working on centering body weight, especially during *demi-pointe* and *pointe,* will decrease the tendency toward hyperextension of the knee. When excessive quadriceps use is noted, the dancer must be taught to initiate *plié* using the short external rotators of the hip, and to end *plié* using adductors of the thigh. Technique can be modified in several ways. Some teachers use terms such as "pull up the thigh," "don't sit in your knees," etc. Other professionals dealing with dancers, including physical therapists, kinesiologists, and movement analysts, have varying approaches to help the dancer find a healthier and more appropriate way of moving. Many dancers have a keen awareness of muscle usage, and are able to change quickly once they are made to realize what they are doing incorrectly. Others utilize imagery techniques or proprioceptive neuromuscular facilitation.

Some dancers require a knee sleeve that incorporates a lateral pad to hold the patella in position. In approximately 10 percent of patients with patellofemoral knee pain due to malalignment, arthroscopic surgery will be indicated to release the lateral retinacular structures pulling the patella laterally. Dancers with extremely anteverted hips should be directed toward types of dance (e.g., tap) that do not demand external rotation.

Subluxating and Dislocating Patellae

Patellar subluxation (partial dislocation) and dislocation usually are due to abnormal rotatory stresses at the knee when the feet are planted. This may occur, for example, when initiating a *pirouette*. Jumps, particularly those associated with turns in midair, are likely to produce abnormal lateral patellar movement, as the torque necessary to produce the lift and rotation comes from the foot pushing against the ground as the body begins to rotate prior to becoming airborne.[28] During the era when the recreational dance "the bump" was popular, many patients came to emergency rooms having suffered patellar dislocations when they bent their knees, then twisted and angled to one side or the other to bump against their partners.

Etiology: These injuries are more common in people whose anatomical alignment is inconsistent with natural turnout—i.e., they have increased femoral anteversion. Whereas we are unlikely to find this degree of malalignment in the professional dancer, it is certainly rampant in the adolescent dancer. In dancers with shallow trochlear grooves, abnormal Q-angles, or excessive ligamentous laxity, abnormal lateral patellar movement is common. In addition, faulty technique, particularly "screwing the knee," produces excessive pull by the iliotibial band on the kneecap and increases the likelihood of patellar subluxation. Dancers whose knees hyperextend also may have subluxing patellae. Hyperextension may be due to excessive ligamentous laxity, or may be compensatory for limited plantar flexion at the ankle or for poor trunk stability. Hyperextension of the knee moves the patella away from the trochlear groove and increases its potential mobility.

Symptoms and Signs: When patellar subluxation occurs, the dancer feels an unpleasant sense of the knee coming apart, and the supporting musculature turning to jelly. This is more dramatic during dislocation, which is usually associated with severe pain. The flatter the trochlear groove, and the looser the medial retinacular structures, the less trauma is suffered during lateral patellar dislocation, because nothing has to tear to allow the patella to dislocate. In most cases, however, for dislocation to occur the patella must ride up and over the lateral trochlear facet. Once the patella is out of its normal position, the quadriceps mechanism in which it resides is useless, as its fulcrum has been displaced.[29] Hence, the dancer usually falls to the ground. During the fall, or often as a reflex, the leg straightens and the quadriceps muscles pull the patella back into position. In some cases a chip of cartilage, with or without bone, is knocked off the underside of the patella on its way out or back into the trochlear groove. When this occurs, or when the medial retinaculum tears, the torn soft tissue or fractured bone ends will bleed into the joint. The dancer then presents with a tensely swollen knee filled with blood. The presence of fat droplets in the blood suggests communication with the fatty bone marrow, i.e., a fracture. The dancer's knee will be tender at the site of damage. In the dancer with marked laxity or a very shallow trochlea, in whom patellar mobility is great, dislocation can occur readily without any damage. These dancers will report a similar history, but will not have much, if any, swelling or tenderness.

Treatment: Immediate care should include rest, ice, compression, and elevation (RICE). Rapid application of ice and compressive wrapping of the injured area will minimize hemorrhage and swelling. Elevation of the leg, preferably above heart level, will also markedly decrease the amount of swelling after injury. If one can minimize swelling and bleeding immediately following an injury, the body will need to do less "clean up" before the healing process begins. The injured area should be rested to avoid further trauma, and a diagnosis should be made as soon as possible so that treatment can proceed quickly.

In the dancer whose knee joint is filled with blood, diagnostic arthroscopy may be done initially to assess the damage. Patellar fracture, chondral injury, or complete medial retinaculum tears may require additional procedures. These might include removal or replacement and fixation of a fragment, drilling the base of a chondral defect to stimulate new cartilage growth, or suture of the retinaculum, respectively. When none of these injuries is found, the patient's knee is placed in a knee immobilizer for about one week to allow resolution of swelling. Rehabilitation is then initiated, and emphasizes strengthening of the vastus medialis obliquus, which is the key to patellar control. Electrical stimulation is especially useful in these patients to initiate quadriceps contractions. Again we progress from isometric contractions of the quadriceps muscle (quad sets) to straight leg raises. The straight leg raises should be done with the limb in external rotation to overwork the vastus medialis and to strengthen the adductors. In dancers, the adductors should control flexion and extension during *plié*, to avoid increasing the compressive forces on the patella. Short arc isotonic exercises are added to the program, but we never recommend full arc isotonic exercises to patients with patellar injury, as these exercises produce additional patellar damage and are poorly tolerated in those patients.

Patients who have suffered patellar dislocation are often found to have tight lateral retinacular structures, particularly the iliotibial band attachment to the patella. Hence, iliotibial band stretching should be added to the quadriceps rehabilitation program. Since hyperextension of the knee also can lead to patellar subluxation or dislocation, hamstring strengthening is recommended to prevent hyperextension. Because of the frequent finding of technical faults, we often recommend the supine *barre*, and learning to use hip short external rotators and thigh adductors. Well-trained movement analysts can be extremely helpful in assessing and correcting poor mechanics that contributed to the injury. Patellar restraining braces, though useful in providing additional support to the returning athlete, can be used by the dancer during class or rehearsal but usually are not worn in performance.

Tendinitis

Inflammation of the patellar tendon is a common problem in the dancer's knee. Patellar tendinitis is also commonly called "jumper's knee" because it is frequently seen in hurdlers and in basketball and volleyball players. Hamstring tendinitis is also common, but is usually located more proximally in the thigh than near the muscles' insertions at the knee.

Etiology: Tendinitis represents an overuse injury. Overuse injuries, by definition, are those that occur from trying to do too much too quickly—i.e., being poorly conditioned. They imply that the musculoskeletal tissues involved may not be strong enough, warm enough, or in the case of soft tissues, flexible enough, to withstand the stresses imposed. Generally the tissues of the musculoskeletal system have a capacity for functionally adapting to loads if these loads are gradually increased.[30] Overuse injuries are caused by relatively low loads that are applied too frequently for normal adaptive and reparative processes to occur.

Recognized causes of overuse injuries include poor training, technique, equipment, and environment. Poor training is probably the most common cause of overuse injuries. Training considerations include frequency of participation, intensity of that participation, and duration of each burst of activity. Obviously the more intense the activity, the shorter the duration needs to be to stress the musculoskeletal system. High intensity activity produces the type of loads seen in traumatic injuries. Duration of activity will be limited by the vascular supply to the involved tissues and by utilization of glucose and glycogen by these tissues, both of which are affected by previous conditioning. Frequency of participation is often the critical factor producing an overuse injury. Practicing new jumps during every class for a week, or adding rehearsals and performances to routine classes, often leads to patellar tendinitis. Many dancers have had the experience of having sore muscles 48 hours after undertaking more activity than usual. The muscle ache is a sign that the metabolic and load-bearing capacities of the involved muscles have been exceeded. By 72 hours, however, recovery generally occurs, and return to activity is possible. Trying to return to the same activity within the first 48 hours, often prior to the appearance of clinical symptoms of overuse, is likely to potentiate the inflammatory response to the initial stress and thereby produce a clinically significant overuse injury with symptoms described in the subsequent section.

Technique is often a factor in overuse injuries as well. Although there are "natural" dancers, one of the important aspects of training is that of developing efficient technique. For the recreational dancer in particular, or for the dancer who has been poorly trained, misuse of various musculotendinous units will cause them to be used unnecessarily and often in ways which are inefficient, thereby producing greater stress on these particular muscle and tendon units.[31] A dancer who uses her rectus femoris muscle to raise her leg to the front is using a muscle which does not have much mechanical advantage across the hip joint, and will ultimately develop rectus femoris tendinitis. In contrast, if she can be taught to use her iliopsoas muscle, a much stronger hip flexor, achieving this particular movement will be much more efficient, will be less likely to produce tendinitis, and will be aesthetically more desirable as there will not be an obvious contraction of thigh muscle. In addition, a dancer often can raise the leg higher using the iliopsoas because the rectus femoris tendon at the hip joint will be more relaxed and therefore can fold into the groin crease without blocking the ability to fold the leg up onto the torso. Similarly, constant use of the quadriceps muscle during *plié*, instead of short external rotator and adductor use, will lead to tendinitis and to the patellar problems previously described.

Equipment and the environment in which a dancer practices or performs often play a role in overuse injuries. Dancers are generally working barefooted, or in shoes with no shock absorption. Hence, the lower extremity muscles must act (usually eccentrically) to decelerate the legs and cushion the impact. Although aerobic dancers wear more shock absorbent shoes, they frequently dance on cement floors or on linoleum or carpeting covering cement. Professional dancers, whenever possible, dance on sprung wood floors that are more shock absorbent.

Symptoms and Signs: Tendinitis is the inflammatory response to a microscopic tear in the tendon, and usually presents as pain during use of the involved musculotendinous unit. One often finds tenderness to palpation of the involved tendon, and pain when the dancer is asked to use the musculotendinous unit against resistance. Stretching the tendon also may produce pain. In the case of patellar tendinitis, straightening the knee against resistance and flexing it beyond 120° produce pain in the patellar tendon. These symptoms are brought about by the components of the inflammatory response. The inflammatory response to a microscopic tear includes the migration of white blood cells to the area with the intent of digesting the damaged tissue. In the process, these cells also contribute to tissue destruction by releasing enzymes and other substances called prostaglandins. The E family of prostaglandins is capable of producing redness, swelling, and pain. The inflammatory response is regulated at the cellular level, and if mild may last only 48 hours. Continued excessive physical activity during this period is likely to induce further microscopic damage to the tendon in its already weakened state. Usually on the third or fourth day following the initiation of the inflammatory response, fibroblasts begin to lay down the substances necessary for aggregation of collagenous protein into collagen fibrils. During the second week following injury, the tendon feels better, but only low levels of activity are tolerated without further injury. At this time the collagen fibers are cross-linking and becoming less soluble, and therefore less liable to further breakdown. Initially these collagen fibrils are laid down in random directions. The tensile forces that can be resisted by multidirectional fibers are limited, thus making newly forming scar more subject to tearing under load. In the third to fourth week after injury, the collagen fibers reorient themselves in line with the tensile force applied to the tissue. Early mobilization of the area, without placing it under resistance, appears to improve tendon tensile strength and excursion.[32] Although there is still a small amount of remodeling that occurs up to one year after injury, most tendons are able to withstand normal stresses by six weeks after injury. One is at risk for injury recurrence during that six week period. In the interim submaximal activity is preferred.

Treatment: Initially the inflammatory process can be kept under control by ice and rest, although not totally eliminated, since it is the inflammatory process which brings to the injured area the cells that will make new collagen. Ice is especially useful in the first few days after injury, as it decreases the swelling and reduces the rate of chemical activity, therefore minimizing the inflammatory response. In addition, cold is effective at relieving pain. Two commonly discussed medications in the treatment of tendinitis are nonsteroidal anti-inflammatory drugs such as aspirin and ibuprofen, and steroids such as cortisone. The nonsteroidal drugs inhibit the synthesis of prostaglandins, thereby reducing some of the components of the inflammatory response. These drugs are useful when the symptoms of inflammation persist beyond four to five days after injury.[33] Injecting corticosteroids into inflamed tendons is frowned upon. Evidence indicates that steroid injection decreases the tensile strength of tendon and inhibits the production of collagen and the matrix between collagen fibers, potentially leading to tendon rupture.[34,35] Ice-friction massage improves circulation to the injured tissue and encourages functional alignment of the newly forming collagen fibers.[36] During the second week following the onset of tendinitis, controlled motion is particularly helpful. This may take the form of warm-up exercises or *barre*, while avoiding impact activities or activity demanding excessive eccentric load.

Because eccentric loading elicits greater force production, greater stress on the tendon is produced during this type of activity, and it is often associated with tendinitis. Therefore treatment should also include eccentric training. For the quadriceps muscle, emphasis should be placed during isotonic short arc exercises on lowering the weight just as slowly as it is raised. Lifting weights and then dropping them produces only concentric strength, and may actually damage the tendon further. In a situation in which the injured dancer is unable to progress with muscle strengthening after an episode of tendinitis, transcutaneous electrical muscle stimulation provides pain relief and the ability to strengthen the muscle without the risk of overloading it.

Torn Cartilage

The medial meniscus is more commonly injured than the lateral meniscus. Many believe that this is due to its shape and attachments. Others believe that the lateral capsular ligaments attached to the lateral meniscus help to pull it out of harm's way during flexion of the knee.

Etiology: Medial meniscal tears are commonly due to twisting the knee while the foot is planted, whereas lateral meniscal injuries are commonly due to hyperflexion of the knee. Previous anterior cruciate ligament injury also can contribute to tears of the meniscus by increasing rotatory instability in the knee. In dancers, the most common mechanism for tearing the medial meniscus is "screwing the knee" to increase turnout. The lateral meniscus is at risk during *plié*, particularly when landing from jumps and, for example, in certain forms of Russian folk dancing, where the forced hyperflexion movement in a squatting position puts a great deal of radial stress on the meniscus.

Symptoms and Signs: The patient with a torn meniscus will usually present with knee pain well localized to either the medial or lateral joint line. Swelling in the knee, if it is present, will have developed a minimum of 12 hours after the injury. The patient may report inability to flex or extend the knee completely. In addition, the patient may report that the knee has "given out." This does not reflect any ligamentous instability, but rather reflex inhibition of the quadriceps muscle secondary to pain.

Physical examination often reveals quadriceps atrophy if the injury is more than a week old. Effusion and tenderness at the site of meniscal tear are usually present. Typically, range of motion is decreased, and pain may be produced by forced flexion or extension of the knee and by twisting maneuvers. Movements that are likely to cause symptoms in a dancer with a torn meniscus might include *pliés*, jumps, or *développé*. True locking occurs when the knee is mechanically limited from full extension or flexion, and when varying amounts of rotation in combination with flexion are required to unlock it. This scenario is different from the ratchety feeling often found in dancers after sitting, and which is relieved by straightening the knee. Persistent pain and swelling in the knee suggests that the torn meniscus is irritating the knee, and may produce damage to the articular cartilage if not removed.

Treatment: Initially, the general rules of first aid pertain. The patient should rest the knee by wrapping it with an Ace bandage or using a knee immobilizer for a few days. During this period frequent applications of ice will decrease the swelling. Quadriceps setting exercises are recommended to avoid atrophy. As the effusion resolves, the patient should attempt to regain range of motion, continue quadriceps strengthening, and gradually return to activity.[37] Injured dancers can try to return to full activity when full range of motion and normal strength are achieved, and when limited participation has resulted in no aggravation of knee pain or swelling. This often takes four to six weeks. If pain or effusion persist or recur, or if the knee locks, further diagnostic evaluation is indicated. The diagnosis can be confirmed using arthrography (dye in the joint and x-rays) or arthroscopy (looking in the joint with a fiber-optic telescope). Arthroscopic excision of the torn part of the meniscus is then recommended, unless the tear is peripheral, in which case the meniscus can be repaired rather than partially excised.[38] The amount of meniscal tissue removed is determined by the pattern and size of the tear.[39] The part left behind must still resemble the original horseshoe shape, in order to retain the normal biomechanical properties of resisting centrifugal stress.

Following surgery, the knee must once again be rehabilitated, including range-of-motion exercises, strengthening, and gradual return to dance, initially omitting torsional activities. When a technical fault such as screwing the knee contributed to the meniscal injury, this fault must be corrected prior to returning to dance. Practicing *barre* exercises while lying on the floor is useful in learning to use the lower extremities correctly. Exercises to encourage using the hip short external rotators for obtaining turnout, and abdominal muscle strengthening and stretching of the hip flexors to control the pelvis, are useful to decrease torsional stresses on the knee.

Torn Ligaments

Ligament injuries are traumatic injuries occurring when a sudden deforming force exceeds the ability of the ligament to lengthen. The ligaments most commonly injured about the knee are the medial collateral and anterior cruciate ligaments. Fortunately, these injuries are uncommon among dancers.

Etiology: Ligament injury in dancers is usually caused by hyperextension of the knee, or improper landing of a jump. Contact injuries are relatively infrequent. Injuries of the collateral ligaments in dancers are distinctly uncommon, as they are usually incurred by forceful contact with another person. The lateral collateral ligament can be injured in a dancer who lands a jump on one leg with his or her body weight to the outside of center, thereby putting greater stress on the lateral collateral ligament. The medial collateral ligament can also be injured, as can the anterior cruciate ligament, from planting the foot and then changing directions, as in initiating a *pirouette* or other turns during which torsional stresses are placed between the leg and the floor. Fortunately, tears of the anterior cruciate ligament are also uncommon in dancers, but can occur during hyperextension of the knee, particularly when landing from jumps.

Symptoms and Signs: Knee ligament injuries present as knee pain following a specific painful incident. It is helpful to know the position of the knee at the time of injury, whether there was an outside force, and whether any sound was heard. An audible pop is often associated with a ligamentous rather than a meniscal injury. Swelling that occurs within 12 hours after injury represents blood in the joint. Seventy percent of the time, blood in the joint is associated with injury of the anterior cruciate ligament, whereas in 20 percent of cases it is associated with fractures, often related to patellar dislocation.[40,41] A collateral ligament tear does not always cause bleeding inside the joint, because only the deep part of the medial collateral ligament is intracapsular. Patients with collateral ligament injuries usually experience swelling similar to that from meniscal injuries—i.e., later than 12 hours after injury—and often are able to bear weight on the injured leg.

The patient with chronic ligament insufficiency often will present with a history of a knee injury producing pain and rapid swelling followed by subsequent episodes of instability and swelling in the knee. This type of instability takes the form of feeling the femur dissociate from the tibia during rotational maneuvers. Instability in a straight-ahead direction is rare because the knee is well controlled by the quadriceps and the hamstring muscles in extension and flexion respectively. Dancers with torn anterior cruciate ligaments have a difficult time turning, as well as landing from jumps. In addition, such jumps as *tour jeté* and *saut de basque* are particularly difficult as they require torque to be developed prior to leaving the ground.[28]

Findings on physical examination of a patient with an acute ligament injury will depend on whether the ligament is a collateral or cruciate ligament. In the case of a collateral ligament the knee is often swollen, and may well have bruising either medially or laterally. Tenderness will be present either at the origin, the insertion, or along the course of the ligament. Applying varus and valgus stress to the knee will often reproduce pain as the injured ligament is stretched (Figure 4.14). Occasionally, stressing a completely torn collateral ligament is painless; however, the examiner will feel abnormal angular joint motion. Applying angular stresses to the fully extended knee tests the integrity of the posterior cruciate ligament, whereas stressing the knee at 20° of flexion tests for collateral ligament damage. A grade 1 injury is manifested by tenderness but no abnormal opening of the joint. When stress testing produces an abnormal opening of between 5 mm and 1 cm, the ligament injury is called a grade 2. A grade 3 exists when the opening exceeds 1 cm or there is no palpable end point. This constitutes a ligament rupture.

In the patient with an acute cruciate ligament tear, one usually finds tense swelling in the knee caused by intra-articular bleeding. Tests of stability will demonstrate abnormal anterior and posterior movement

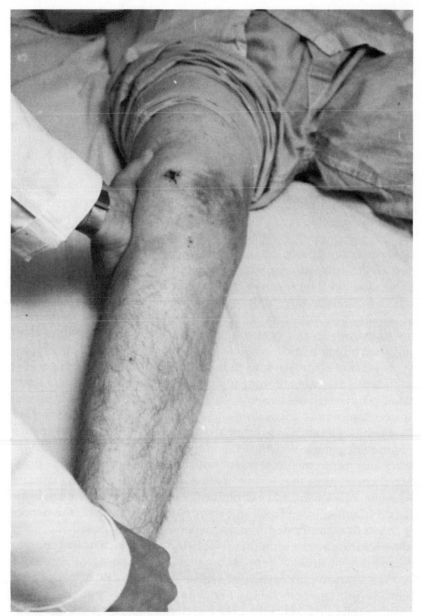

Figure 4.14. Valgus stress testing in a patient with a medial collateral ligament injury
From Teitz, C.C. (1983). Office management of common knee problems. *Current Concepts in Pain,*
1(4), 13. Reprinted by permission.

of the tibia on the femur (Figures 4.15-A and 4.15-B), and provocative rotatory tests will demonstrate abnormal rotational movement of the tibia on the femur.

Treatment: The treatment of collateral ligament injuries is a function of the injury grade. Grade 1 injuries can usually be treated symptomatically using immobilization and ice in the first three to four days, quadriceps exercises, and weight bearing as tolerated. Generally, full flexion of the knee is not possible for four to six weeks because it creates increased tension on the ligament and is painful. Grade 2 and grade 3 ligament injuries are treated using a knee brace with bilateral metal hinged stays. These stays allow flexion and extension, but protect the knee from abnormal angulatory forces medially and laterally. The ligaments are thus shielded from abnormal strains that would stretch the newly forming collagen and make the knee permanently lax. At the same time, mobilization provides a better environment for creating stronger new collagen tissue.[42,43] A patient with a grade 2 injury is weaned from the brace gradually over a two- to three-week period. Patients with a grade 3 injury use these braces for six weeks. Quite often the dancer can be kept in class doing *barre* exercises within a pain-free range, but should avoid jumping and turning.

The situation with cruciate ligaments is entirely different. Torn cruciate ligaments do not heal, because once they have ruptured they untwist and are bathed inside the joint in synovial fluid, which prevents healing of collagenous tissue. A great deal of controversy surrounds the treatment of these injuries. Direct repair yields poor functional results. Debates between surgeons advocating immediate reconstruction and those advocating a trial of rehabilitation and bracing are based on factors such as functional demands of the patient, the chance of future degenerative arthritis, and the likelihood of functional instability and future meniscal tears. Athletes in many sports wear functional knee braces that restrict motion of the knee following cruciate ligament injuries and allow continued performance. Unfortunately for dancers, although a brace can be worn during rehearsal, the dancer is still at risk during performance, when costuming usually does not allow wearing a brace. Another issue in the dancer is that most cruciate ligament reconstructive procedures, particularly those for the anterior cruciate ligament, are associated with a loss of 5° to 10° of knee extension. In most people this is perfectly acceptable, but the dancer requires full extension of the knee both for stability on *pointe* and *demi-pointe* and for aesthetic reasons. Hence, most orthopaedic surgeons taking care of dancers agree that reconstruction, particularly of the

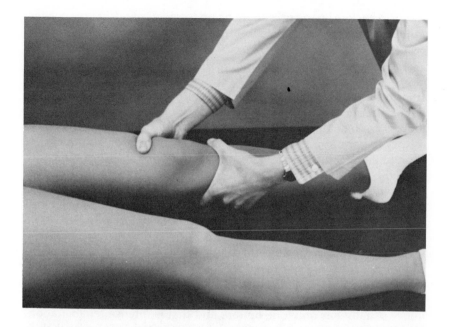

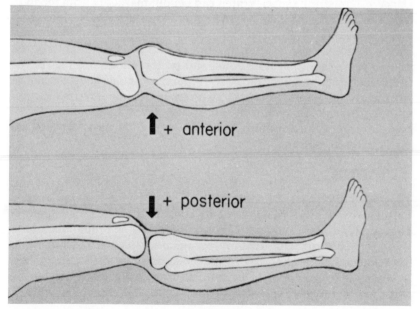

Figures 4.15 A & B. Lachman's test demonstrates anterior or posterior instability
(Figure 4.15-A) From Teitz, C.C. (1983). Office management of common knee problems. *Current Concepts in Pain, 1*(4), 14. Reprinted by permission.
(Figure 4.15-B) From Teitz, C.C. (1988). Ultrasonography in the knee: clinical aspects. *Radiologic Clinics of North America, 26*(1), 55. Reprinted by permission.

anterior cruciate ligament, should be undertaken only after the conservative approach to rehabilitation using hamstring strengthening and proprioceptive training has failed.

The principal goal of rehabilitating a patient with a cruciate ligament injury is to produce a stable knee. To my knowledge a posterior cruciate ligament injury has not been reported in a dancer. In the case of an anterior cruciate ligament injury, hamstring strengthening is utilized because the hamstrings insert on the back of the tibia and will restrict it from abnormal forward sliding motion. Despite muscular strengthening and repair or reconstruction of a torn ligament, the knee often is perceived to be less stable than before injury. This perception may be due to the lack of proprioceptive input in the scar or reconstructed ligament. When proprioceptive fibers have been torn with the ligament, the recruitment of muscles is often too late to be protective.[44,45] Training dancers in proprioceptive exercises during which they practice turning and changing directions may help prevent further episodes of knee instability.

Unlike the athlete who can choose from rehabilitation, bracing, and operative reconstruction, the dancer with an anterior cruciate ligament injury usually has only one option, and that is intense rehabilitation. Dancers' hamstring muscles often can benefit markedly from rehabilitation because they are lax due to frequent knee extension. Hamstring muscles are strengthened utilizing isotonic exercises as well as isokinetic exercises. Prior to returning to full activity, the strength of the injured knee should at least equal and preferably exceed that of the uninjured knee by approximately 10 percent. If the knee cannot be sufficiently stabilized using a rehab program, ligament reconstruction must be considered within the constraints mentioned above. Obviously cruciate ligament injuries are devastating. Fortunately they are uncommon in dancers.

Summary

The above discussion has dealt with knee problems seen in dancers. Fortunately, the most common problems are those of patellofemoral pain and tendinitis, and for the most part, following proper diagnosis, these can be dealt with utilizing proper principles of rehabilitation. These must include analysis of any predisposing factors such as weakness, tightness, or poor technique, so that those problems can be corrected and recurring injury avoided.

References

1. Garrick, J.G., Gillien, D.M., Whiteside, P. (1986). The epidemiology of aerobic dance injuries. *American Journal of Sports Medicine, 14,* 67-72.

2. Rovere, G.D., Webb, L.X., Gristina, A.G., Vogel, J.M. (1983). Musculo-skeletal injuries in theatrical dance students. *American Journal of Sports Medicine, 11,* 195-198.
3. Washington, E.L. (1978). Musculoskeletal injuries in theatrical dancers: site, frequency, and severity. *American Journal of Sports Medicine, 6,* 75-98.
4. Quirk, R. (1983). Ballet injuries: the Australian experience. *Clinics in Sports Medicine, 2,* 507-514.
5. Teitz, C.C. (1988). Gymnastics and dance athletes. In: Mueller, F.E., Ryan, A., eds. *The sports medicine team and athletic injury prevention.* Philadelphia: F.A. Davis.
6. Harty, M., Joyce, J. (1977). Synovial folds in the knee joint. *Orthopaedic Review, 6,* 91-92.
7. Hardaker, W.T., Whipple, T.L., Bassett, F.H. (1980). Diagnosis and treat-ment of the plica syndrome of the knee. *Journal of Bone and Joint Surgery, 62A,* 221-225.
8. Goodfellow, J., Hungerford, D.S., Zindel, M. (1976). Patellofemoral joint mechanics and pathology. 1. functional anatomy of the patellofemoral joint. *Journal of Bone and Joint Surgery, 58B,* 287-290.
9. Arnoczky, S.P., Warren, R.F. (1982). Microvasculature of the human meniscus. *American Journal of Sports Medicine, 10,* 90-95.
10. Reiman, P.R., Jackson, D.W. (1987). Anatomy of the anterior cruciate ligament. In: Jackson, D.W., Drez, D., eds. *The anterior cruciate deficient knee.* St. Louis: C.V. Mosby.
11. Laros, G.S., Tipton, C.M., Cooper, R.R. (1971). Influence of physical activity on ligament insertions in the knees of dogs. *Journal of Bone and Joint Surgery, 53A,* 275-286.
12. Czerniecki, J.M., Lippert, F., Olerud, J.E. (1988). A biomechanical evalua-tion of tibiofemoral rotation in anterior cruciate deficient knees during walking and running. *American Journal of Sports Medicine, 16,* 327-331.
13. Markolf, K.L., Graff-Radford, A., Amstutz, H.C. (1978). In vivo knee stability: a quantitative assessment using an instrumented clinical testing apparatus. *Journal of Bone and Joint Surgery, 60A,* 664-674.
14. Kaufer, H. (1971). Mechanical function of the patella. *Journal of Bone and Joint Surgery, 53A,* 1551-1560.
15. Huberti, H.H., Hayes, W.C. (1984). Patellofemoral contact pressures. *Journal of Bone and Joint Surgery, 66A,* 715-724.
16. Reilly, D.T., Martens, M. (1972). Experimental analysis of the quadriceps muscle force and patellofemoral joint reaction force for various activities. *Acta Orthopaedica Scandinavica, 43,* 126-137.
17. Perry, J., Antonelli, D., Ford, W. (1975). Analysis of knee-joint forces during flexed-knee stance. *Journal of Bone and Joint Surgery, 57A,* 961-967.
18. Barfred, T. (1971). Experimental rupture of the achilles tendon: compari-son of various types of experimental rupture in rats. *Acta Orthopaedica Scandinavica, 42,* 528-543.
19. Newham, D.J., Mills, K.R., Quigley, B.M., Edwards, R.H.T. (1983). Pain and fatigue after concentric and eccentric muscle contractions. *Clinical Science, 64,* 55-62.

20. Woo, S.L., Matthews, J.V., Akeson, W.J., Amiel, D., Convery, F.R. (1975). Connective tissue response to immobility. *Arthritis and Rheumatism, 18,* 257-264.

21. Krause, W.R., Pope, M.H., Johnson, R.J., Wilder, D.G. (1976). Mechanical changes in the knee after meniscectomy. *Journal of Bone and Joint Surgery, 58A,* 599-604.

22. Walker, P.S., Erkman, M.J. (1975). The role of the menisci in force transmission across the knee. *Clinical Orthopaedics and Related Research, 109,* 184-192.

23. Arnoczky, S., Adams, M., DeHaven, K., Eyre, D., Mow, V. (1988). Meniscus. In: Woo. S.L.-Y., Buckwalter, J.A., eds. *Injury and repair of the musculoskeletal soft tissue.* Parkridge, Illinois: American Academy of Orthopaedic Surgeons, 489-537.

24. Teitz, C.C. (1983). Sports medicine concerns in dance and gymnastics. *Clinics in Sports Medicine, 2,* 571-593.

25. Insall, J. (1982). Current concepts review: patellar pain. *Journal of Bone and Joint Surgery, 64A,* 147-152.

26. Lieb, F.J., Perry, J. (1968). Quadriceps function. *Journal of Bone and Joint Surgery, 50A,* 1535-1548.

27. Laughman, R.K., Youdas, J.W., Garrett, T.R., Chao, E.Y.S. (1983). Strength changes in the normal quadriceps femoris muscle as a result of electrical stimulation. *Physical Therapy, 63,* 494-499.

28. Laws, K. (1984). *The physics of dance.* New York: Schirmer Books.

29. Ariel, G. (1988). Biomechanics. In: Teitz, C.C., ed. *Scientific foundations of sports medicine.* Burlington, Ontario: B.C. Decker.

30. Teitz, C.C. (1989). Overuse injuries. In: Teitz, C.C., ed. *Scientific foundations of sports medicine.* Burlington, Ontario: B.C. Decker.

31. Solomon, R.L., Micheli, L.J. (1986, Aug.). Technique as a consideration in modern dance injuries. *The Physician and Sportsmedicine, 14,* 83-92.

32. Woo, S.L., Gelberman, R.H., Cobb, N.G., Amiel, D., Lothringer, K., Akeson, W.H. (1981). The importance of controlled passive mobilization on flexor tendon healing. *Acta Orthopaedica Scandinavica, 52,* 615-622.

33. Almekinders, L.C., Gilbert, J.A. (1986). Healing of experimental muscle strains and the effects of nonsteroidal anti-inflammatory medication. *American Journal of Sports Medicine, 14,* 303-308.

34. Kennedy, J.C., Willis, R.B. (1976). The effects of local steroid injections on tendons: a biochemical and microscopic correlative study. *American Journal of Sports Medicine, 4,* 11-21.

35. Halpern, A.A., Horowitz, B.G., Nagel, D.A. (1977). Tendon ruptures associated with corticosteroid therapy. *Western Journal of Medicine, 127,* 378-382.

36. Chamberlain, G.J. (1982, Summer). Cyriax's friction massage: a review. *Journal of Orthopaedic and Sports Physical Therapy, 4,* 16-22.

37. Teitz, C.C. (1986). First aid, immediate care, and rehabilitation of knee and ankle injuries in dancers and athletes. In: Shell, C.G., ed. *The dancer as athlete.* Champaign, Illinois: Human Kinetics.

38. DeHaven, K.E. (1985). Meniscus repair—open versus arthroscopic. *Arthroscopy, 1,* 173-174.
39. McGinty, J.B., Geuss, L.F., Marvin, R.A. (1977). Partial or total meniscectomy. *Journal of Bone and Joint Surgery, 59A,* 763-766.
40. Noyes, F.R., Bassett, R.W., Grood, E.S., Butler, D.L. (1980). Arthroscopy in acute traumatic hemarthrosis of the knee. *Journal of Bone and Joint Surgery, 62A,* 687-695.
41. DeHaven, K.E. (1980). Diagnosis of acute knee injuries with hemarthrosis. *American Journal of Sports Medicine, 8,* 9-14
42. Tipton, C.M., James, S.L., Mergner, W., et al. (1970). Influence of exercise on strength of medial collateral knee ligaments of dogs. *American Journal of Physiology, 218,* 894-902.
43. Woo, S.L.-Y., Gomez, M.A., Sites, T.J., et al. (1987). The biomechanical and morphological changes in the medial collateral ligament of the rabbit after immobilization and remobilization. *Journal of Bone and Joint Surgery, 69A,* 1200-1211.
44. Schultz, R.A., Miller, D.C., Kerr, C.S., Micheli, L. (1984). Mechanoreceptors in human cruciate ligaments: a histological study. *Journal of Bone and Joint Surgery, 66A,* 1072-1076.
45. deAndrade, J.R., Grant, C., Dickson, A.S. (1965). Joint distension and reflex muscle inhibition in the knee. *Journal of Bone and Joint Surgery, 47A,* 313-322.

5

Biomechanical Considerations in Turnout

Karen Clippinger-Robertson, M.S.P.E.

Turnout presents a unique challenge in many dance forms. Turnout refers to external rotation of the femur at the hip such that the knees and feet face as close to directly side as possible. Correct turnout involves appropriate strength, flexibility, and neural activation patterns at the hip. Although anatomical constraints are an important underlying limiting factor, many dancers can improve their turnout with a better understanding of proper biomechanics and with supplemental exercises. Correct turnout is essential not only for skill development but also for injury prevention. Many of the overuse injuries that occur in dance are related to improper turnout and the resultant excessive stresses at the back, hip, knee, and foot.

Anatomical Constraints

Perfect or ideal turnout requires that the feet and knees face directly sideways (180 degrees), such that a straight line could be drawn between the first and second toe of the right foot, right heel, left heel, and between the first and second toe of the left foot. Theoretically, this rotation should be accomplished at the hip joint rather than by rotating the lower leg out relative to the upper leg (Figure 5.1). Although few dancers actually possess perfect turnout, most dancers strive to get as close to the ideal as their bodies will allow. Range of motion at the hip, and hence potential proper turnout, is most fundamentally determined by anatomical constraints including bony, ligamental, and musculotendinous factors.

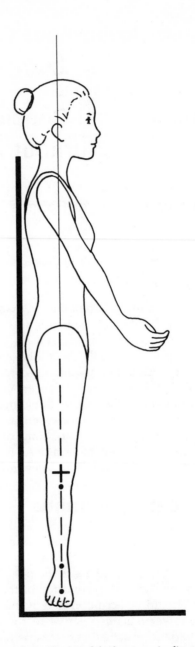

Figure 5.1. With correct turnout the midpoint of the knee-cap is aligned over the long axis of the foot, while the torso remains vertical and the longitudinal arches of the foot are maintained. With perfect turnout the knees would be facing directly side so that a straight line is formed by the feet.

Illustration: Mary Cosenza.

Bony and Ligamentous Constraints

The orientation of the acetabulum, the socket of the pelvis in which the head of the femur sits, is important in determining potential turnout (Figure 5.2-A). The angle of the neck of the femur relative to the long shaft of the femur (angle of femoral neck anteversion or retroversion) is also crucial in determining the amount of external rotation possible at the hip.[1] Excessive femoral neck anteversion (Figure 5.2-B) is commonly associated with the tendency to toe-in, and is considered undesirable for dance. In contrast, femoral neck retroversion (Figure 5.2-C) is commonly associated with the tendency to toe-out, and will allow much greater external rotation at the hip. Hence, it is considered desirable for dance forms emphasizing turnout.

It is commonly held that most children are born with femoral neck anteversion, and that this angle decreases with maturation.[2] In normal adult skeletons the range is approximately 38 degrees anteversion to 20 degrees retroversion, with an average of 8 degrees anteversion.[3] It used to be believed that the starting angle and degree of change were in large part structurally determined. However, there is now good evidence to suggest that function can play a powerful role. It appears that dancers who begin training before 11 years of age can significantly alter the actual angle of the femoral neck to enhance turnout.[2] Careful stretching in the commonly used "frog position" (prone, double *passé* position), as well as dynamic technique training, may effect structural changes in young dancers.

After approximately 11 years of age it seems unlikely that the femoral neck can be molded; changes are restricted to the joint capsule, ligaments, and musculotendinous structures. The strong hip ligaments form thickened bands of the hip joint capsule, and both structures play important roles in limiting joint mobility. One particularly important ligament for the dancer is the iliofemoral ligament. This is the strongest ligament in the body, and it limits how far the femur can turn out, as well as how far the leg can be brought behind the body (hip extension/hyperextension).[4] So, early stretching of this ligament and the closely associated capsule may be important for achieving maximal turnout. Dancers who genetically have extreme ligamental laxity may have excellent turnout even with a less than optimal angle of femoral neck retroversion.

This early plasticity of key anatomical structures provides rationale for early dance training, particularly for the aspiring classical ballet dancer. Potential improvements in turnout in the older dancer are probably limited to gains allowed by the musculotendinous complex.

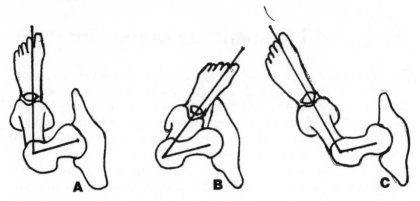

Figure 5.2. Femoral neck anteversion and retroversion with associated rotation: A. Normal hip; B. Femoral neck anteversion with associated femoral internal rotation; C. Femoral neck retroversion with associated femoral external rotation.

Certainly the femoral neck can no longer be molded. The degree to which capsule and ligaments can be stretched, how this distensibility is influenced by age, and whether rigorous stretching of these structures can have long term negative effects are controversial issues which require further scientific investigation.

Musculotendinous Constraints

The muscles and their adjoining tendons also limit motion at the hip. Increases in flexibility of the musculotendinous complex can be produced through dance movements which require a large range of motion at the hips, strengthening exercises which use a full range of motion, or through stretching.

Methods of Stretching

Recommended methods of stretching include static and Proprioceptive Neuromuscular Facilitation (PNF) techniques utilized when the muscles are already warm (i.e., after *barre*, center floor warm-up, or at the end of class). With static techniques, a position which places the desired muscle and related connective tissue in a position of elongation is maintained for 30 seconds to 1 minute. The magnitude of the stretch should be moderate, so that a sensation of stretch but not pain is experienced. An effort should be made to "relax" the muscle which is undergoing the stretch. It appears that better gains in flexibility can be achieved by repeating the same stretch about three times.

PNF techniques attempt to alter neural input influencing muscle extensibility in order to improve flexibility. One common version (contract-relax) utilizes a 10-second contraction of the muscle followed by 10 seconds of "relaxation" during which the same muscle is passively stretched. This procedure is generally repeated three times, and a static stretch of 30 seconds or more is added at the end. For example, using the hamstring stretch shown in Figure 5.3,[5] the dancer first contracts the hamstring for 10 seconds by attempting to bring the right leg down toward the ground (hip extension) while the arms resist that motion. This contraction is followed by a conscious relaxation of the hamstrings as the arms are used to pull the leg closer to the chest, effecting a passive hamstring stretch. This procedure is repeated three times, each time attempting to bring the leg slightly closer to the chest. The third passive stretch should be maintained for a duration of 30 seconds to a minute. PNF techniques can be particularly useful for dancers who are having difficulty improving their flexibility.

Ballistic stretching involves bouncy movements where momentum is dynamically used to stretch a muscle. An example is "flat-back bounces" commonly used in jazz classes. Although ballistic stretches appear to be effective, the risk for muscle injury and muscle soreness is much greater than with other methods of stretching. Therefore, it is advisable (at least until further research clarifies this issue) to substitute static or PNF stretch variations which are potentially as effective and less dangerous.

Specific Stretches

For improving turnout it is particularly important to stretch the hip internal rotators, hamstrings, hip adductors, and hip flexors. Although the latter three muscle groups may not directly limit external rotation of the hip, proper execution of many high movements to the front (e.g., *grand battements* or *développés*) requires tremendous hamstring flexibility. The hamstring stretch shown in Figure 5.3 should be performed in a turned-out position as well as the parallel position shown. This variation is particularly relevant to the needs of dance, and will also help stretch the hip internal rotators. The more flexible dancer can perform this stretch in a standing position with the leg up and against a wall, or in a split position on the floor.

Correct performance of many high movements to the side not only require great hamstring flexibility, but also marked hip adductor flexibility. The adductors can be included in the stretch shown in Figure 5.3 by turning the leg out and carrying it to the side (second position). This stretch can also be performed in a side-lying position as shown

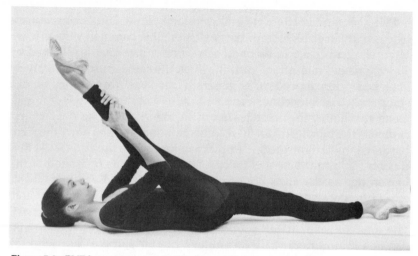

Figure 5.3. PNF hamstring stretch. The hamstrings are actively contracted by attempting to bring the leg away from the chest as the arms resist the motion. This 10 second contraction is followed by relaxation of the hamstrings as the arms are used to pull the leg closer to the chest. This sequence is repeated three times, and the final stretch is sustained for 30 seconds or longer. (Model: Maurya Kerr)

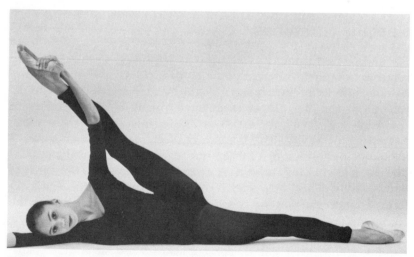

Figure 5.4. Hamstring and adductor stretch. The leg is pulled towards the head in a full externally rotated position. To add PNF techniques the arm can be used to resist knee flexion, internal hip rotation, or adduction.

in Figure 5.4. This latter variation offers another opportunity to use PNF techniques. The arms can be used to resist knee flexion, hip internal rotation, or movement of the leg towards the front. Another way of stretching the hip adductors is the straddle stretch (sitting with the legs in second position). To add greater resistance the stretch can be carefully performed with the feet widely separated against a wall in either a sitting or supine position. Again, PNF techniques can be easily added by pulling the legs together as the wall resists and prevents this motion. On the relaxation phase, a greater stretch can be applied by carefully bringing the pelvis closer to the wall.

Most dance movements to the back will be limited by the extensibility of the hip flexors, the hip capsule, and the iliofemoral ligament. Two stretches to improve hip flexor flexibility are shown in Figures 5.5-A and 5.5-B. To achieve effective gains with these stretches, particular emphasis on correct form is essential.

The most powerful hip flexor (iliopsoas) attaches onto the sides of the spine and the inside of the pelvis (ilium). Several of the other primary hip flexors (sartorius and rectus femoris) attach onto the front of the pelvis. Due to this anatomical arrangement, either letting the low back arch or the top of the pelvis tilt forward (anterior pelvic tilt) will slacken the muscles which the dancer is attempting to stretch. So, to be effective, the dancer must learn to use the abdominal muscles to prevent these undesired movements. In the first stretch (Figure 5.5-A) the dancer should concentrate on using the abdominal muscles to pull the pubic bone forward and closer to the ribs until a stretch is felt across the front of the hip (of the extended leg). As flexibility improves, the back leg can be moved further backwards and the front knee can be further bent such that the stretch is intensified. The dancer should continue to concentrate on keeping the torso vertical (rather than leaning forward) and bringing the bottom of the pelvis forward (posterior pelvic tilt). To enhance the transfer to dance, this stretch should also be performed with both legs turned out.

As correct form is mastered, the more rigorous stretch shown in Figure 5.5-B can be added. Again, the abdominals should be used to prevent an anterior pelvic tilt, and emphasis should be on bringing the bottom of the pelvis forward to create the stretch. This stretch can be done with the back knee either straight or bent, and should be performed in both parallel and turned-out positions.

Stretching of the hip internal rotators will have the most direct effect on improving turnout. This can be fostered by inclusion of an externally rotated position in each of the stretches just described. Internal rotator flexibility can also be improved with the external rotator strengthening exercise shown in Figure 5.8. The end position of

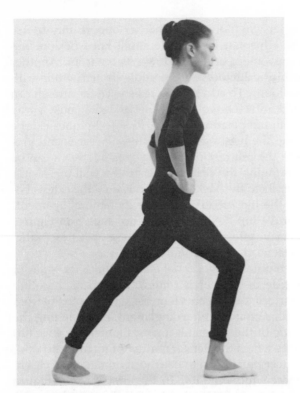

Figure 5.5-A. Standing hip flexor stretch. As the abdominals are used to stabilize the pelvis, the dancer brings the bottom of the pelvis forward until a stretch is felt across the front of the hip.

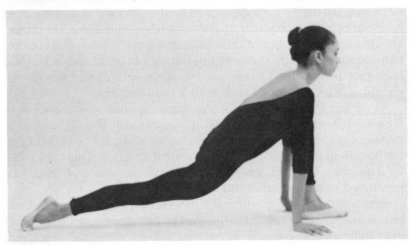

Figure 5.5-B. Lunge hip flexor stretch.

full external rotation used in this exercise will stretch the internal rotators as well as strengthen the external rotators. Another option is to add PNF techniques to either a standing or supine *passé* stretch. The standing variation can best be performed in a doorway with the knee of the bent leg against the wall. The dancer contracts the *passé* leg by attempting to bring the knee forward and down (hip horizontal adduction and internal rotation) as the wall resists the motion. After relaxing the muscles, the torso and support leg are rotated slightly further away from the *passé* leg as the gesture leg is further externally rotated (i.e., greater trochanter brought closer to ischial tuberosity). The abdominals should be used to keep a neutral pelvis and prevent the low back from arching.

To perform the supine variation, the dancer uses her arm for resistance rather than the wall. It is easier to keep the hips square if a double *passé* position is used, or if the support leg is bent with the foot pressing against the ground to lend stability. The abdominals should again be firmly contracted to prevent the low back from arching. If the dancer has difficulty maintaining a neutral pelvis, a towel can be rolled and placed under the bottom of the pelvis to create a slight posterior pelvic tilt (tuck). Later, as form is perfected, the exercise can be adjusted to a neutral pelvis without the towel, using abdominal stabilization.

When these positions are used to stretch the hip internal rotators or hip flexors it is important to realize that the hip capsule and ligaments often are stopping further movements rather than the musculotendinous complex. To avoid injury it is therefore important that these stretches be performed slowly and gently, and that no hip joint pain is experienced.*

Measurement of Turnout

An estimate of how much turnout a dancer has can be obtained by passively measuring external rotation of the hip. Two methods are shown in Figure 5.6. These measures will be primarily determined by the bony, ligamentous, and musculotendinous constraints previously discussed. To obtain accurate results, it is essential for the pelvis to be in a neutral position, not tilted anteriorly. An anterior pelvic tilt will

---

*Because the focus of this chapter is on improving turnout, stretches for the hip extensors, hip adductors, hip flexors, and hip internal rotators have been described. However, for a rounded flexibility program for the hip, and from a perspective of injury prevention, stretches for the hip abductors and hip external rotators should also be included in the dancer's routine.

slacken the hip capsule and iliofemoral ligament and give a falsely high measure of external rotation.

The first measure (Figure 5.6-A) is performed with the knees straight and the hip extended (straight down versus flexed). This measure will best reflect the potential turnout of the dancer when standing with the knees straight, and is considered the most meaningful reflection of the usual definition of turnout. When performing this measurement it is important to realize that many dancers have marked ligamental laxity, which allows significant external rotation of the lower leg (tibia) relative to the upper leg (femur), and of the foot relative to the tibia. To avoid an inaccurate measurement it is important to rotate the hip by movement of the femur rather than the foot. A more reflective measure can also be achieved if the ankle is fully dorsiflexed with one hand to help lock the foot, while the other hand of the examiner is placed on the inner thigh above the knee to help fully rotate the femur externally at the hip. Some examiners prefer to do this test supine with the knee flexed and hanging over the edge of a table, or prone with the knee flexed to about 90 degrees.[3] This offers the examiner better leverage for externally rotating the hip. However, even more care must then be taken that movement of the tibia relative to the femur is minimized and not included in the measure of rotation at the hip.

The second technique, shown in Figure 5.6-B, is performed with the hip and knee flexed to 90 degrees. Flexing the hip slackens the hip capsule and iliofemoral ligament. This measure is more reflective of turnout possible in movements such as a front *attitude* (i.e., rotation possible with the hip in flexion). It can be performed with the dancer sitting at the edge of a table with both knees flexed (as shown) or lying supine with the other limb extended. To achieve an accurate measurement it is again essential to try to isolate the rotation to the hip and limit accessory rotation or adduction of the tibia relative to the femur. Placing one hand of the examiner above the knee to effect the external rotation of the hip will help improve measurement accuracy.

It is helpful to perform both of these measures of hip external rotation because the results are often quite different, and the information from both is useful in teaching students how best to maximize their potential turnout. For example, many students may be lower than desired in the first measure (Figure 5.6-A), yet quite good with the second measure (Figure 5.6-B). In such cases, the aesthetics of the dancers' work can often be significantly improved by teaching them to fully utilize their turnout in the gesture leg in the many movements

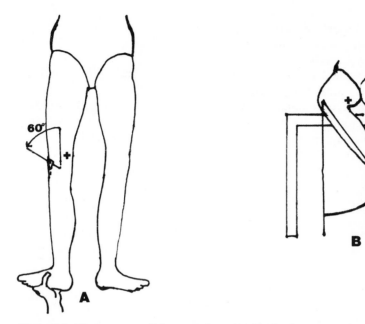

Figure 5.6. Measurement of hip external rotation ("+" indicates sites for placement of examiner's hands to produce external hip rotation). A. Hip external rotation with the hip extended; B. Hip external rotation with the hip in flexion.

performed with the hip flexed, or abducted (i.e., front *attitudes*, extensions, kicks, *rond de jambes*. . .).

Biomechanical Constraints

Many dancers exhibit greater external rotation at the hip when passively measured with the tests just described than they use functionally. In other words, many dancers have greater turnout than they have learned to use during dancing. This finding demonstrates that factors other than bony, ligamentous, and musculotendinous constraints are involved in determining functional turnout. Two other important factors are adequate strength of key muscles, and appropriate activation patterns of these muscles for optimization of correct mechanics.

Strength

The deep outward rotators and gluteus maximus are considered prime movers for hip external rotation, while the sartorius, biceps femoris, and gluteus medius (posterior fibers) can assist with external rotation in some positions. Although more controversial, some anatomists also hold that the iliopsoas and some of the hip adductors may aid slightly with external rotation.[6,7,8]

When focusing on turnout in dance, special attention should be given to the six deep outward rotators (Figure 5.7). These six muscles are capable of producing the desired external rotation with minimal accessory motions. This capability is important both for optimizing range of motion and for achieving the desired dance aesthetic.

For example, since the gluteus maximus causes hip extension as well as external rotation, when the muscle contracts it will tend to produce both of these actions. In movements such as a front *attitude,* where the desired action is hip flexion and external rotation, the undesired opposite action of hip extension of the gluteus maximus can limit range of motion (i.e., how high the leg can be lifted). Similarly, the sartorius and gluteus medius produce hip abduction as well

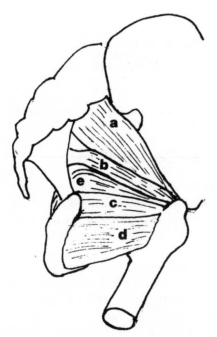

Figure 5.7. Deep outward rotators of the hip. The six deep outward rotators of the hip span the pelvis and the femur, and are comprised of the following muscles: A. Piriformis; B. Gemellus superior; C. Gemellus inferior; D. Quadratus femoris; E. Obturator internus; F. Obturator externus (located behind quadratus femoris and not visible in this view).

as external rotation, and so their unbalanced use can often produce a slight undesired abduction of the hip instead of the desired isolated external rotation. In dance terminology this slight abduction is frequently termed "lifting the hip," or "hip-hiking," and is considered an undesired aesthetic by most schools of dance.

As specific use and strengthening of the deep outward rotators can be helpful for enhancing turnout, an exercise for strengthening these muscles is shown in Figure 5.8. When performing this exercise it is important that the movement occurs at the hip; that there is no twisting of the lower leg relative to the upper leg. The abdominal muscles should be used throughout the exercise to prevent the pelvis from tilting forward and the spine from arching. The dancer should focus on relaxing the outer gluteus maximus and on using the deep outward rotators. This muscle emphasis can sometimes be aided by having the dancer place her hand at the base of the buttocks while concentrating on tightening the lower muscles under the gluteus maximus.

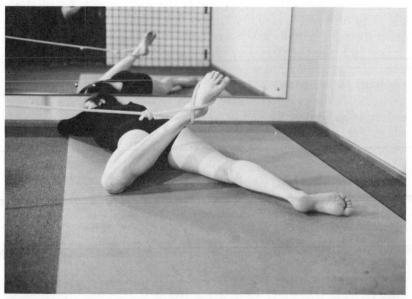

Figure 5.8. Deep outward rotator strengthening. While lying prone with the knee bent to 90 degrees, rotate outwards at the hip, bringing the heel toward the opposite knee. Use surgical tubing for resistance with a "Figure 8" wrapped around the ankle and the opposite end tied to something stable. Perform 10 repetitions, holding a three count with the thigh at 30, 60 and 90 degrees. Allow a rest of 30 seconds to 2 minutes between sets. Be careful to keep the angle of the knee constant and rotate from the hip, rather than twisting the knee by leading with the heel. Maintain a posterior pelvic tilt and try to relax the outer gluteal muscles while emphasizing the use of the deep outward rotators.

If any discomfort is felt at the knee, an alternative exercise with the knee extended should be substituted. The dancer lies on his or her side and lifts the upper leg (hip abduction) while the knee is facing the ceiling (i.e., full external rotation at the hip). The heel of the top leg should be kept one or two inches behind the bottom heel (i.e., the femur of the top hip should be in about five degrees of hyperextension) throughout the exercise. To achieve the desired emphasis of the deep outward rotators the following sequence is often helpful: 1) The dancer raises the rotated leg about 10 degrees and holds this position for 3 counts. 2) The dancer then attempts to add further outward rotation without letting the leg come forward (i.e., focus on rotating along the long axis of the leg to bring the heel further around). Maintaining this additional rotation, the leg is raised another 10 degrees and held 3 counts. 3) The dancer adds further rotation, raises the leg 10 more degrees, and holds a final 3 counts. The emphasis in this particular exercise is on maximizing the degree of rotation while limiting how high the leg is raised. Throughout the exercise the abdominals should be used to help maintain correct pelvic/torso alignment. As strength and isolation improve, ankle weights, elastic bands, or surgical tubing can be used to provide additional resistance.

As with flexibility exercises, muscle groups in addition to the deep rotators become important for optimizing turnout in common dance movements. Movements to the front require adequate hip flexor strength. Movements to the side require adequate strength of the hip abductors as well as the hip flexors. Movements to the back require adequate hip extensor strength. Examples of strengthening exercises for a few of these key muscles follow.

Specific Muscle Activation Patterns

When performing various dance movements which use turnout, specific selection of appropriate muscles, the timing of their activation, and the relative magnitude of their activation are all important for maximizing turnout.

Second Position Grand Plié

Pliés are one of the most fundamental vocabulary elements of dance, and so are a good place to begin working on improving turnout. When performing *pliés*, turnout can often be enhanced by emphasizing use of the deep outward rotator muscles and hip adductors while maintaining a vertical torso and pelvis. This technique modification is usually easiest to achieve using a second position (Figure 5.9-A). A helpful exercise is to perform second position *grand pliés* with the back against a wall and the heels one to two inches away from the wall. The mid-thoracic spine and mid-sacrum should remain in contact with the wall throughout the exercise. Use of the deep outward rotators can be encouraged by such techniques as: 1) Putting the fingertips at the base of the buttocks and feeling the muscles contract; 2) attempting to pull the outside of the thigh (greater trochanter) closer to the bottom of the back of the pelvis (ischial tuberosity); or 3) pulling the knees as close to the wall as possible throughout both the down- and up-phase of the *plié*.

Since with proper turnout motion occurs as close to a frontal plane as the dancer's structure will allow, the hip adductors are also in an appropriate location to provide important assistance (Figure 5.9-B). The adductors work eccentrically on the down-phase of the *plié* and concentrically on the up-phase. Most dancers seem to be able to cue into the concentric or shortening phase of a muscle more easily. Therefore, another helpful hint is to encourage dancers to pull the inner thighs together on the up-phase of the *plié*. Once they have cued into the use of these muscles on the up-phase, they can usually transfer the muscle use to the down-phase. On the down-phase, cues such as "reach the knees directly side rather than allowing them to fall forward and inside the feet," or "stretch the inner thighs away from each other" can sometimes help emphasize the desired adductor use. Use of the adductors can also be encouraged by performing these second position *pliés* immediately following adductor strengthening exercises, while awareness is heightened.

The adductors can be strengthened by lifting the lower leg while in a side-lying position. The top leg is in a *passé* position with the toes just touching the ground behind the bottom knee, to aid with balance. A weight can be added at the ankle or just above the knee of the lower leg to increase resistance. The hip adductors can also be strengthened by using surgical tubing to resist bringing the leg towards the midline while in a turned-out supine position. For less isolated but more functional strengthening, second position turned out *pliés* can be performed in a shuttle, or using a leg press.

Maintaining a vertical torso can also enhance turnout. During this exercise (second position wall *pliés*) the vertical position is ensured by sliding the back against the wall, keeping the mid-thoracic spine and mid-sacrum constantly in contact as the knees bend and straighten. This procedure can help counter the common tendency that many dancers have to lean forward (slight hip flexion) during *pliés*. Leaning forward is often accompanied by an anterior tilt of the pelvis, decreased turnout, and greater use of the quadriceps femoris muscles.

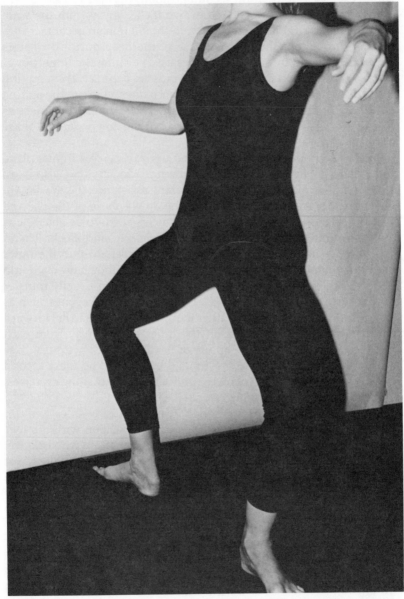

Figure 5.9-A. Use of the hip adductors in second position *grand plié*. The adductors are in an appropriate position to work eccentrically on the down-phase, and concentrically on the up-phase, of the *plié*.

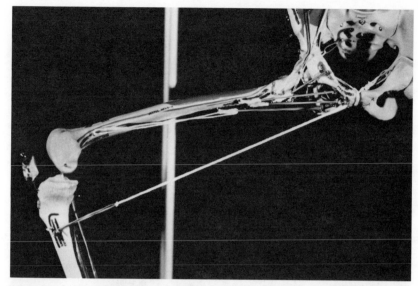

Figure 5.9-B. Line of pull of the adductors, showing how the use of turnout puts these muscles in an appropriate position to assist with *pliés*.

Although further investigation is necessary, preliminary findings suggest that a balanced co-contraction of the hip adductors, hamstrings and quadriceps (versus quadriceps dominance) is desirable for optimizing turnout.[9]

Développé à la Seconde

As with *pliés*, proper activation patterns are essential for optimizing turnout during movements involving lifting the leg to the side. For example, when performing a *développé à la seconde*, specific use of the deep outward rotators is necessary to enhance elevation and minimize undesired lifting of the hip (see Figures 5.10-A-D).[10] Dance teachers often describe this as "dropping the hip under before lifting the leg up" in a *développé*. The anatomical correlate to this directive is to bring the projection on the outer part of the upper femur (greater trochanter) "down"—closer to the bottom of the pelvis (ischial tuberosity)—through use of the deep outward rotators and appropriate use of the other hip muscles. With proper activation and timing, these muscles can work to rotate the femur externally and pull the greater trochanter down, so that the process clears and maximum elevation of the leg to the side can be achieved (Figure 5.11-A). To help dancers achieve this proper mechanics it is often helpful to focus on the lower rotators, working to rotate the leg fully and bring the trochanter down at the

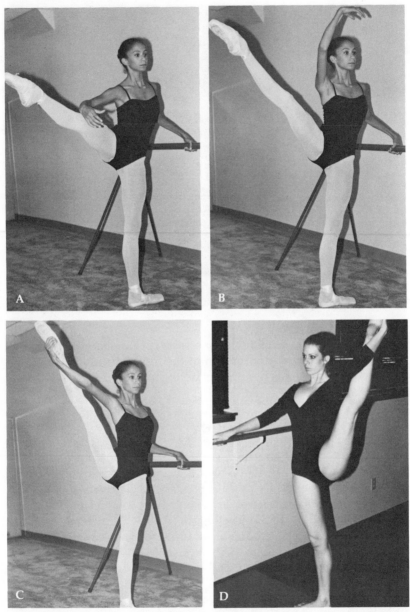

Figures 5.10-A-D. *Développé à la seconde:* A. Incorrect execution with the hip lifted; B. More correct position, with the greater trochanter of the femur coming closer to the ischial tuberosity. Height of the leg is limited by current strength levels; C. More correct position and greater height when assisted with hand, showing potential turnout as strength develops; D. Ideal position. (Model: Patricia Barker)

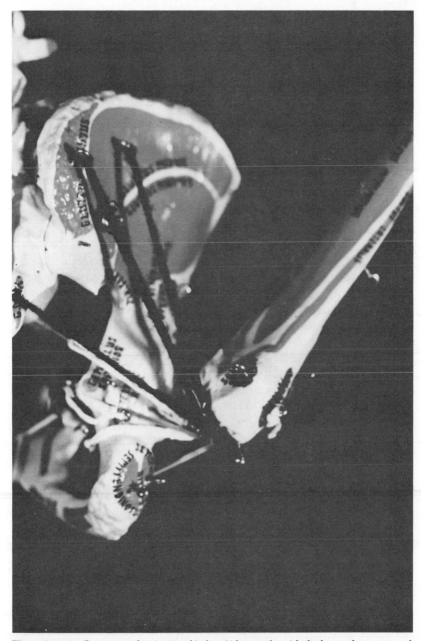

Figure 5.11-A. Correct mechanics in a *développé à la seconde*, with the lower deep outward rotators working to bring the greater trochanter down, resulting in greater external rotation and elevation of the leg.

very beginning of the *développé*. This can help counter the upward pull of the gluteal muscles (Figure 5.11-B). After this, the focus can be shifted to bringing the knee close to the chest and reaching the foot towards the ceiling as the knee is extended. As the correctness of execution of the *développé* improves (Figures 5.10-A-D), the knee faces further backwards (i.e., there is greater femoral external rotation), there is less lifting of the hip (i.e., lateral pelvic tilt), and more of the desired elevation of the leg is achieved.

Often when dancers attempt to change their mechanics as described above they find they can bring the leg higher, but have inadequate strength to hold it in the fully extended position. This change in mechanics requires a use of muscles different from that which has been developed with years of training. To aid in this transition it is important to strengthen the deep outward rotators and the iliopsoas. Exercises for strengthening the deep outward rotators have already been described (Figure 5.8). The iliopsoas is a powerful hip flexor which is also very important in the upper ranges of hip abduction. Many of the other muscles of the hip lose their ability to produce much force by 90 degrees, so the iliopsoas becomes important when lifting the leg to either the side or front. Furthermore, using an externally rotated position shifts the line of pull of the muscles such that the hip flexors become important in producing movement which in parallel position would be carried out primarily by the hip abductors.

An exercise for strengthening the iliopsoas is shown in Figure 5.12. When first performing this exercise, the dancer should sit in a tucked position (posterior pelvic tilt). This increases the ability of the iliopsoas to produce force (length-tension principle), and often helps to isolate the muscle. An effort should be made to relax the quadriceps and use the deeper, higher muscle (iliopsoas). As strength improves, one set with a neutral pelvis (sitting straight up versus tucked) and one set using a turned-out position can be added. After about six weeks of performing the exercise, increase the number of sets to both the side and the front. This will help strengthen the needed combination of hip flexors and abductors. Although the variation to the side can be done as before while sitting in a chair, it is often easier for dancers to begin by performing the exercise while lying on the side. The surgical tubing should be anchored directly below the body, with the other end looped above the knee. These variations will help develop the specific strength needed when working to the side with *développés*, *grand battements*, etc., while the initial variation (Figure 5.12) will best transfer to frontal movements.

To help make the strength aspect of these exercises directly applicable to dance technique, a position can be used with the knee extended

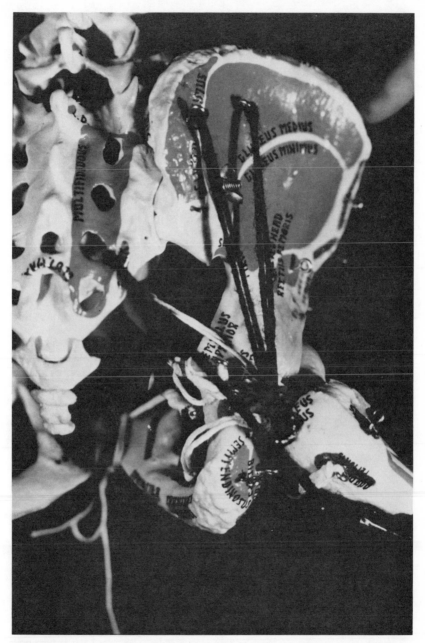

Figure 5.11-B. Incorrect mechanics with the gluteal muscles pulling the greater trochanter upwards.

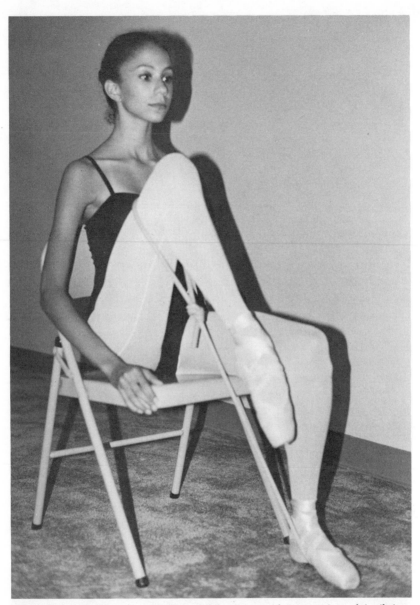

Figure 5.12. Hip flexor strengthening. While sitting with a posterior pelvic tilt in a chair, bring the knee towards the armpit. Use surgical tubing for resistance with a loop around the thigh and the other end stabilized under the opposite foot. One hand can be placed on the loop on the thigh to keep it from sliding. Perform 2 sets in the upper 30 degrees of hip flexion, and 1 set in the full arc from the chair. Use a 3 count hold at the top of the arc. As strength and muscle isolation improves, a turned-out position can be added. Since these exercises use a restricted range of motion, they should be followed by a stretch for the hip flexors.

and a weight on the ankle for resistance while sitting, standing, or side-lying. To work in higher ranges it is helpful to use the hands to raise the leg slightly higher than it can go unaided, then let go of the leg and either hold the position for three to five counts or control the lowering back down to the *barre* (standing) or floor (sitting).[11] In this latter exercise the weight of the leg provides adequate resistance, so no additional weight is needed.

General Principles

Each dance movement involves a different combination of muscles with optimal timing and activation to maximize turnout and correct technique. However, some common principles apply: 1) Emphasize use of a neutral pelvis with its center of gravity appropriately placed over the feet. Avoid the common errors of linking an excessive anterior pelvic tilt, posterior pelvic tilt, lateral pelvic tilt, or rotation of the pelvis with movements of the legs. 2) When performing any type of *plié*, emphasize using the deep outward rotators and hip adductors and keeping the knees reaching as far side as the dancer's turnout allows. 3) Begin movements involving lifting the leg by emphasizing use of the deep outward rotators first to fully rotate the femur externally in the socket (without linked pelvic compensations), and then lift the leg in the desired direction. 4) With movements to the front or side, emphasize use of the iliopsoas with the outside of the thigh "wrapping under" rather than lifting or rotating forward. 5) For a dancer who is having difficulty making these technique modifications, perform strengthening exercises for improving both strength and awareness of the muscle and its use. For all directions, strengthening of the deep outward rotators should be included. For movements to the front add exercises for the hip flexors (especially iliopsoas). For movements to the side (where the leg is raised in the air) include hip abductors. For movements to the back include exercises for the hip extensors (especially hamstrings).

Implications of Improper Turnout

In an attempt to approach perfect turnout, some dancers make the error of emphasizing the position of the feet without adequate external rotation at the hips. This improper technique is sometimes termed "turning out from below the knees," or "forced turnout." Years of such training combined with the ligamental laxity present in many dancers can produce extreme torsion (Figure 5.13-A). This tendency to twist the lower leg out relative to the femur can be even more pronounced if the knees are bent. Because the knee is a modified rather than true hinge joint, with 90 degrees of knee flexion as much as 40-50 degrees of external rotation of the tibia is possible.[12] Hence, it is easy to bring the heels forward when the knees are bent (i.e., at the base of a *grand plié*), which results in greater turnout of the feet, but also an extreme torsional stress to the knees when the knees are straightened.[10] This improper turnout is conducive to injury of the knee and knee-cap. It also alters the mechanics above and below the knee, and so can contribute to injuries of the spine, hip, shin, ankle, and foot. In my clinical experience with dancers, a large percentage of the overuse injuries occurring in the lower body are related to improper turnout.

In addition to increasing the risk for injury, improper turnout can interfere with skill development. The dance student using improper turnout often develops undesired compensations in order to maintain balance. For example, a common pattern accompanying forced turnout includes pronated feet (arches rolling-in), hyperextended knees with relative internal rotation, an anterior pelvic tilt, and the ribs sticking forward (arched spine with torso in front of the desired plumbline). Such compensations not only distort proper alignment and the desired aesthetic, but can make it hard to develop the difficult technical skills required of the advanced and professional dancer. In addition, such poor habits do not develop necessary muscles in a manner which will allow improved turnout or proper biomechanics.

With correct turnout the midpoint of the knee cap should fall over the long axis of the foot (line between the first and second toes, Figure 5.13-B). Since the natural toe-out of the foot relative to the tibia is generally about 15 degrees,* one can probably turn the feet out about 15 degrees more than the knee without creating potentially dangerous torsion stresses at the knee. However, when working with young dancers and at the *barre*, it is often helpful to use the "knee-cap over foot" positioning so that development of hip external rotation is

---

*This measure refers to the degree of tibial torsion or malleolar torsion present. There appears to be a marked individual variation with this measure, and researchers differ in average values given to it, probably due to different measurement methods, age of subjects, and the populations studied. Thomasen[3] uses 15 degrees of tibial torsion as an average measure and Gray[13] uses 13-18 degrees as average adult values. For the purpose of this chapter, 15 degrees was chosen as average. It is interesting to note that when the femoral condyles are held in a neutral plane, Gray considers values as high as 30 degrees of external rotation (measured relative to the malleolar axis) as normal.[14]

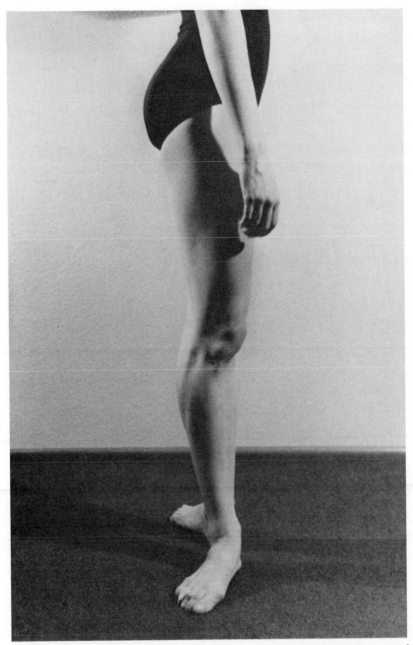

Figure 5.13-A. Incorrect or "forced" turnout in first position, with greater turnout of the feet than the hips and marked twisting of the tibia relative to the femur.

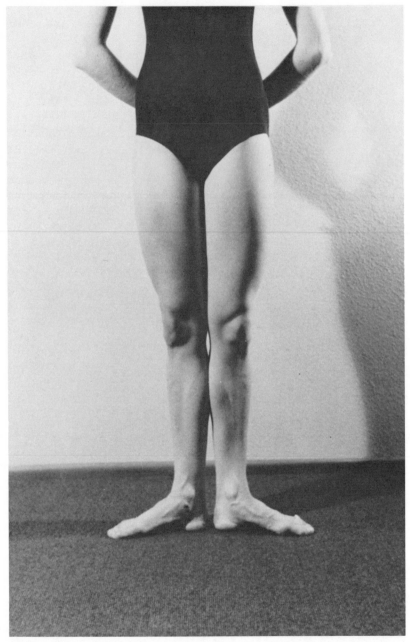

Figure 5.13-B. Correct turnout, with appropriate relationship between hip external rotation and knee and foot alignment.

encouraged and further improper stretching of the knee and ankle-foot complex discouraged.

Using the criteria listed above, the external rotation possible at the hip will determine the placement of the feet. For many dance forms, including modern and jazz, this approach is acceptable. However, for many professional training schools in classical ballet a 180 degree position of the feet (or very close to it) is an aesthetic prerequisite. Thomasen holds that since the lower leg is generally rotated out about 5 degrees at the knee, and the normal ankle joint has an axis with external rotation of 15 degrees, external rotation of 70 degrees at the hip is needed to achieve classical turnout.[3] He recommends that dancers with less than 60 degrees of hip external rotation (measured prone with the hip extended and knee bent) after age 15 be advised to stop classical ballet training. This perhaps harsh approach points to the difficulty of achieving the desired dance aesthetic and avoiding repetitive injuries if inadequate hip turnout is present. In my experience there are certainly dancers whose artistry and other technical expertise allows them to be successful professional ballet dancers with less turnout than this. However, it is probably wise to counsel "ballet hopefuls" with very limited turnout of other options for dance or dance-related careers. Those with moderate turnout should be carefully evaluated and recommendations for training based on a composite of artistry, talent, functional considerations, and structural characteristics. It is important to remember that dance is an art form, and there is more to the form than turnout.

Summary

Turnout is influenced by the orientation of the acetabulum, the angle of femoral neck anteversion or retroversion, capsular constraints, ligamental constraints, and musculotendinous constraints. These anatomical factors can be improved by early training which emphasizes proper turnout from the hip and careful stretching. However, additional areas whose importance is frequently underestimated include strength and appropriate muscle activation patterns to optimize biomechanics. In my clinical experience most dancers can improve their use of turnout by 15 to 30 degrees through specific strengthening of the deep outward rotators and refined muscle use. Successful optimization of turnout often requires correct mechanics, specific flexibility and strengthening exercises, and appropriate use of the needed muscles.

References

1. Hoppenfeld, S. (1976). *Physical examination of the spine and extremities.* New York: Appleton-Century-Crofts.

2. Sammarco, G.J. (1983, Nov.). The dancer's hip. *Clinics in Sports Medicine,* 2, 485-498.
3. Thomasen, E. (1982). *Diseases and injuries of ballet dancers.* Denmark: Universitetsforlaget I. Arhus.
4. Gray, H., Pickering, P., Howden, R. (1974). *Gray's anatomy.* Philadelphia: Running Press.
5. Clippinger-Robertson, K. (1987). *Flexibility for aerobics and fitness.* Seattle: Seattle Sports Medicine. (Available from Seattle Sports Medicine, 501 First Ave. S., Seattle, WA 98104.)
6. Basmajian, J.V. (1978). *Muscles alive.* 4th ed. Baltimore: Williams and Wilkins.
7. Brunnstrom, S. (1972). *Clinical kinesiology.* Philadelphia: F.A. Davis.
8. Rasch, P.J., Burke, R. (1978). *Kinesiology and applied anatomy.* 5th ed. Philadelphia: Lea & Febiger.
9. Clippinger-Robertson, K.S., Hutton, R.S., Miller, D.I., Nichols, T.R. (1986). Mechanical and anatomical factors relating to the incidence and etiology of patellofemoral pain in dancers. In: Shell, C.G., ed. *The dancer as athlete.* Champaign, Illinois: Human Kinetics.
10. Clippinger-Robertson, K. (1986, Mar.). Increasing functional range of motion in dance. *Kinesiology for Dance, 8,* 8-10.
11. Clippinger-Robertson, K. (1988). Principles of dance training. In: Clarkson, P.M., Skrinar, M., eds. *Science of dance training.* Champaign, Illinois: Human Kinetics.
12. Frankel, V., Nordin, M. (1980). *Basic biomechanics of the skeletal system.* Philadelphia: Lea and Febiger.
13. Gray, G. (1984). *When the feet hit the ground everything changes.* Toledo: American Physical Rehabilitation Network, 98.
14. Gray, G. (1988). [Personal Communication, Gary Gray Associates, Adna, Michigan].

Acknowledgements: The author wishes to express gratitude to Patricia Barker and Maurya Kerr of Pacific Northwest Ballet School for modeling for the photographs in this chapter.

Illustrations for Figures 5.2, 5.6, 5.7, and photography: Karen Clippinger-Robertson

6

Spinal Problems in the Dancer

Elly Trepman, M.D.
Arleen Walaszek, P.T.
Lyle J. Micheli, M.D.

Injury to the spine accounts for 7-18% of all dance injuries.[1-5] The percentage of dancers who have a past history of back injury ranges from 8-11% of aerobic dancers[4] to 60-80% of ballet and modern dancers.[5] The majority of spinal injuries in dancers involve the lumbar region, but cervical and thoracic injury is not uncommon.[2] Other spinal conditions such as scoliosis are prevalent in dancers.[6] Furthermore, poor spinal posture and technique can contribute to pelvic and lower extremity malalignment and injury.[7] Therefore, attention to the anatomy and biomechanics of the spine during dance training should be a top priority for both student and teacher. Such attention should decrease the incidence and severity of spinal and lower extremity dance injuries.

Anatomy and Biomechanics of the Spine

Skeletal Structure

The skeletal framework of the spine consists of an undulated arrangement of 7 cervical, 12 thoracic, and 5 lumbar vertebrae perched on the sacrum (Figure 6.1). The vertebrae are separated by intervertebral discs, which absorb impact and allow for motion between the vertebrae. The normal spinal column is curved into lordosis (concave posterior) in the cervical and lumbar regions, and into kyphosis (convex posterior) in the thoracic region (Figure 6.1). The magnitude of the

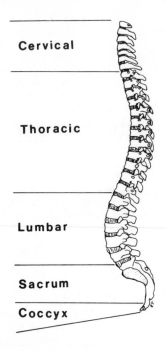

Cervical

Thoracic

Lumbar

Sacrum

Coccyx

Figure 6.1. The spinal column viewed from the side. The cervical and lumbar regions are curved into lordosis (concave posterior), balancing the kyphosis (convex posterior) of the thoracic spine.

lumbar lordosis and pelvic tilt are interrelated: a greater degree of lumbar lordosis is associated with more pelvic extension relative to the spine, with the coccyx tipped backwards and upwards.

The spinal curves themselves are determined by a balance of the action of the supporting muscles of the spine, and allow for impact absorption. However, when the curves are exaggerated in magnitude, as with excessive lumbar lordosis ("swayback"), undue stresses are placed on the spinal elements (as described below), which may lead to injury. The development of excessive lumbar lordosis and thoracic kyphosis may be a result of muscle imbalance, which in dancers can often be traced to errors in posture and technique.

The Vertebrae

Each vertebra is a complex bone, analogous in basic structure to a padlock, consisting of an anterior cylindrical body and a posterior bony arch (Figure 6.2-A). The vertebrae surround and protect the dural sac containing the spinal cord, which sends branches (nerve roots) to the trunk and extremities for control of motion and other bodily functions (Figure 6.2-B). The vertebral arch consists of the laminae and pedicles, which connect the arch to the body. Each arch

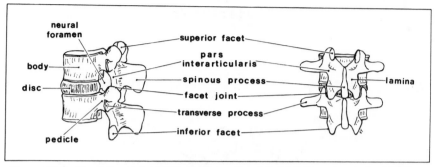

Figure 6.2-A. Normal anatomy of the lumbar spine. Lateral (left) and posterior (right) views of two adjacent lumbar vertebrae and intervertebral disc.

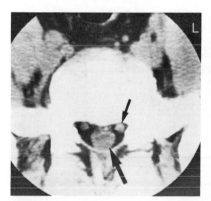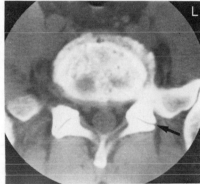

Figures 6.2-B and 6.2-C. Normal horizontal cross section of the lumbar spine as viewed by computed tomography (CT) scanning. Radiographic information is processed to highlight either soft tissue (6.2-B) or bony (6.2-C) structures. The spinal canal (6.2-B) protects the dural sac (large arrow), which contains the spinal cord and origin of the nerve roots, and the nerve roots (small arrow) prior to exit from the spine. The bone view (6.2-C) reveals the normal facet joint (arrow).

has seven bony projections: two transverse processes and one posterior spinous process, which provide attachment for ligaments and muscles; and two superior and two inferior facets, which articulate with facets of the adjacent vertebrae above and below to form the facet (apophyseal) joints (Figure 6.2-C and 6.2-D). These are true synovial joints, consisting of articular cartilage, joint fluid, and a surrounding capsule. Motion between adjacent vertebrae occurs at the intervertebral disc and the two facet joints. The superior and inferior facet on each side of the vertebral arch is separated by a supporting bar of bone known as the pars interarticularis (Figure 6.2-A). A foramen formed between the pedicles, disc, and facet joint of two adjacent vertebrae allows passage of the nerve root from the spine, and injury to any of

ANTERIOR

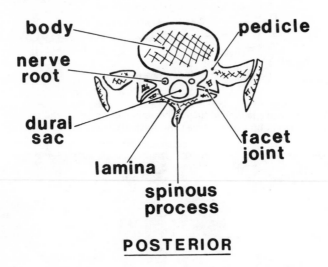

POSTERIOR

Figure 6.2-D. The detailed anatomy is clarified in the corresponding line drawing (one pedicle is not seen because the cross section is slightly oblique from the horizontal plane).

these structures can result in nerve root irritation, as in certain types of sciatica (Figure 6.2-A).

The regional differences in vertebral structure partially account for the differences in motion characteristics of the regions (Figure 6.3). The plane of orientation of facet joints in the cervical spine is more horizontal than in the other regions, and allows for more rotation of the neck in the horizontal plane. The lumbar facet joints are more vertical, thus limiting rotation while allowing flexion and extension of the lumbar spine. The thoracic spine is restricted by rib attachments and longer, more vertical posterior spinous processes, and this partly explains the relatively smaller range of motion in this region.[8]

Excessive lumbar lordosis or repetitive hyperextension of the lumbar spine results in increased stresses on the facet joints and the pars interarticularis, and may lead to facet arthritis or stress fracture of the pars. Sudden flexion of the spine results in compressive stress on the vertebral bodies, and may cause compression fracture and loss of body height.

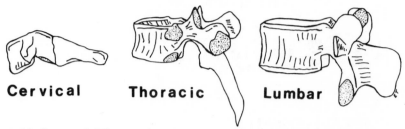

Figure 6.3. Structural differences between cervical, thoracic, and lumbar vertebrae partially account for the different ranges of motion of the neck, upper back, and lower back.

The Intervertebral Discs

The bodies of adjacent vertebrae are separated by intervertebral discs, which consist of a fibrous ring (annulus fibrosus) enclosing a pulpy center (nucleus pulposus), analogous in cross section to a jelly donut (Figure 6.4). The discs act as cushions which absorb impact and allow for motion between adjacent vertebrae. Flexion of the spine, either in the sitting or standing position, results in an increase in load on the disc.[9] This may explain the contribution of flexion injury to disc herniation, as discussed below. Tightness associated with excessive lumbar lordosis may also increase the risk of injury to the disc.

Muscular and Ligamentous Support

The ligaments of the spine connect and stabilize the vertebral bodies, transverse processes, posterior spinous processes, laminae, and facet joint capsule. They allow for normal motion in the physiological range, and provide a static, protective constraint to abnormal motion.[8]

The spine is extremely unstable in the absence of active muscular control.[8] The many muscles which provide stability and control movement can be grouped into categories based on anatomic location and function.

A. The paraspinal muscles (erector spinae) are long muscles located posterior and lateral to the vertebrae (Figure 6.5). They arise from the sacrum, and attach to the posterior spinous processes and ligaments of the lumbar and lower thoracic vertebrae. They then branch into three major muscle groups—the iliocostalis, longissimus, and spinalis muscles—which insert on vertebrae, ribs, and the skull. These muscles extend the spine when both right and left sides are working in synchrony, and laterally flex the spine when acting unilaterally.

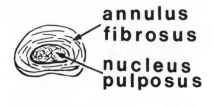

annulus
fibrosus

nucleus
pulposus

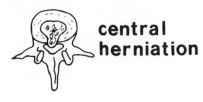

central
herniation

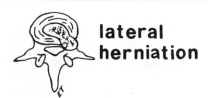

lateral
herniation

Figure 6.4. The normal intervertebral disc (top) consists of a fibrous annulus which encloses a pulpy central nucleus. Central disc herniation (middle) may result in pressure on the dural sac, whereas lateral herniation (bottom) may compress a nerve root as it exits the neural foramen.

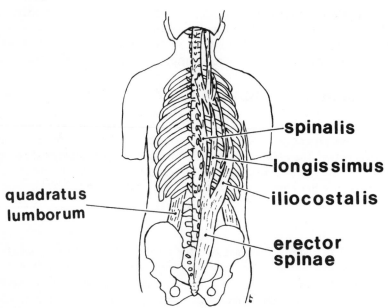

spinalis

longissimus

iliocostalis

quadratus
lumborum

erector
spinae

Figure 6.5. The paraspinal muscles and quadratus lumborum. The erector spinae arise from the sacrum, and branch into the iliocostalis, longissimus, and spinalis groups. The quadratus lumborum is an abdominal muscle which originates from the posterior iliac crest and inserts on the twelfth rib and transverse processes of the lumbar vertebrae.

B. The deep back muscles connect the posterior elements of vertebrae (for example, transverse process of one vertebra to spinous process of another) over shorter distances than the erector spinae. The
main function of the deep muscles, such as the multifidus, semispinalis, and rotatores, includes spinal extension, rotation, and stabilization.

C. The abdominal muscles, consisting of the rectus abdominis,
external oblique, internal oblique, and transversus abdominis, join the
rib cage to the pelvis (Figure 6.6). This muscle group assists in flexion
of the lumbar spine, and when acting unilaterally causes lateral flexion
or rotation of the trunk. Furthermore, by increasing intraabdominal
(hydrostatic) pressure, the abdominal muscles facilitate the support
of the erect body, thereby decreasing the supportive work required of
the erector spinae muscles. Weakness of the abdominal muscles may

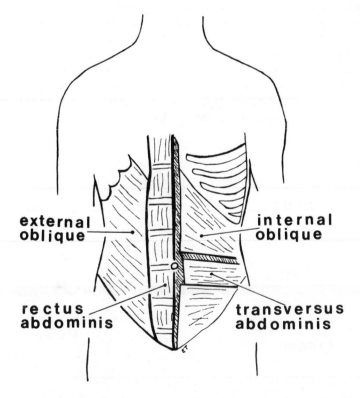

Figure 6.6. The abdominal muscles originate from the ribs and insert on the pelvis. The
rectus abdominis is located adjacent to the midline. The external oblique, internal
oblique, and transversus abdominis muscles are arranged as three layers, with muscle
fibers of each oriented in different directions.

result in excessive lumbar lordosis, and therefore may contribute to spinal and lower extremity dance injury.

The quadratus lumborum, which originates from the posterior iliac crest and inserts on the twelfth rib and the transverse processes of the lumbar vertebrae, is also classified as an abdominal muscle (Figure 6.5). It laterally flexes the lumbar spine when working unilaterally.

D. The iliopsoas, one of the most powerful muscles of the body, is the only muscle which attaches to the spine, pelvis, and femur.[10] The two components of the iliopsoas are the iliacus, which originates from the inside of the iliac crest, and the psoas, which takes origin from the vertebrae between the twelfth thoracic (T12) and fifth lumbar (L5) vertebrae (Figure 6.7). The iliacus and psoas are joined in the common iliopsoas tendon, which inserts on the lesser trochanter of the femur. This insertion is on the posteromedial aspect of the proximal femur (Figure 6.7); therefore, iliopsoas contraction with shortening of the muscle (concentric contraction) would appear primarily to cause hip flexion, with possibly some associated adduction and external rotation.[10, 11] There is controversy regarding the effect of the iliopsoas on hip rotation.[12] Some authors believe that in certain circumstances it may act as an internal rotator of the hip.[13,14] Nevertheless, the effect of the iliopsoas on hip rotation is probably small in comparison with other hip rotators. Bilateral concentric iliopsoas contraction results in flexion (forward bending) of the lumbar spine and pelvis. Unilateral

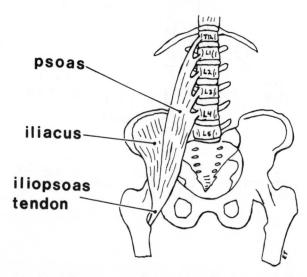

Figure 6.7. The iliopsoas consists of the iliacus and psoas muscles. The iliopsoas tendon inserts on the lesser trochanter of the femur.

concentric iliopsoas contraction results in lateral bending (scoliosis) of the lumbar spine.[10]

The iliopsoas is important in stabilizing the lumbar spine and pelvis, and is a major determinant of posture and movement.[15] The psoas has been shown by electromyography to be active in the upright sitting and standing positions, thereby contributing to the stability of the lumbar spine.[16]

Stabilization of the lumbar spine by bilateral eccentric (lengthening) or isokinetic (constant length) iliopsoas contraction may decrease lumbar lordosis.[17] Weakness of the psoas and peripheral abdominal muscles is associated with hyperlordosis.[18] An exercise program which improves iliopsoas strength and flexibility may reduce lumbar hyperlordosis and associated technical errors which can lead to dance injury.[17,18] A further benefit of such a program is an increase in postural stability centrally, which may free peripheral muscles for finer control of extremity movement.[17,18]

Anatomic and Technical Factors which Contribute to Lumbar Hyperlordosis

Lumbar hyperlordosis may contribute to many dance injuries because of the associated increased stresses on the posterior elements and discs (Figure 6.8-A, 6.8-B). Therefore, it is important to determine the etiology of this posture in the individual dancer (Table 6.1).[7,19] With appropriate attention to technical errors and rehabilitation, hyperlordosis can often be corrected, and this may prevent injury and prolong the career of the dancer. The young dancer is especially at risk for the development of lumbar hyperlordosis because of the tightening of the lumbar fascia and hamstrings which occurs during the adolescent growth spurt.[20]

Dynamics of the Spine and Muscular Control in Dance Movement

There are no available electromyographic studies of spinal muscle function in dance movement. Furthermore, quantitative estimates of individual muscle strength, such as those available for the muscles about the knee,[21] are difficult to obtain for the musculature of the spine. Therefore, the current understanding of the muscular control of the spine in dance is based on the astute clinical observations of dance instructors, therapists, physicians, and dancers themselves.

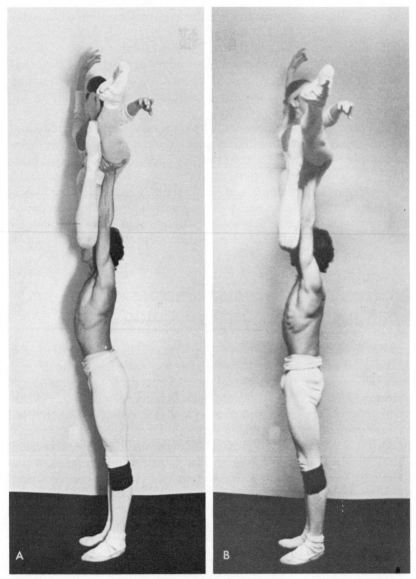

Figure 6.8-A. Incorrect lifting posture, with excessive lumbar lordosis, may contribute to disc herniation.

Figure 6.8-B. Proper lifting posture, with stabilization of the lumbar spine, is promoted by an anti-lordotic strengthening and flexibility program and postural awareness.

TABLE 6.1
Factors Associated with Lumbar Hyperlordosis

Anatomic factors
    Thoracic hyperkyphosis
    Weak psoas
    Tight hip flexors (ex. iliopsoas)
    Hip flexion contracture
    Femoral anteversion
    Weak abdominal muscles
    Tight lumbar fascia
    Tight hamstrings
    Genu recurvatum ("swayback knees")

Technical errors
    Compensation for limited hip turnout (i.e., flexing the pelvis on the hip to
        allow for greater turnout in the flexed hip)
    Arabesque or *attitude* with extension from the lumbar spine instead of the hip
    Poor lifting posture
    Lack of postural awareness

Other factors
    Decreased flexibility during the growth spurt

Concentric muscle contraction, in which the muscle shortens as it contracts, is only one of several mechanisms by which muscles control the dynamics of spinal movement. Isometric contraction, in which the length of the muscle remains constant during contraction, is important for the stability of the spine. The concept of eccentric muscle contraction, in which the muscle contracts as it lengthens ("controlled letting go"), has resulted in an improved understanding of the importance of antagonist muscle function and strength in movement.

A specific muscle may work in any of these varied manners during different dance movements. For example, a powerful concentric contraction of the abdominal muscles provides the impulse for movement in a Graham contraction or return from a back arch; in contrast, during a back arch, control is accompanied by eccentric contraction of the abdominal muscles.[22] Isometric contraction of the abdominal muscles provides stability to the lumbar spine during a lift. Therefore, it may be important to strengthen the abdominal muscles in these three different modes in order to optimize function and minimize risk of injury.

Differences in flexibility of the cervical, thoracic, and lumbar regions may also affect the dynamics of spinal movement in dance. The thoracic spine is intrinsically less flexible because of the orientation of the facet joints and posterior spinous processes, as well as rib attachments.[8,23] Therefore, the long graceful arch of the classical *arabesque* may be difficult to achieve, and a compensatory exaggeration of the cervical and lumbar lordosis may occur, resulting in increased stress and risk of injury.[22] This problem may be corrected by the use of a program directed at increasing thoracic extension flexibility and cervical and lumbar strength.[22,24]

Spinal motion and stability are also influenced by the muscles of the extremities. The hip extensors, including the gluteus maximus and hamstrings, may stabilize the hip in extension and assist in reducing lumbar lordosis.[22] However, as noted above, use of the iliopsoas for stabilization of the lordosis may be more advantageous, as the extensors can then be used primarily for movement.[17]

Overuse Injuries of the Spine

Although single impact trauma is the cause of some injuries to the spine in dancers, many others result from overuse.[25] The stresses and strains of repetitive dance training may lead to microscopic injury; if the rate of occurrence of this microtrauma exceeds that of tissue healing, then macroscopic overuse injury will occur.[26,27]

Several risk factors have been identified as contributors to overuse injury of the spine in dancers (Table 6.2).[28] Abrupt increases in dance intensity or changes in choreographic technique may not allow musculoskeletal adaptation to the increased rate or altered pattern of stresses on the bones, discs, ligaments, and muscles of the back. This may occur when a dancer returns from a layoff period or begins intensive

TABLE 6.2
Risk Factors for Overuse Injuries of the Spine

1. Abrupt changes in training style, intensity, duration, or frequency	
2. Technical errors:	excessive dynamic lumbar hyperextension (lordosis) *attitude* *arabesque* lifting a partner increasing hip flexion to force turnout
3. Anatomic malalignment:	lumbar hyperlordosis femoral anteversion limb length discrepancy other
4. Shoe wear:	spiked heels
5. Dance surface	
6. Growth factors:	decreased flexibility with growth spurt growth cartilage
7. Hormonal factors:	delayed menarche amenorrhea hypoestrogenism

training in an unfamiliar style of dance. Overuse injuries are also seen in students who suddenly increase classes from two hours per day during the school year to six or eight hours per day at a summer program.

As noted above, excessive lumbar lordosis resulting from anatomic causes or technical errors may result in increased stresses on the discs, pars interarticularis, and facet joints. Therefore, hyperlordosis is a major risk factor for overuse injury to the spine, such as stress fracture or ligament sprain. Muscle imbalance, weak abdominal muscles, or femoral anteversion may contribute to lumbar hyperlordosis and overuse injury.

The use of high spiked heels in jazz dance may increase lumbar lordosis and strain.[28] Poor impact absorption by the dance surface may result in increased stress on the lower extremities and lumbar spine.[29]

Adolescents have growth-dependent risk factors which may contribute to overuse injury. The decrease in flexibility during the adolescent growth spurt[20] may result in tight lumbodorsal fascia and increased lumbar lordosis. Traction injury to growth cartilage may also cause back or pelvic pain, as with ischial apophysitis associated with tight hamstrings.[30] Furthermore, delayed menarche may predispose the young female dancer to stress fractures and scoliosis.[6]

The treatment of overuse injuries begins with an accurate diagnosis and removal of contributing risk factors. The dancer is prescribed alternate activities which do not exacerbate the injury, in order to maintain aerobic and musculoskeletal fitness during the recovery period. Inflammatory conditions such as tendinitis may respond to a short course (one to two weeks) of oral anti-inflammatory medication. Physical therapeutic modalities, such as ice, heat, ultrasound, and electrical stimulation may also accelerate healing.[31] Braces may be useful in specific situations such as disc herniation or spondylolysis (see below).

The cornerstone of any good therapeutic program for overuse injuries of the spine is a directed, progressive, strengthening and flexibility exercise program. A program of exercises to improve iliopsoas strength and flexibility may be especially useful in the overall rehabilitation of overuse injuries of the spine.[17] The use of floor work may minimize stresses on the lower back during the gradual return to dance activity after overuse injury.[17]

Specific Problems

Spondylolysis

Spondylolysis is a defect in the normal bony structure of the pars interarticularis which is present in 6 percent of adults.[32] This condition usually occurs at L4 or L5, unilaterally or bilaterally, and is believed to have a hereditary predisposition.[32,33] When separation at a bilateral defect occurs, spondylolisthesis may result, in which the upper vertebra slips forward over the lower one. If the amount of slippage is severe, spinal instability may result, requiring surgical fusion of the two levels. Fortunately, the degree of spondylolisthesis is usually mild, and progression is unusual.[32]

Spondylolysis may be more common in the dancer than in the general population. Repetitive hyperextension of the lumbar spine in *arabesque* or *attitude* can result in stress at the pars interarticularis, and this may be exacerbated by excessive lumbar lordosis or poor technique (Table 6.1). The dancer with this condition may notice a gradual onset of localized low back pain, which is often in a discrete location on the side of the involved pars. The pain is increased by lumbar hyperextension, particularly while standing on the leg of the affected side. The physical examination may also be notable for paraspinous muscle spasm, hyperlordosis, and limitation of forward bending due to tightness of the hamstrings and lumbar fascia. Radiographs of the lumbar spine may reveal a frank bony pars defect which has the appearance of a stress fracture (Figure 6.9). A technetium pyrophosphate radionuclide bone scan, which is more sensitive than radiography, may show increased activity at the involved pars, even if no pars defect is detected on radiographs.[34] An occasional dancer with this condition will nonetheless have normal radiographs and bone scan.

Treatment of spondylolysis includes the discontinuation of dance activity and immobilization of the low back with an anti-lordotic brace for six months (Figures 6.10-A, 6.10-B, 6.10-C). This must be supplemented with a program of abdominal and pelvic strengthening exercises, and a stretching program for the hamstrings and lumbodorsal fascia, to prevent atrophy, weakness, and tightness which may otherwise be associated with immobilization.

Such a treatment regimen may result in bony and radiographic healing of the pars stress fracture.[35] However, failure to heal radiographically does not preclude return to dance activity. In this situation, fibrous healing may have occurred, or the symptoms may have been due to mechanical back pain or strain with a coincident old spondylolysis. Frequently, avoidance of painful technique and institution of the anti-lordotic rehabilitation program without bracing may eliminate pain and allow return to full dance activity. Spinal fusion is only rarely required for treatment of painful spondylolysis that interferes with dance activity despite bracing and exercises.[28]

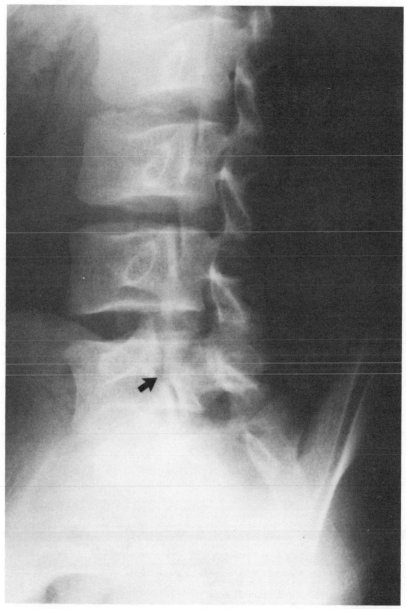

Figure 6.9. Spondylolysis is a defect in the pars interarticularis (arrow) which may be seen on the oblique radiograph of the lumbar spine.

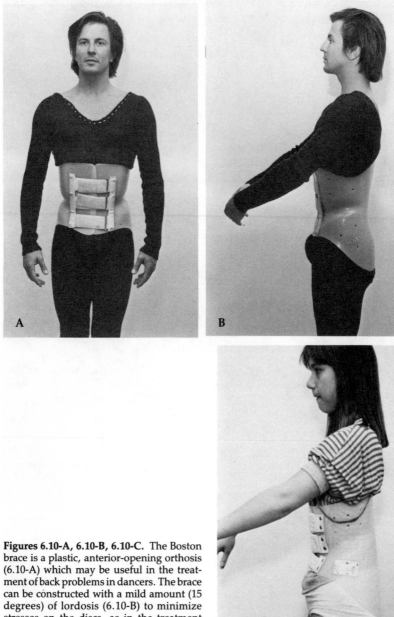

Figures 6.10-A, 6.10-B, 6.10-C. The Boston brace is a plastic, anterior-opening orthosis (6.10-A) which may be useful in the treatment of back problems in dancers. The brace can be constructed with a mild amount (15 degrees) of lordosis (6.10-B) to minimize stresses on the discs, as in the treatment of disc herniation. Alternatively, the anti-lordotic (zero degree lordosis) version (6.10-C) is used to treat posterior element conditions such as spondylolysis or facet arthrosis.

The older dancer with intermittent episodes of low back pain associated with spondylolysis may be helped by a short period of full-time bracing, followed by part-time use of the brace, thus enabling dance activity to be continued. Healing of the spondylolytic defect is not expected in this instance, but use of the brace appears to speed clinical recovery.

Injury to the lumbar pedicle is rare in the dancer. Stress fracture of the pedicle, resulting from repetitive flexion and hyperextension of the lumbar spine, has been reported in only one dancer.[36] Occasionally, stress fracture of the pars is associated with reactive hypertrophy of the contralateral pedicle and lamina, which may be difficult to differentiate from benign bone conditions such as osteoid osteoma.[37]

Scoliosis

Scoliosis is a spinal deformity which consists of a structural curvature of the spine sideways, with an associated rotational deformity of the vertebrae (Figure 6.11). The curvature of scoliosis is usually associated with a flexible compensatory curve in the opposite direction (Figure 6.11) in order to maintain trunk balance. The rotational component is manifested by the characteristic unilateral thoracic rib hump or lumbar asymmetry observed when the affected individual bends forward to touch the floor.

Scoliosis is significantly more common in dancers than in the general population.[6] The most common type of scoliosis is the adolescent idiopathic type, which may progress from a small to a large curve during growth. This may be a result of a relative decrease in rate of bone growth on the concavity of the curve, because of the greater pressure on the growth cartilage on this side of the spine. Adolescent idiopathic scoliosis occurs in up to 10-16 percent of the general population.[38,39,40] In most cases specific treatment is not required other than observation until growth is completed, after which progression of curve magnitude is unlikely for small curves. Above the age of 10-11 years, scoliosis is more common in females,[39] and risk of progression is greater prior to menarche.[40] The higher prevalence of scoliosis in ballet dancers (24%) has been attributed to hypoestrogenism secondary to delayed menarche and prolonged intervals of amenorrhea.[6]

Screening children for scoliosis, which can be accomplished by a school nurse, physical education teacher, or dance instructor, can lead to early detection and non-operative treatment of mild curves which may otherwise progress in severity and require spinal fusion.[41] In the screening examination, the child is observed as she bends forward to 90 degrees at the hips with the knees straight, arms dangling, and the

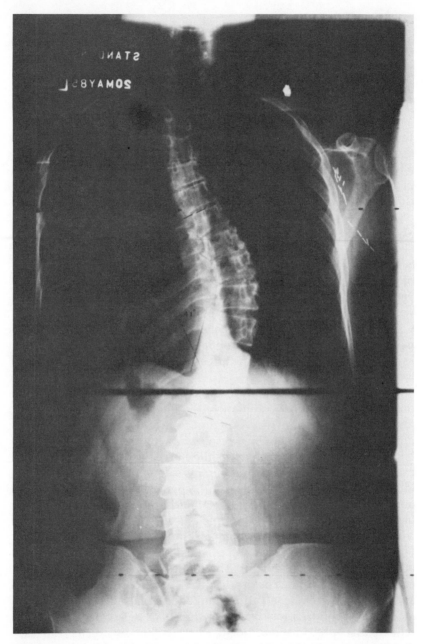

Figure 6.11. Scoliosis in a professional dancer. This curve (41 degrees) is balanced, with the head, shoulders, and torso centered over the pelvis. It has not interfered with her thirty-year career of modern dance performance, choreography, and teaching.

feet and hands together. An asymmetric prominence of one side of the thoracic or lumbar region compared with the other side, resulting from vertebral rotation, is an early sign of scoliosis.[41] In the upright standing position, asymmetry of shoulder height or scapular prominence, unequal arm height, pelvic obliquity, unequal waist line, and lower limb length inequality should be noted, and are indications for orthopaedic referral.[41]

The most accurate determination of magnitude of scoliosis is from a standing radiograph of the spine (Figure 6.11). Individuals with small curves (less than 20 degrees) who do not show signs of radiographic progression are followed until growth is completed. If progression by 10-15 degrees does occur, or if the curve is larger than 20 degrees, then a plastic brace, similar to that used for spondylolysis, may prevent further progression. The brace may be removed for dance activities, and is worn the rest of the day and night.[42] We do not use electrical stimulation or exercise alone for progressive scoliosis. If the severity of the curve progresses despite bracing, or if it is greater than 40 degrees, spinal fusion may be required.

A well balanced curve, even if large, does not necessarily preclude a successful dance career (Figure 6.11). Problems such as diminished pulmonary function, back pain, neurological compromise, or loss of self esteem, which may occur with very large curves, are not generally observed with curves of up to 40-50 degrees.[43] Therefore, low back pain in the dancer should not be attributed to scoliosis, and a thorough investigation of other potential causes should be performed.

Facet Arthrosis

The repetitive lumbar hyperextension in dance technique places enormous stresses on the facet joints as well as the pars. After many years of dance these stresses may result in degenerative changes of the facet joints characteristic of osteoarthritis, including erosion of the cartilage surface of the facets and secondary joint space narrowing and irregularity, with osteophyte formation ("bone spurs") at the edges of the joints.

Although the degenerative changes of facet arthrosis may develop over many months or years, the symptoms can appear in a relatively short period of time. During a vigorous schedule, a fracture of an osteophyte at the edge of the facet, or of the facet itself, may occur with hyperextension of the lumbar spine in *attitude* or *arabesque*. The pain may be localized to the low back on the side of the lumbar facet involved, or may radiate down the lower extremity because of irritation of the nerve root adjacent to the facet. The pain may be exacerbated by lateral bending towards the involved side, or by hyperextension of the lumbar spine while standing on the ipsilateral lower extremity.

Radiographs may reveal irregularity of the facet joint, and a bone scan may show an area of increased activity if a fracture has occurred (Figures 6.12-A, 6.12-B). A computed tomography (CT) scan may demonstrate the facet joint irregularity in better detail (Figures 6.12-C, 6.12-D).

Initial treatment consists of rest, anti-inflammatory medication, and anti-lordotic exercises. If the pain continues, immobilization of the facet joint with an anti-lordotic brace (Figure 6.10-C) may encourage healing of the injury. Rarely, surgical exploration of the facet joint and excision of the osteophyte may be considered if nonoperative treatment fails. As a last resort, limited spinal fusion may provide relief.

The dancer with this condition usually has been performing for many years, and is often among the older members of the company. Depending on the severity of the pain, he/she may be faced with the difficult decision of whether to dance in pain, undergo surgery which may yield limited improvement, accept technical limitations secondary to the arthrosis, or retire from professional performance.

Disc Herniation

Discogenic back pain may result from inflammation of a disc, disc protrusion, or frank disc herniation or rupture ("slipped disc"). These problems are more common in male dancers because of the stresses imposed by lifting. Forward flexion of the lumbar spine results in a major increase in the load on the lumbar discs compared with that during neutral upright stance, and this load is further increased when a weight is held in the arms, or when the flexed spine is rotated.[9,44] This may be exacerbated by the presence or accentuation of lumbar hyperlordosis (Figure 6.13-A). Poor lifting technique, with outstretched arms away from the body, may increase disc pressure and hence, disc-related pain, or even result in herniation.[45] Lifting with hyperlordosis of the lumbar spine may also place extensive stress on the discs and cause herniation (Figure 6.8-A).

With herniation, the pulpy disc center (nucleus) extrudes through a tear in the fibrous annulus, and causes pain because of pressure on the neural elements of the spine (Figures 6.4, 6.13-B, 6.13-C). If the herniation is in the midline, the extruded nucleus presses on the central neural sac, and the pain is felt in the low back; if the nucleus herniates more laterally, it may press on the nerve roots which run to

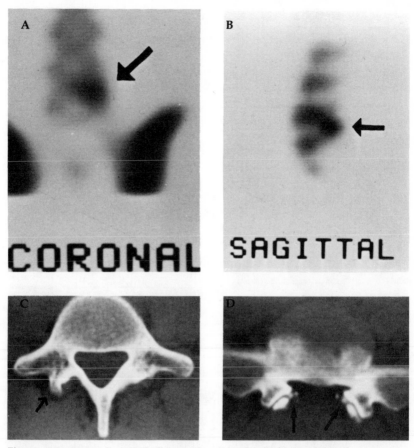

Figures 6.12-A, 6.12-B, 6.12-C. Facet arthrosis in the professional dancer.
This 36 year old ballet dancer developed left lumbar back pain following a vigorous summer program. The pain was exacerbated by lateral bending and hyperextension towards the left side, including *arabesque*, and was associated with left lumbar spasm. There were no lower extremity symptoms or signs. A bone scan (6.12-A and 6.12-B) showed increased activity of the posterior elements of the left L4-5 region, and a computed tomography (CT) scan (6.12-C) demonstrated left L4-5 facet arthrosis, with osteophyte ("bone spur") and fracture of the inferior L4 facet. Despite over one year of conservative treatment, including relative rest, bracing, rehabilitation, and injection of the facet joint with cortisone, she continued to have pain which limited dance activity. Surgical exploration of the left L4-5 facet joint revealed an old fracture of the superior margin, and a loose osteophyte at the inferior margin of the inferior facet of L4; otherwise, the joint cartilage was healthy. Debridement of the arthrosis resulted in some improvement of pain, but persistent symptoms have limited performance.
Figure 6.12-D. This 32 year old ballet dancer had intermittent low back pain radiating to the back of her left lower extremity associated with *arabesque* and *développé*. The physical examination revealed pain with extension testing and lateral bending. The bone scan of the lumbar spine was unremarkable, but CT scan revealed arthrosis (arrows) of the L5-S1 facet joints. Despite episodes of the recurrent pain, she has done well with rehabilitation, and has been able to continue performance.

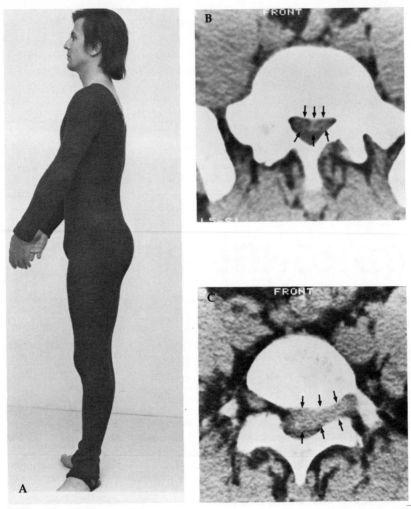

Figure 6.13-A. Disc herniation.

This 30 year old ballet dancer developed acute low back pain during a performance. Examination revealed lumbar spasm, with inability to reverse his lumbar curve, and irritability with sciatic nerve stretching maneuvers. His posture was remarkable for a moderate hyperlordosis.

Figure 6.13-B. The pain was later exacerbated during a lift, and a CT scan (6.13-B) demonstrated a disc herniation at L5-S1 (arrows). He was treated with relative rest, a Boston brace (see Figures 6.10-A and 6.10-B), and an anti-lordotic and postural rehabilitation program. Within 6-7 months he was able to return to class, and his lumbar lordosis was improved.

Figure 6.13-C. CT scan of a patient with left low back pain, sciatic pain, plantarflexion weakness, and loss of the ankle jerk reflex. A large central and lateral L5-S1 disc herniation is present (arrows), with compression of the dural sac and left S1 nerve root.

the lower extremity on that side, and pain may radiate down this extremity (Figures 6.4, 6.13-C).

Discogenic back pain is exacerbated by forward bending, sitting, coughing, sneezing, or straining, because these activities increase disc pressure. In addition to pain, disc herniation may result in numbness or paresthesias ("pins and needles") radiating down the lower extremities as a result of pressure on specific nerve roots. Passively flexing the hip with the knee extended may cause pain and spasm because of stretch on an irritated nerve root. A detailed neurological examination is important because pressure on the nerve roots may result in muscle weakness or loss of a reflex. Rarely, pressure on the nerves to the bladder or bowel may result in incontinence, which requires emergency attention.

Most disc herniations resolve over several weeks or months, possibly because the extruded nucleus fragment shrinks as its water content is resorbed. Therefore, treatment usually consists of rest, analgesics, anti-inflammatory medication, and muscle relaxants, followed by a progressive anti-lordotic strengthening and flexibility rehabilitation program. A plastic brace or corset in conjunction with the exercise program may immobilize the lumbar spine, prevent further lordosis, and improve comfort during the first four to six months after injury (Figures 6.10-A, 6.10-B, 6.10-C).[46] The dancer may be able to continue limited dance classes, perform character roles, and maintain fitness with swimming and gentle, directed exercises.

Every attempt is made to manage disc herniation nonoperatively. Surgical excision of a herniated disc is indicated if bowel or bladder symptoms or signs are present. If pain and spasm is severe, and is associated with specific neurological loss such as muscle weakness or loss of a reflex, disc excision can be considered if there is no improvement with nonoperative treatment. However, the dancer may not be able to perform for a full year following discectomy, and extensive rehabilitation is required. Further professional dancing may not be possible, depending on the extent of recovery.

Mechanical Low Back Pain

Mechanical low back pain is a syndrome in which localized aching low back pain is exacerbated by motion, turns, lifts, or prolonged standing or sitting, but no definite anatomic cause can be defined. The dancer with mechanical low back pain usually has lumbar hyperlordosis, and the pain may be a reflection of facet joint stress, muscular strain, or ligament sprain secondary to the lordotic posture. The pain may be reproduced by motion of the lumbar spine, possibly in more than one direction. The hamstrings and lumbodorsal fascia may be tight, but neurological examination is normal. The diagnosis of mechanical low back pain can only be made after other specific causes of low back pain, such as spondylolysis, disc herniation, infection, or tumor, have been excluded by appropriate studies such as radiography, bone scans, and computed tomography scans.[47,48]

Management of mechanical low back pain begins with attention to technical errors which contribute to hyperlordosis. A directed anti-lordotic rehabilitation program may result in improvement of pain and hyperlordosis. In cases refractory to an exercise program alone, anti-lordotic bracing has been helpful in accelerating pain relief and improving a tight hyperlordosis.[48] When used for mechanical back pain, the brace is worn full-time initially except during dance activity, and pain is often relieved after 6-12 weeks of bracing. The dancer is then weaned of the brace over the next 3-4 months, with emphasis on the exercise program throughout the entire period of bracing. Recurrence rate after bracing is low if anti-lordotic strengthening and flexibility are maintained.

Sciatica

The term sciatica does not refer to a specific diagnosis, but rather to the symptom of pain along the course of the sciatic nerve, the largest peripheral nerve in the body. The pain of sciatica may radiate from the back to the buttock and down the posterior aspect of the lower extremity.

Any condition which causes mechanical or inflammatory irritation of the nerve roots which join to form the sciatic nerve, or of the sciatic nerve itself, may cause sciatic pain. The possible causes of sciatica are manifold, including disc herniation, facet arthrosis, low back strain, spondylolisthesis, or pressure on the nerve by muscles at the back of the hip (piriformis syndrome). The treatment of these problems may differ. Therefore, it is important to define the etiology of the pain, rather than to simply attribute the pain to "sciatica."

Upper Back Injuries

Upper back and periscapular injuries in dancers usually consist of muscle strains or ligament sprains. They may occur while lifting a partner, as a result of weakness or being off balance. Periscapular strains can result from repetitive elevation and rotation of the upper arm.

First aid includes ice massage or cold spray, which may enable completion of a performance. Massage may minimize muscle spasm and stiffness. Physical therapeutic modalities, including ice, heat, ultrasound, massage, and electrical stimulation, may accelerate recovery. Anti-inflammatory medications can be useful. A strengthening and flexibility exercise program may also promote healing and prevent recurrence.

Injury to the bony elements and discs of the thoracic spine is unusual in the dancer. The most common problem of the thoracic vertebrae in the adolescent is a variant of Scheuermann's disease, or dorsal kyphosis ("roundback") deformity. This condition is caused by increased stress on the vertebral bodies of the thoracic spine, leading to stress fracture and wedging. Contributing factors include repetitive flexion of the thoracic spine, loss of flexibility associated with the growth spurt, and increased lumbar lordosis with compensatory thoracic kyphosis. Dorsal back pain may be present, and there is usually a tight lumbar hyperlordosis and tightness of the hamstrings. Treatment consists of dorsal extension and lumbar anti-lordotic strengthening and flexibility exercises, hamstring stretching, and occasionally, bracing for 9-12 months.[47,48]

Neck Injuries

Injury to the neck and cervical spine is less common in the dancer than lumbar spine injuries. Cervical spondylosis, brachial plexus injury, and thoracic outlet syndrome in the dancer are considered elsewhere.[49]

Rehabilitation of the Injured Back in the Dancer

The goals of rehabilitation include return to pain-free performance and prevention of recurrent injury.[50] Rehabilitation begins with an accurate diagnosis of the injury and/or anatomic malalignment. Specific exercise programs for different injuries, as noted above, are planned and modified as pain and spasm improve. The dancer's awareness of body mechanics and alignment facilitates the rehabilitation process.

In addition to rest, directed exercises, and bracing for the specific injury, it is important to prescribe a program to maintain cardiovascular and musculoskeletal fitness. Swimming is particularly useful because it minimizes stresses of gravity on the injured spine and provides water resistance for strengthening. Floor work is also useful because gravitational stresses can be minimized, and dance exercises maintain interest.[17] Progression to chair exercises[24] and *barre* work may be modified to minimize stresses on the back and preserve good technique.

The contribution of lumbar hyperlordosis to many injuries has been noted above. The mainstay of rehabilitation for this postural malalignment is a program of abdominal muscle and psoas strengthening, including gentle sit-ups and pelvic tilts, and flexibility exercises for the low back and hamstrings. Attention to concentric, eccentric, and isometric exercises may be important. Postural awareness in daily life, both in and out of the classroom, is emphasized throughout rehabilitation. Vocalization is particularly useful as a means of monitoring effort and tension in movement.[17] Breathing and relaxation techniques may also be useful in rehabilitation, and may help improve lumbar expansion and awareness.[50]

The modalities, including ice, heat, ultrasound, and massage, may be useful in decreasing spasm and pain, and improving passive stretch and relaxation. Postural mechanics may be improved with techniques such as those based on the Alexander principle.[51] Sleeping posture with the low back maximally flexed may allow a passive anti-lordotic stretch, whereas prone positions should be discouraged because they may exacerbate tight lumbar lordosis.

The upper back muscles can be strengthened with directed weight training. This will improve upper extremity control while lifting a partner.

For the purposes of rehabilitation, the standard elements of a dance class can be thought of as separate units. The importance of warm-up should be emphasized, and the dancer with back problems can progress from *barre* to center work as recovery proceeds.

If surgery has been necessary, the return to dance participation is individualized. Successful resumption of training and performance will depend on the nature of the injury, type of surgery, level of the spine involved, extent of spinal fusion if any, and the potential for subsequent instability or neurological injury.[52]

(Authors' Note: This chapter is dedicated to Elaine Bauer, Principal Dancer for the Boston Ballet Company, in honor of her retirement from the stage.)

References

1. Washington, E.L. (1978). Musculoskeletal injuries in theatrical dancers: site, frequency, and severity. *American Journal of Sports Medicine, 6*(2), 75-98.

2. Rovere, G.D., Webb, L.X., Gristina, A.G., Vogel, J.M. (1983). Musculo-skeletal injuries in theatrical dance students. *American Journal of Sports Medicine, 11*(4), 195-198.

3. Francis, L.L., Francis, P.R., Welshons-Smith, K. (1985, Feb.). Aerobic dance injuries: a survey of instructors. *The Physician and Sportsmedicine, 13*:105-111.

4. Garrick, J.G., Gillien, D.M., Whiteside, P. (1986). The epidemiology of aerobic dance injuries. *American Journal of Sports Medicine, 14*(1), 67-72.

5. Solomon, R., Trepman, E., Micheli, L.J. (1989). Foot morphology and injury patterns in ballet and modern dancers. *Kinesiology and Medicine for Dance, 12*(1), 20-40.

6. Warren, M.P., Brooks-Gunn, J., Hamilton, L.H., Warren, L.F., Hamilton, W.G. (1986). Scoliosis and fractures in young ballet dancers: relation to delayed menarche and secondary amenorrhea. *New England Journal of Medicine, 314*(21), 1348-1353.

7. Gelabert, R. (1986). Dancers' spinal syndromes. *Journal of Orthopaedic and Sports Physical Therapy, 7*, 180-191.

8. White, A.A., Panjabi, M.M. (1978). *Clinical biomechanics of the spine.* Phila-delphia: J.B. Lippincott.

9. Nachemson, A. (1966, Mar.-Apr.). The load on lumbar disks in different positions of the body. *Clinical Orthopaedics and Related Research, 45*, 107-122.

10. Michele, A.A. (1960). The iliopsoas muscle: its importance in disorders of the hip and spine. *CIBA Clinical Symposia, 12*(3), 66-101.

11. McKibbin, B. (1968). The action of the iliopsoas muscle in the newborn. *Journal of Bone and Joint Surgery, 50-B*, 161-165.

12. Williams, P.L., Warwick, R., eds. (1980). *Gray's Anatomy.* 36th ed. Phila-delphia: W.B. Saunders.

13. Ranney, D.A. (1979, Sept.). The functional integration of trunk muscles and the psoas. *Kinesiology for Dance, 9*, 10-12.

14. Bachrach, R.M. (1987, Mar.). Dance injuries of the low back. *Kinesiology for Dance, 9*, 4-8.

15. Michele, A.A. (1962). *Iliopsoas: development of anomalies in man.* Springfield, Illinois: C.C. Thomas.

16. Nachemson, A. (1968). The possible importance of the psoas muscle for stabilization of the lumbar spine. *Acta Orthopaedica Scandinavica, 39*(1), 47-57.

17. *Anatomy as a Master Image in Training Dancers* [Video-recording]. Santa Cruz, California: Ruth Solomon [1988]. 1 videocassette; 59 minutes; color; 1/2 inch, VHS or Beta, 3/4 inch U-matic. (Available from Ruth Solomon, Arts Business Office, Porter College, University of California, Santa Cruz, CA 95064).

18. Micheli, L.J., Solomon, R. (1987). Training the young dancer. In: Ryan, A.J., Stephens, R.E., eds. *Dance medicine: a comprehensive guide.* Chicago and Minneapolis: Pluribus Press/*The Physician and Sportsmedicine*, 51-72.

19. Howse, J., Hancock, S. (1988). *Dance technique and injury prevention.* New York: Theatre Arts Books/Routledge.

20. Gurewitsch, A.D., O'Neill, M.A. (1944). Flexibility of healthy children. *Archives of Physical Therapy, 25,* 216-221.
21. Minkoff, J., Sherman, O.H. (1987). Considerations pursuant to the rehabilitation of the anterior cruciate injured knee. *Exercise and Sport Sciences Reviews, 15,* 297-349.
22. Ryman, R. (1979). Training the dancer IX: the spine in motion. *Dance in Canada, 21,* 14-18.
23. Ryman, R. (1979). Training the dancer VIII: the spine. *Dance in Canada, 20,* 19-22.
24. Dowd, I. (1984, Apr.). Technique and training: how to arch your back. *Dancemagazine, 58,* 118-119.
25. Stanish, W. (1987, Apr.). Low back pain in athletes: an overuse syndrome. *Clinics in Sports Medicine, 6,* 321-344.
26. Trepman, E., Micheli, L.J. (1988). Overuse injuries in sports. *Seminars in Orthopaedics, 3,* 217-222.
27. Hunter-Griffin, L.Y., ed. (1987, Apr.). Overuse injuries. *Clinics in Sports Medicine, 6,* 225-470.
28. Micheli, L.J. (1983, Nov.). Back injuries in dancers. *Clinics in Sports Medicine, 2,* 473-484.
29. Seals, J.G. (1983, Nov.). A study of dance surfaces. *Clinics in Sports Medicine, 2,* 557-561.
30. Micheli, L.J. (1987, Apr.). The traction apophysitises. *Clinics in Sports Medicine, 6,* 389-404.
31. Gieck, J.H., Saliba, E.N. (1987, Apr.). Application of modalities in overuse syndromes. *Clinics in Sports Medicine, 6,* 427-466.
32. Fredrickson, B.E., Baker, D., McHolick, W.J., Yuan, H.A., Lubicky, J.P. (1984). The natural history of spondylolysis and spondylolisthesis. *Journal of Bone and Joint Surgery, 66-A,* 699-707.
33. Pizzutillo, P.D. (1985). Spondylolisthesis: etiology and natural history. In: Bradford, D.S., Hensinger, R.M., eds. *The pediatric spine.* New York: Thieme, 395-402.
34. Jackson, D.W., Wiltse, L.L., Dingeman, R.D., Hayes, M. (1981). Stress reactions involving the pars interarticularis in young athletes. *American Journal of Sports Medicine, 9(5),* 304-312.
35. Steiner, M.E., Micheli, L.J. (1985). Treatment of symptomatic spondylolysis and spondylolisthesis with the modified Boston brace. *Spine, 10,* 937-943.
36. Ireland, M.L., Micheli, L.J. (1987). Bilateral stress fracture of the lumbar pedicles in a ballet dancer: a case report. *Journal of Bone and Joint Surgery, 69-A,* 140-142.
37. Sherman, F.C., Wilkinson, R.H., Hall, J.E. (1977). Reactive sclerosis of a pedicle and spondylolysis in the lumbar spine. *Journal of Bone and Joint Surgery, 59-A,* 49-54.
38. Brooks, H.L., Azen, S.P., Gerberg, E., Brooks, R., Chan, L. (1975). Scoliosis: a prospective epidemiological study. *Journal of Bone and Joint Surgery, 57-A,* 968-972.

39. Edmonson, A.S. (1987). Scoliosis. In: Crenshaw, A.H., ed. *Campbell's Operative Orthopaedics*, Vol 4. 7th ed. St. Louis: C.V. Mosby, 3167-3236.
40. Bunnell, W.P. (1988, Apr.). The natural history of idiopathic scoliosis. *Clinical Orthopaedics and Related Research, 229*, 20-25.
41. Renshaw, T.S. (1988, Apr.). Screening school children for scoliosis. *Clinical Orthopaedics and Related Research, 229*, 26-33.
42. Micheli, L.J., Marotta, J.J. (1989, Mar/Apr.). Scoliosis and sports. *Your Patient and Fitness, 2*, 5-11.
43. Winter, R.B. (1987). Natural history of spinal deformity. In: Bradford, D.S., Lonstein, J.E., Moe, J.H., Ogilvie, J.W., Winter, R.B., eds. *Moe's textbook of scoliosis and other spinal deformities*. 2nd ed. Philadelphia: W.B. Saunders, 89-95.
44. Nachemson, A.L. (1981). Disc pressure measurements. *Spine, 6*, 93-97.
45. Andersson, G.B.J., Ortengren, R., Nachemson, A. (1976). Quantitative studies of back loads in lifting. *Spine, 1*, 178-185.
46. Micheli, L.J. (1985, Autumn). The use of the modified Boston brace system (B.O.B.) for back pain: clinical indications. *Orthotics and Prosthetics, 39*, 41-46.
47. Micheli, L.J. (1979). Low back pain in the adolescent: differential diagnosis. *American Journal of Sports Medicine, 7*(6), 362-364.
48. Micheli, L.J., Hall, J.E., Miller, M.E. (1980). Use of modified Boston brace for back injuries in athletes. *American Journal of Sports Medicine, 8*(5), 351-356.
49. Nixon, J.E. (1983, Nov.). Injuries to the neck and upper extremities of dancers. *Clinics in Sports Medicine, 2*, 459-472.
50. Walaszek, A. (1982). Physical therapy rehabilitation for dance injuries. In: Cantu, R.C., Gillespie, W.J., eds. *Sports medicine, sports science: bridging the gap*. Lexington, Massachusetts: Collamore Press, 151-159.
51. Jones, F.P. (1979). *Body awareness in action: a study of the Alexander technique*. Revised ed. New York: Schocken.
52. Micheli, L.J. (1985, Sept.). Sports following spinal surgery in the young athlete. *Clinical Orthopaedics and Related Research, 198*, 152-157.

Illustrations: Elly Trepman, M.D.

7

Stress Fractures In Dancers

Lyle J. Micheli, M.D.
Professor Ruth Solomon

Doctors who have incorporated dance medicine into their practice and research are well aware that most injuries to dancers occur as a result of repetitive microtrauma, and therefore fall into the classification of overuse injury. The endless repetition of prescribed movements which is so basic to the study and performance of dance makes the dancer's body particularly susceptible to these injuries. There are often additional etiologic factors which contribute to the occurrence of overuse injury in the case of each individual dancer, but repetitive movement is generally the mechanism of injury.

Overuse injuries may affect a number of different tissues, including bone, articular cartilage lining the joints, tendons, or ligaments. A stress fracture (also known as "fatigue" or "insufficiency" fracture) is the overuse injury of bone. Like an acute fracture it involves an interruption of the continuity and structure of a bone, but it presents in different ways. When someone falls on an outstretched arm or receives a severe impact to the leg and has a frank, acute fracture of the arm bones or leg bones, there is usually pain, swelling, and obvious deformity at the site of injury. With stress fracture, however, the onset is often insidious. The fracture may present itself as simply a low-grade aching which is activity-related. With continuation of activity, the hairline crack in the bone, which is really what the stress fracture is, may deepen, or promulgate into additional small cracks in the same bone, resulting in more pain. Throughout this process, the body is attempting to heal the stress fracture site, but is unsuccessful. A repetitive cycle of microfracture-partial healing, microfracture-partial healing, etc. is established. Rarely, the stress fracture may suddenly develop into a frank fracture through the bone following a particular dance movement, as in one of our cases reported below. More typically, the pain persists and worsens until the activity which has gradually caused the injury becomes almost impossible. It is usually at this point that medical assistance is sought.

The diagnosis of stress fracture is seldom a simple matter. Certain ailments which don't even involve the bones *per se*—tendinitis, bursitis, strains and sprains, and even tumors—can produce much the same symptomology, and need to be ruled out. In the lower leg, which is the most common site of stress fractures, shin splints, a frequent precursor of stress fracture, can be confused with the real thing.

Obviously the business of diagnosis must be placed in the hands of a qualified medical person. This is true not only because of the medical knowledge required to make an accurate judgment, but even more so because these are the people who have access to the various imaging technologies which are crucial to diagnosing problems of the bones. In addition to the standard x-rays, specialized techniques such as tomography or bone scans are available, which may allow early diagnosis even before plain x-rays demonstrate a problem. The earlier this diagnosis is made, the sooner corrective action can be initiated, lessening the period of disability.

Of course not only dancers suffer from stress fractures; any segment of the population that is regularly involved in repetitive activities is at high risk for this injury. The first published report of this type of injury was by a German military physician named Briethaupt in 1855. He discovered a high incidence of what came to be called "march fractures" in Prussian Army soldiers who were experiencing painful feet following long marches.[1] Subsequent publications have continued to associate stress fractures with military training systems. In 1975, Dr. Angus McBryde reviewed the current literature on stress fractures. "In the military," McBryde noted, "the inciting activity is standard for that particular service or installation, causing a group injury and permitting a group diagnosis. . . . The military experience has been, by far, the primary contributor in the understanding of stress fractures."[2] That is, because the military tends to subject groups of men to standardized physical regimens for which they have had no prior training, the physiological reactions of those groups—e.g., a predisposition to stress fractures of the feet after sustained marching—provide a particularly pure measure of the effects of physical activity on the body.

McBryde pointed out certain similarities between the military and the typical sports training situation as regards susceptibility to stress fracture. Further review of sports-related stress fractures was done by Dr. Carl Stanitski. "Interestingly," Stanitski observes, "in only three animals have stress fractures been documented: thoroughbred racing horses, racing greyhounds, and man. These all have been systematically trained to produce maximum performance with certain types of repetitive physical exertion. Sufficient time is often not allowed for the normal reparative processes of bone to withstand the relentless forces demanded by the athlete."[3] Stanitski uses brief case studies of subjects involved in various sports activities to speculate on the nature of stress fractures. Ultimately he theorizes that "It is the rhythmic repetitive muscle action [required in the practice of most sports] that causes subthreshold mechanical insults which summate beyond the stress-bearing capacity of the bone."[3]

Sports which involve running, jumping, or repetitive throwing have been particularly indicted. Our own early work on stress fractures encompassed a number of sports, but focused most often on running. In a review of stress fractures of the lower extremities in runners, we found stress fractures in every major bone of the lower extremity. We presented the following checklist which we believe represents risk factor categories to be considered in analyzing the etiology of these injuries (Table 7.1).[4] In every stress fracture site studied, training error was the most frequently associated etiology, followed by tendinous imbalance and so on down the list to those factors which are rarer or more difficult to assess.

This list points to a close correlation between the causes of stress fractures in runners and in dancers. Not only do they experience many of the same injuries in much the same ratio to the number of participants in the activity studied (actually, dancers seem to have a slightly higher percentage of stress fractures than runners),[5,6] but it is

TABLE 7.1
Factors to Check in Overuse Syndrome

1. TRAINING ERRORS: abrupt changes in intensity, duration, or frequency of training.
2. TENDINOUS IMBALANCE: of strength, flexibility, or bulk.
3. ANATOMICAL MALALIGNMENT OF THE LOWER EXTREMITIES: femoral anteversion, patella alta or lateral alignment, genu valgum, tibia vara, pes planus or cavo varus.
4. FOOTWEAR: improper fit, inadequate impact absorbing material, excessive stiffness of sole, and/or insufficient support of hindfoot.
5. RUNNING SURFACE: concrete pavement versus asphalt, versus running track, versus dirt or grass.
6. ASSOCIATED DISEASE STATE OF THE LOWER EXTREMITY: osteoarthritis, neuromuscular disease, vascular insufficiency, or old fracture.

obvious that the mechanics that at least in part precipitate the injury are similar. Simply put, if you train and perform regularly in an activity which requires that your lower extremities repetitively exchange energy with a hard surface for prolonged periods of time, you are a prime candidate for stress fractures.

Since we made our original list, several other probable risk factors have come to our attention. In our study of injuries in modern dancers we found differences in the techniques studied to be of significance.[7] Modern dance encompasses many different techniques, each of which makes unique demands on the dancer's body, thereby creating its own stress patterns. More recently, authors in this field have suggested additional factors which have to do with nutrition and gender. In female dancers and athletes a correlation between menstrual irregularities and bone disorders has been observed. Dr. Michelle Warren, for example, suggests that the very high incidence of fractures in the group of young ballet dancers she studied (46 fractures in 75 dancers, or 61 percent) may be related to hypoestrogenism as reflected in delayed menarche and prolonged amenorrhea.[5] Similarly, a study of female distance runners reported in *The American Journal of Sports Medicine* indicates that "female distance runners who have a history of irregular or absent menses and who have never used oral contraceptives [i.e., artificially altered their estrogen balance] may be at an increased risk for developing a stress fracture."[6] Both articles go on to draw eating disorders into an equation which might be expressed as follows: extreme concern with physical fitness (and, perhaps, with body image) yields exercise and eating patterns which produce hypoestrogenism (and resulting menstrual irregularities), which in turn contributes to bone disorders such as stress fractures (Table 7.2).

Perhaps these more recent considerations in explaining the etiology of stress fractures can be assimilated to produce a more complete picture. In order to remain healthy, bones require certain nutrients which result from proper food intake and the maintenance of normal hormone balances. If the bones are not receiving these nutrients—as a result of such classic eating disorders as anorexia nervosa or bulimia, or excessive dieting, or the loss of appetite that can accompany heavy

TABLE 7.2
Additional Risk Factors in Overuse Syndrome in Dancers

1. Specific Dance Technique Training
2. Gender
3. Nutrition

physical training—they lose their normal ability to "remodel," or rebuild, themselves, and are hence particularly prone to injury. This condition in itself can produce what we sometimes call (when we split stress fractures into sub-groups) insufficiency fractures. If at the same time these bones are being asked to do hard, repetitive work, they may well develop fatigue fractures.

Concerning treatment: the dancer who develops a stress fracture must anticipate a fairly substantial period of time away from dancing. When a stress fracture is recognized early and diagnosed properly we normally treat it with "relative rest," by which we mean a period of approximately three weeks during which dancing is discontinued and replaced with such nonimpact activites as swimming, cycling, or floorwork. Whatever alternate activity is used, it should not involve impacting on the already fatigued site; inherent in the injury we call stress fracture is an attempt by the bone to restructure itself, and it can do this healing work only when the stress that has caused the injury is removed. Initially, we may use crutches, a cane, casting, or pneumatic bracing (air cast) to augment the nonweight-bearing approach to treatment. It is important to keep the patient (dancer) functioning for both physical and psychological reasons, but unfortunately the dance activity which caused the stress fracture must be temporarily suspended.

With this brief introduction in mind we turn now to some case studies from our practice, which should help to exemplify the subject of stress fracture. The dancers reported in these cases are all professionals who were thoroughly involved in taking classes, rehearsing, and performing during the time their injuries materialized.

Case 1. A 24-year-old jazz dancer came in with persistent pain at the ball of her foot. This is a common complaint of dancers, and one that does not necessarily raise the prospect of stress fracture; quite often it is diagnosed as a "bone bruise." In this case, the x-ray taken after her initial visit *did* give clear indication of stress fracture, although still in an early stage, of one of the two small bones at the base of the first toe, the sesamoid bones (Figure 7.1). We recommended no classes for four weeks, substituting careful stretching and strengthening exercises, and the use of a special rigid shoe insert. The injury healed. Other cases of this sort, when not treated promptly, have gone on to nonunion fractures, which may then require surgical fusion or resection.

Case 2. This 29-year-old female ballet dancer presented with pain in the forefoot. She had a long history of stress fractures involving both fibulas and bi-lateral fractures of the first and third metatarsals. This proven predisposition increased our suspicion of stress fracture.

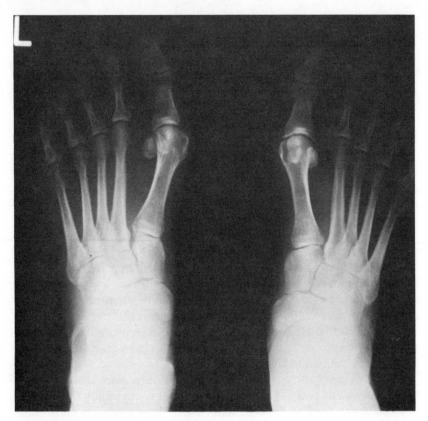

Figure 7.1. Radiograph: Sesamoid fracture.

X-rays were inconclusive, showing only a cortical thickening of the second and third metatarsals, but a subsequent bone scan confirmed our diagnosis through increased uptake, or "hot spots" (unexpectedly in *both* feet), at the base of the metatarsals and adjacent tarsal bones, including the cuneiform bones (Figure 7.2).

It should be noted that ballet dancers who perform on *pointe* are at high risk for another apparently unique stress fracture of the metatarsal bones. This involves the Lisfranc joint, at the proximal end of the second metatarsal (Figure 7.3). In such cases pain usually occurs not in the forefoot, but in the middle portion of the foot, at or near the point where the second metatarsal articulates with all three cuneiforms. The mechanism of this injury is of particular interest: When the foot goes on *pointe* the proximal head of the second metatarsal essentially locks in place, becoming rigid in its socket and therefore vulnerable to injury. This is not an easy injury to diagnose (it was not reported in

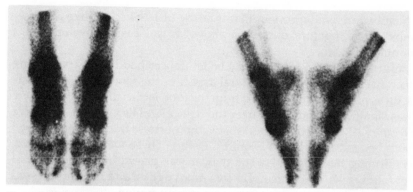

Figure 7.2. Bone Scan: Bilateral stress fracture 2nd metatarsal.

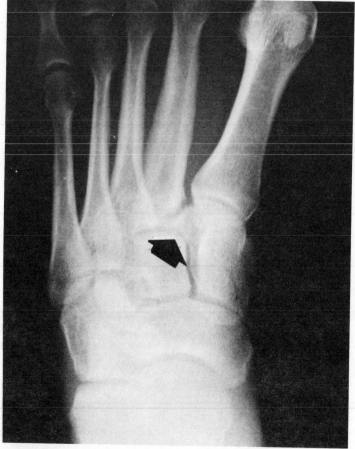

Figure 7.3. Radiograph: Lisfranc fracture proximal head of 2nd metatarsal.

the literature on dancers until our article of 1985),[8] and, like the sesa-moid stress fracture described above, it can easily develop into a nonunion fracture.

Case 3. This 22-year-old male ballet dancer had been experiencing pain over the dorsum and lateral aspect of the foot for 3-4 weeks, as soon as pressure was released from the foot, especially after *plié.* There was significant tenderness over the navicular. His x-ray was negative (Figure 7.4), yet we remained suspicious of stress fracture and ordered both bone scan (Figure 7.5) and CT scan. These were both positive, confirming the diagnosis. The dancer was placed in a short leg cast for four weeks, on crutches for two more weeks, and then progressed to *barre* and center work over a one-month period.

Case 4. A 24-year-old female ballet dancer experienced generalized pain in her right foot during an intense run of "The Nutcracker."

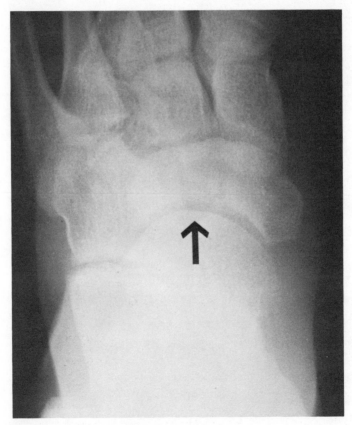

Figure 7.4. Radiograph: Negative navicular fracture.

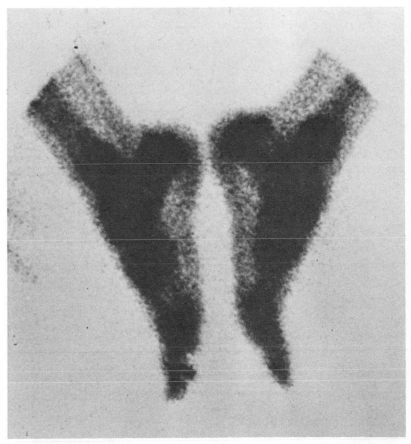

Figure 7.5. Bone Scan: Showing stress fracture of the navicular along with additional areas of increased uptake.

Although the pain was quite persistent, she waited two months after the run had ended before seeking medical help. The x-ray taken at her initial visit showed suspicious cortical thickening of her distal fibula, above the ankle (Figure 7.6). A bone scan four days later confirmed increased uptake over the right fibular shaft (Figure 7.7). Diagnosis of right fibular stress fracture was made, and the patient was given an air cast and taken off all physical activity except swimming. Two and one-half weeks later she was allowed to do a gentle *barre*, and one week thereafter she resumed across-the-floor work. However, pain over the fibula recurred. Four more weeks of total rest were prescribed, followed by a gradual, pain-free return to full dance work.

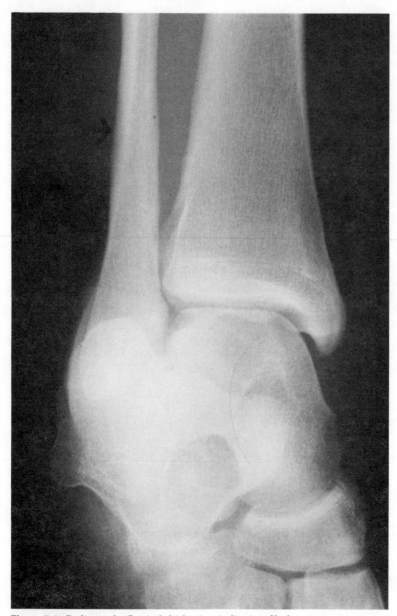

Figure 7.6. Radiograph: Cortical thickening indicating fibular stress.

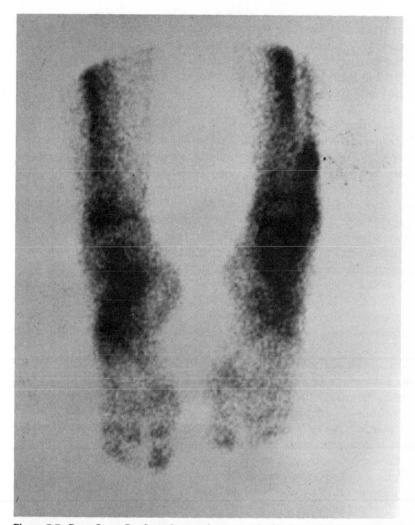

Figure 7.7. Bone Scan: Confirmed stress fracture right fibular and stress reaction over left tarsal bones.

Case 5. This 22-year-old female ballet dancer presented with pain suggestive of stress fracture in the tibia. First x-rays showed a clear-cut but incomplete fracture, with a dense margin across the tibial cortex. She was removed from dancing and given electro-stimulation to encourage bone formation. Two months later there was little pain, swelling, or tenderness, and she was returned to partial dance activity. However, an x-ray taken one month thereafter showed incomplete healing, so she was not allowed to dance full-out (Figure 7.8). Six months later there was still some pain in the area, and the x-ray taken at that time indicated that whereas the original fracture was healed, she had at some point had bi-lateral stress fractures in the mid-third of the tibias (Figure 7.9).

Case 6. This is a case referred to in passing above. It involves both tibia and fibular fracture in a male ballet dancer that occurred during a rehearsal from the sudden explosive force of jumping while in an extreme turned out position. This was obviously a macrotrauma injury, but review of his x-rays suggested multiple stress fracture sites of the tibia, doubtless of variable chronicity. The spiral fracture of the mid-shaft of the left tibia was initially treated with closed reduction and placed in a long-leg cast. Over the next few weeks there was progressive loss of reduction (separation of the bone fragments), and an exacerbation of the varus position of the bones (Figure 7.10). Hence, an open (surgical) reduction of the fracture was performed, and fixation with stainless steel lag screws was accomplished. An x-ray taken a month later shows the screws in place, and significant healing underway (Figure 7.11). It goes without saying that this is an extreme example of what can happen if stress fractures are not attended to promptly.

Case 7. Finally, we turn to the case of a 35-year-old ballerina who, also during a run of "The Nutcracker," was experiencing unrelenting pain in the area of the femur. An x-ray taken at that time showed new bone formation (Figure 7.12), and a bone scan supported the diagnosis of stress fracture of the femur. Three months later the pain persisted, there was a sense that the bone damage was not healing, and additional x-rays confirmed this. The patient was then taken off all dance activities and given a cane to limit weight-bearing. Swimming was recommended, and she was allowed to do Pilates exercises. Two months later the pain was gone, and she was able gradually to resume dancing.

This survey of case studies has intentionally moved up the foot and leg, reflecting the pattern in which stress fractures in dancers are most frequently seen. It should be understood, however, that like active people in all walks of life, dancers may experience stress fracture in virtually any part of the body. Stress fractures in the spine, especially, occur with increased frequency in dancers.

By far the majority of spinal stress fractures are what we call spondylolysis—tiny (sometimes not so tiny) cracks in the bone at the site of the pars interarticularis, most often in the lumbar spine (Figure 7.13). If not dealt with properly the loss of continuity at the pars interarticularis can weaken the spinal structure and contribute to low back pain,

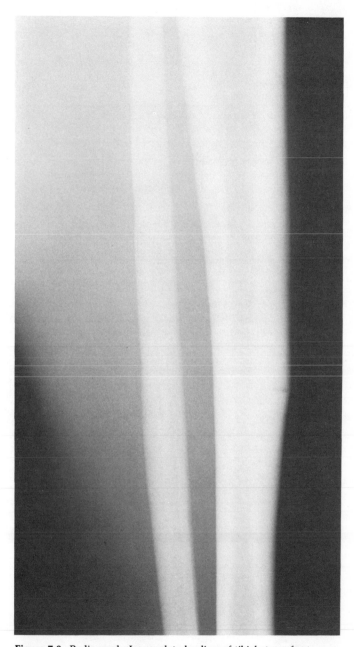

Figure 7.8. Radiograph: Incomplete healing of tibial stress fracture.

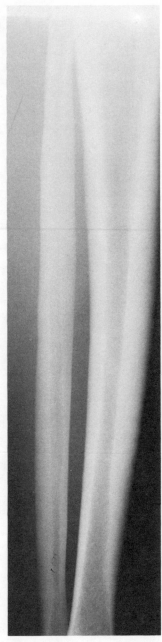

Figure 7.9. Radiograph: Original tibial fracture healed, but x-ray shows past stress fracture in mid-third of tibia.

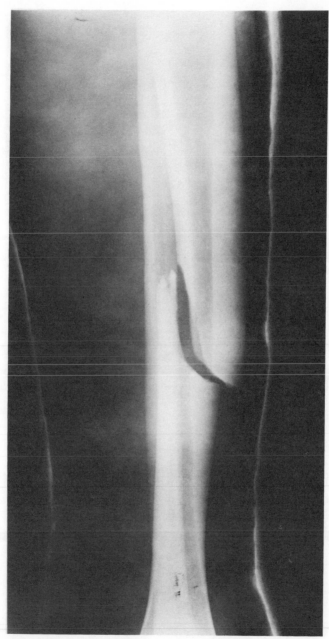

Figure 7.10. Pre-operative radiograph: Taken in cast, fracture showing loss of reduction and exacerbation of varus position.

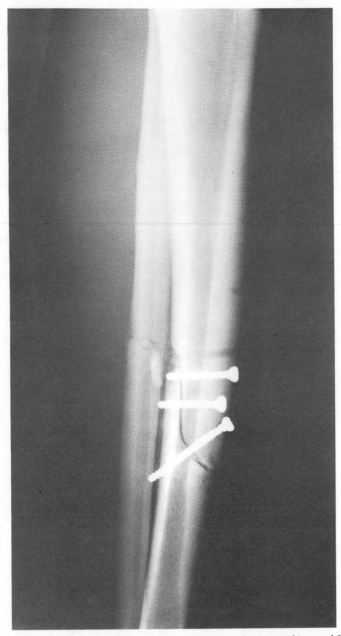

Figure 7.11. Post-operative radiograph following open reduction and internal fixation.

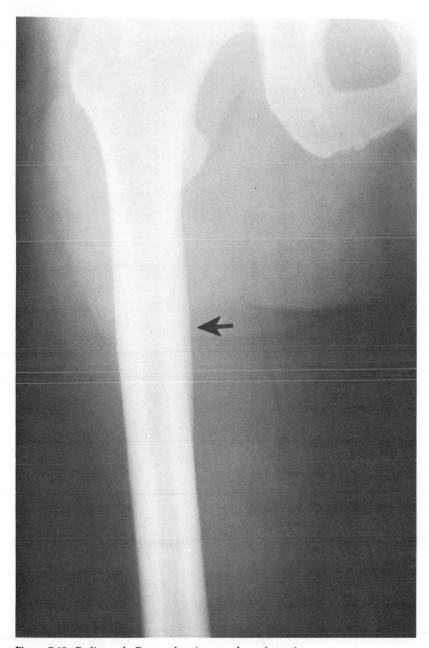

Figure 7.12. Radiograph: Femur showing new bone formation.

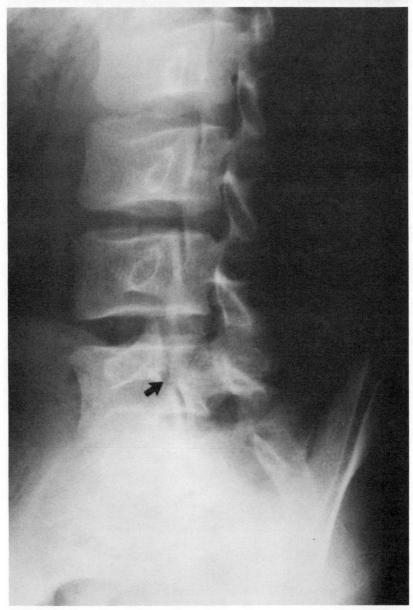

Figure 7.13. Spondylolysis: radiograph of lumbar spine, demonstrating fracture defect in the pars interarticularis of L-5.

particularly with movements involving extension to the rear, such as the *arabesque*. Whenever a dancer—or, for that matter, a gymnast—presents with pain upon performing back extension, this injury must be suspected. One study of female gymnasts found spondylolysis in over 11 percent of its subjects upon x-ray, whereas no more than 2.3 percent of the female population at large might be expected to have it.[9] Another study of two ballet companies found spondylo in over 7 percent of the members x-rayed.[10] Bracing for a period of months, often in combination with pelvic strengthening exercises, has proven a very successful method of treating this particular fracture.[11]

The pars interarticularis is clearly the most vulnerable site in the spine, but stress fractures have also been found in the lumbar pedicles (Figure 7.14). This is another possibility that must be considered in diagnosing and treating lower back pain in dancers.[12]

We close with a word about prevention. Virtually everything in the way dancers are trained, and much, we suspect, in the lifestyle they

P T. O.

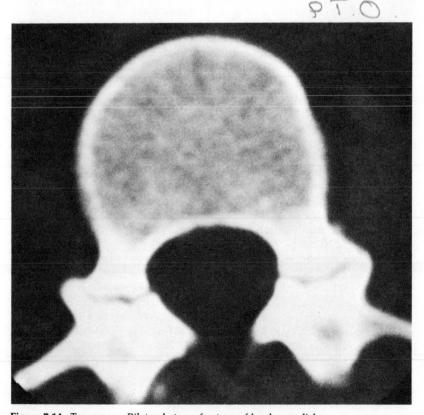

Figure 7.14. Tomogram: Bilateral stress fracture of lumbar pedicles.

share as a group, predisposes them to stress fractures. In order to gain and maintain the skills required for their art, dancers have to subject their bodies to very severe, and repetitive, extremes of motion. However, this regimen *can* be pursued in ways which minimize the risk. The keys to prevention of stress fractures, we believe, lie in such factors as: a slow, progressive approach to training, with careful attention to avoiding rapid changes of style or technique; a reasoned attempt to match the anatomical characteristics of the individual dancer to the demands of the technique he/she is practicing; and, a general awareness of body mechanics, especially as they pertain to avoiding excessive fatigue. Maintaining proper nutrition may be another important factor. Attention to these matters by dancers, and those who are responsible for their training, can reduce the incidence of stress fracture.

References

1. Breithaupt, M.D. (1855). Zur Pathologie des menschlichen fusses. *Medicinische Zeitung, 24,* 169-171, 175-177.
2. McBryde, A.M. (1975). Stress fractures in athletes. *Journal of Sports Medicine, 3*(5), 212-217.
3. Stanitski, C.L., McMaster, J.H., Scranton, P.E. (1978). On the nature of stress fractures. *American Journal of Sports Medicine, 6*(6), 391-396.
4. Micheli, L.J., Santopietro, F., Gerbino, P., Crowe, P. (1980, Apr./June). Etiologic assessment of overuse stress fractures in athletes. *Nova Scotia Medical Bulletin, 59,* 43-47.
5. Warren, M.P., Brooks-Gunn, J., Hamilton, L.H., Warren, L.F., Hamilton, W.G. (1986). Scoliosis and fractures in young ballet dancers: relation to delayed menarche and secondary amenorrhea. *New England Journal of Medicine, 314*(21), 1348-1353.
6. Barrow, G.W., Saha, S. (1988). Menstrual irregularity and stress fractures in collegiate female distance runners. *American Journal of Sports Medicine, 16*(3), 209-216.
7. Solomon, R., Micheli, L.J. (1986, Aug.). Technique as a consideration in modern dance injuries. *The Physician and Sportsmedicine, 14,* 83-92.
8. Micheli, L.J., Sohn, R.S., Solomon, R. (1985, Dec.). Stress fractures of the second metatarsal involving Lisfranc's joint in ballet dancers: A new overuse injury of the foot. *Journal of Bone and Joint Surgery, 67A,* 1372-1375.
9. Jackson, D.W., Wiltse, L., Cirincione, R.J. (1976). Spondylolysis in the female gymnast. *Clinical Orthopaedics and Related Research, 117,* 68-73.
10. Garrick, J.G. (1986). Ballet Injuries. *Medical Problems of Performing Artists, 1*(4), 123-127.
11. Steiner, M.E., Micheli, L.J. (1985). Treatment of symptomatic spondylolysis and spondylolisthesis with the modified Boston brace. *Spine, 10*(10), 937-943.

12. Ireland, M.L., Micheli, L.J. (1987, Jan.). Bilateral stress fracture of the lumbar pedicles in a ballet dancer: a case report. *Journal of Bone and Joint Surgery, 69A,* 140-142.

PART III:

Prevention

8

Physical Screening of the Dancer:
General Methodologies and Procedures

Janice Gudde Plastino, Ph.D.

Introduction

This chapter is intended to introduce a basic screening model to teachers, choreographers, directors, and health professionals who care for the well-being of dancers. The procedure described here can also be used to increase the aesthetic/artistic ability of dancers in any technique or at any level in the dance world.

Evaluation of the student or professional dancer before actual physical participation is virtually unknown in the United States. In the U.S.S.R., on the other hand, dancers are carefully screened and chosen at a young age before they enter the rigorous training programs that lead to performance in the very competitive world of ballet. In addition, most schools and all companies in that country have medical care and other appropriate modalities of therapy and treatment available for all dance participants, whether at the professional or student level.[1]

Physical screening is the process of evaluating dancers for general health and welfare, as well as for existing and/or previous injuries that might eventually affect their dancing career. The process is a requirement in the athletic world, and no self-respecting amateur or professional sports program would begin a training or performance season without a pre-participation examination of all performers.

There are numerous reasons for this involved, multifaceted, and time-consuming procedure in the athletic world. Athletic directors want to be covered in case of lawsuit if the athlete is injured; coaches want the strongest and hardiest athlete possible, who is able to give the maximum amount to the team; trainers hope to have fewer injured athletes in the training room; and the athletes themselves want to give the best performance possible at all times. The most prevalent complaint about the screening process for athletes is that it is often perfunctorily completed, without careful consideration of the whole athlete. Too often it is done simply to satisfy the NCAA recommendation or individual school requirements.

The pre-participation screening program in dance at the University of California, Irvine, has been developed with the hope that dance injuries can be lessened, and student dancers taught more about their own bodies. The screening process was the original idea of this author (who is a kinesiologist), the Athletic Department trainer and his staff, and an orthopedic surgeon who, as a sports medicine specialist, was seeing all the injured dancers at the University Student Health Service. With the cooperation of the physician in charge of the Student Health Service and qualified faculty and students in the dance department, the actual physical exam is completed in one intense afternoon session at the beginning of the university year, before the students begin technique classes. Auditions are held the previous day, so that the results of the screening and the placement audition can be used to place each student at the proper level of technique class for the upcoming quarter.

The main problem facing the faculty, given the very large population of dancers at Irvine (130 majors and minors and 1,100 participants overall quarterly), is the amount of time needed to advise the dancers based upon the audition/placement exam and the results of the screening. At the present time the last station of the screening process is a consultation with the dance kinesiologist, who is also a technique teacher, choreographer, and ex-professional performer. Any problem that has been found by the examiners is specifically brought to the attention of the kinesiologist, who in turn brings it to the attention of the dancer. The kinesiologist informs each dancer of potential problems, and recommends alternative or additional training procedures

and/or alteration of the level or number of technique clas
taken. For the student dancer, rehearsal and performance s
are an integral part of the evaluation, though the pressing ....u to
complete University requirements for graduation often takes priority
over other considerations. In the private school or professional company situation the dancer's immediate rehearsal and performance
schedule must be a major factor in the evaluation. Regardless of the
level of the dancer, the appropriate teacher/advisor must have access
to the findings of the screening and follow the progress of his/her
advisees. The most pressing problem with all levels and types of dance
is the follow-up and proper advising of each individual dancer about
physical and aesthetic progress combined with any associated problems.

Proper pre-participation screening can be time-consuming and labor
intensive. It takes less time to evaluate each individual body than it
does to assess each examination and then advise each dancer. Yet
there is no doubt that the time spent can help dancers to know what
they can do about their own bodies, and how they might help themselves to become better and stronger in their craft.

The large professional and regional ballet companies employ full-
time therapists or have access to a network of therapists and qualified
physicians who treat and advise their dancers. Peter Marshall, therapist for American Ballet Theatre, has seen an enormous increase in
the number of practitioners available to professional and regional
ballet companies in the past year.[2] However, screening is not a part
of that world; most therapists work with members of those companies
after they are hurt. They are able to direct dancers in special conditioning
programs to keep them dancing, and often they can bring a potential
problem to the attention of the directors. L.M. Vincent in *The Dancer's
Book of Health,* states that on average some 15 to 20 dancers out of 90
members of the New York City Ballet Company are unable to perform
at any given time.[3] This percentage changes as repertory, length of
season, and numbers of choreographers vary. Elizabeth Larkin, Dance
Medicine Specialist at St. Francis Hospital in San Francisco, reports
that 25 percent is probably a conservative estimate of dancers injured
during a San Francisco Ballet performance season. Probably 15-18
percent of those injured could not perform.[4]

Analogously, university dancers are more likely to be injured during
performance and final examination time. In the beginning of the fall
quarter, 1988, at the University of California, Irvine, two major performances were scheduled during the fourth and sixth weeks of classes.
Forty-six student and off-campus professional dancers performed. Ten
of those performers had been screened and advised about potential

problems, and no new injuries from that group occurred during that period. There were, of course, no records for the nonscreened performers, but a total of 51 dancers were seen in the training room with injuries during that time. Of those, 33 were involved in one or both of the performances.

History Form

The most important aspect of the screening process is the health and injury history form that is completed by each dancer. The form should be as brief as possible and organized in such a manner that it can be completed by the dancer in a short period of time. It should contain questions that reveal all aspects of the dancer's present health that might affect performance either now or in the future. The form should contain the following information, organized in such a manner that it is easily interpreted by the dance professional who advises the dancer:

1. Name, current and permanent address and telephone number; the identification and appropriate information about someone who is responsible for the dancer (parent, spouse, significant other, friend); the dancer's age, date of birth, status in the school (e.g., junior) or the company (e.g., corps member three years).
2. The next section should briefly question the dancer, requiring simple yes or no answers, about histories of heart disease, diabetes, bladder problems, epilepsy, extraordinary menstrual irregularities, or recent surgeries. This type of information is usually available in more detail at the Student Health Service or from the dancer's private physician, and is needed in case of emergency only.
3. The most important part of the form asks for identification of specific injuries, date, recurrence, treatment, specific diagnosis, person who identified the injury, and current status of the injury. This is most easily accomplished by a form that lists the specific parts of the body (toes, foot, ankle, etc.) and has appropriate boxes to be checked by the dancer to indicate the injuries and the care received.

An additional, crucial aspect of the form asks for the number of hours spent in technique class, rehearsal and performance in the last two months, and the type and level of technique practiced. The amount of time spent in any other specific, regular physical activity is also identified.

Few, if any, high schools, colleges, private studios, or regional companies have free access to a physician, physical therapist, or

trainer for consultation in their dance program, a
certainly not available for a pre-participation scree
following procedures are suggested with this realiza
may seem incomplete or inadequate to those who a
complete medical team at their disposal. They are a
dance teacher rather than the physician or therapist.

Actual Screening

The following parts of the screening are easily completed by any
dance teacher with minimum specific expertise: weight, height, body
composition (Figure 8.1), flexibility, general posture, body type as it
relates to certain types of dance, and general evaluation of the feet,
ankles, knees, hips and spine. An exam progresses faster if the examiner has a recorder; also, for liability protection, more than one person
should be present during the process. Height and weight can be
measured in the school nurse's office or the training room. The other
tests can be carried out in the studio, with exceptional problems
referred to the health professional (Table 8.1).

The flexibility of dancers is easily tested with a square box (so the
dancers can place their heels against it) and a ruler to measure the
length of the arms (Figure 8.2). There are commercial devices that can
be purchased to measure flexibility, but dancers tend to be extremely
well stretched, and the devices available (which are calibrated for the
general population) are not usually adequate to record the dance
population.

It is important that the same tester complete the measurements
for each specific test, to ensure some degree of consistency. This is
especially true for the body composition testing, since it requires
experience and knowledge of the instrument used for the measurement. This test and the recording of weight are most stressful for
dancers, and should be done by the teacher, nurse, or another person
the dancers trust, and where other dancers cannot see the results.

Two parts of the screening are the most crucial: the basic postural
evaluation as it applies to dance, and the specificities of the toes, feet,
ankles, legs, hips and spine as they apply to the dancer.

For testing, the women should be dressed in a two-piece bathing
suit, the men in trunks, and both should be barefoot. It is also desirable
that the dancers bring any shoes and orthotics used daily and/or in
class, rehearsal, and performance.

Posture Exam

Be sure to scan the history form before starting the exam. Any current,
former, or recurrent injury should be inquired about and any existing

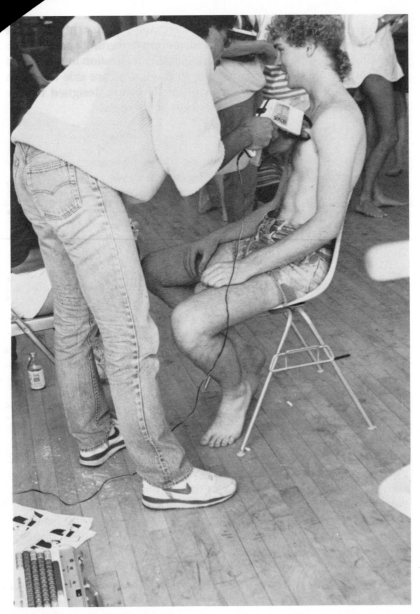

Figure 8.1. Body composition testing

TABLE 8.1.
The Screening Exam

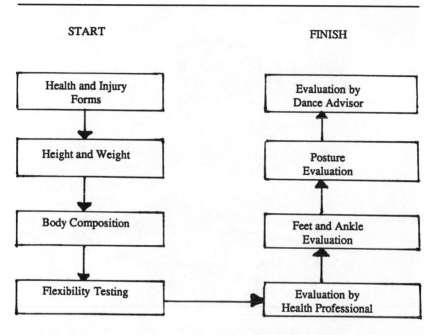

medical protocol noted. Any other medical problem, such as diabetes, should be briefly discussed and noted. It is also important to be aware of the amount of time the dancer has spent in dance activities and associated physical exercise in the past six weeks. This indicates how fast the dancer can get into "performing shape."

Each dancer should be viewed from the side in the "normal stance." This exam reveals potential or existing problems, and is the easiest way to bring them to the attention of the dancer. It must be completed by a teacher or health professional who is trained in dance and understands proper dance alignment. If a posture grid is available, this part of the exam can proceed faster and more accurately. As few places have these, however, the trained dance eye is the most often used device.

The imaginary (plumb) line that is used to evaluate posture as seen from the side descends as follows: from the mastoid process just in front of the ear, through the center of the shoulder joint, just in front of the greater trochanter of the hip, slightly behind the center of the knee joint, and just slightly anterior to the lateral malleolus. Perhaps the greatest single problem facing dancers is some degree of spinal

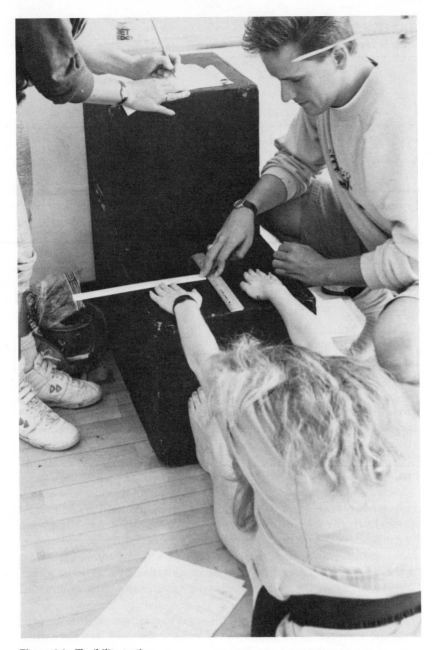

Figure 8.2. Flexibility testing

lordosis (sway back), and it can readily be seen in relation to this plumb line. Verbal and manipulative instructions can then be used to indicate how the problem is to be corrected.

Although dance teachers commonly concentrate on the back in evaluating posture, hyperextension of the knee must also be considered. It is actually a desirable trait in some styles of ballet, yet the dancer needs to be made aware of the condition, and told that it can contribute to a weak knee if not properly strengthened. The dancer in Figure 8.3 is only slightly exaggerating the posture with which she came to dance four years ago as a freshman. By now she has mastered advanced ballet, modern, and jazz techniques, and assumed a new alignment (Figure 8.4).

Following evaluation from the side, the dancer is viewed from the back. A discrepancy in the height of the two shoulders can be an indication of scoliosis (curvature of the spine), though we must bear in mind that many humans have one shoulder higher than the other (Figure 8.5). After observing the level of the shoulders and noting it either mentally or verbally to the recorder, have the dancer bend forward toward the knees with the hands touching in front of the body and the feet together in parallel position. One side of the back may disclose a slight hump, which would indicate some degree of curvature. Usually the hump will be more pronounced on the side where the shoulder is higher (Figure 8.6). In the young dancer this curvature may indicate problems of sufficient degree to have the student referred to an orthopedic physician before proceeding with technique classes. The dancer should be made aware that one side is likely to be stronger and/or preferred over the other.

To continue with the exam, the dancer is asked to face the evaluator with the feet in parallel position. The anterior superior iliac crests can be palpated and should be level. If the teacher has noticed a spinal curvature, the iliac crests may not be level. By measuring with a small steel tape measure from the iliac spines to the medial malleolus, the discrepancy can usually be pinpointed. If this measurement shows that both legs are the same length, the evaluator can have the dancer lie flat on his or her back, with knees bent, and check to see if the knees are level. If the knees are not level, a difference in length of the femurs may be indicated. The addition of an orthotic in the street shoe, character, or jazz shoe, and in extreme cases the soft ballet shoe, can help balance the dancer. These devices are prescribed by an orthopedist or podiatrist, and must be professionally and individually built for each dancer (Figure 8.7). In most cases, orthotics cannot be worn on stage in *pointe* or soft ballet shoes, or with bare feet for modern dance. Hence, the use or nonuse of orthotics in the training process

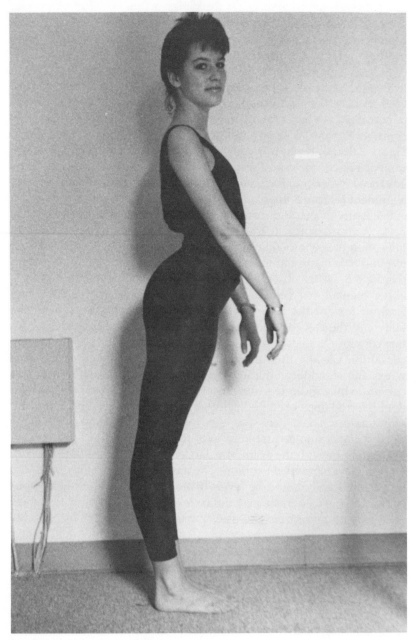

Figure 8.3. Exaggerated posture

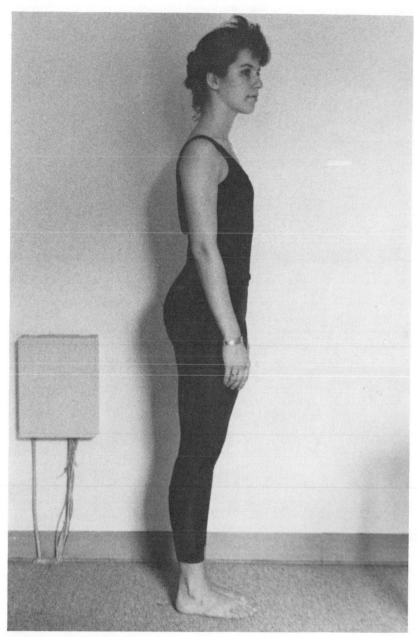

Figure 8.4. Corrected posture

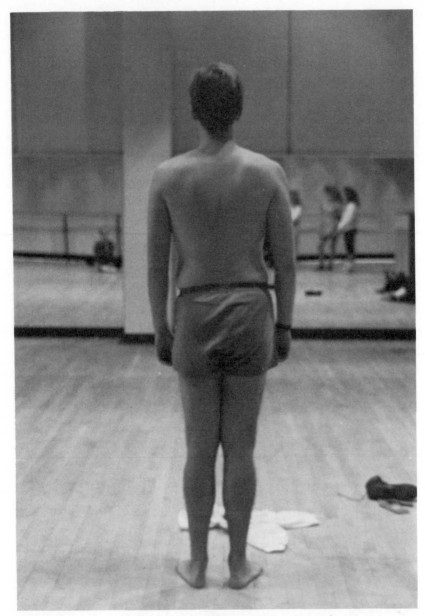

Figure 8.5. Unequal shoulder height: left shoulder higher than right

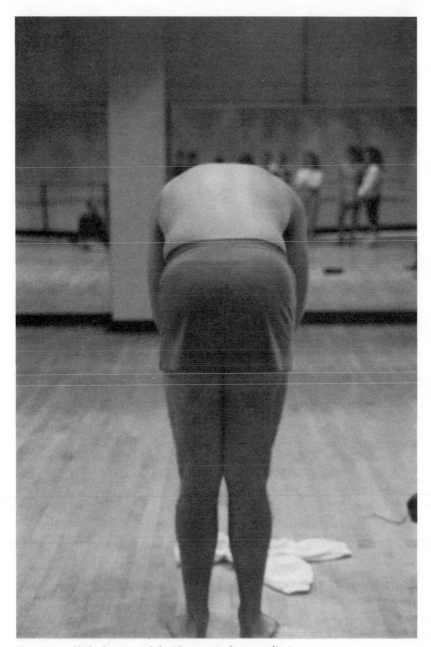

Figure 8.6. Slight hump on left side, may indicate scoliosis

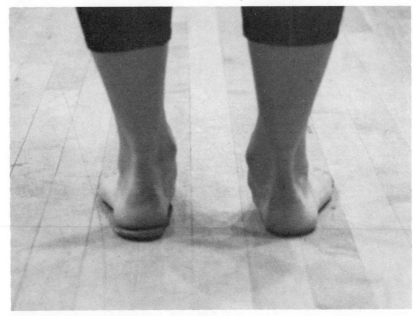

Figure 8.7. Use of orthotic

must be carefully weighed when preparing for performance, as balance and technique may be affected.

Knees are one of the easiest areas to evaluate because the dance population understands knock knees (genu valgus), bowlegs (genu varum), hyperextended knees (genu recurvatum) and femoral anteversion. In this author's experience, many advanced students and professional female dancers have bowlegs. Whether this results from training or from genetics is unknown, but it is common (Figure 8.8). This outward (lateral) curvature of the femur and/or tibia must be brought to the attention of the dancer, as it can be helped if not completely corrected. With genu varum the natural weight of the body descends through the lateral side of the foot rather than through the tarsus bones, where it should end in line with the second toe (Figure 8.9). This alignment problem can lead to lateral tendinitis, which is a relatively common injury in dance.

The propensity to knock knees is more natural in females because of the width of the hip, and can lead to poor turn out, as can the problem of femoral anteversion (lack of external rotation). Often, "squinting kneecaps" can indicate a lack of hip external rotation (Figure 8.10). These are common occurrences in the less-trained dancer, and may require additional strength training of the lower body.

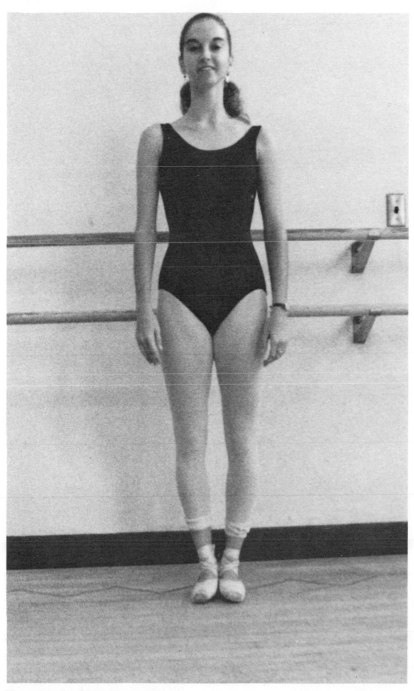

Figure 8.8. Bowlegs (genu varum)

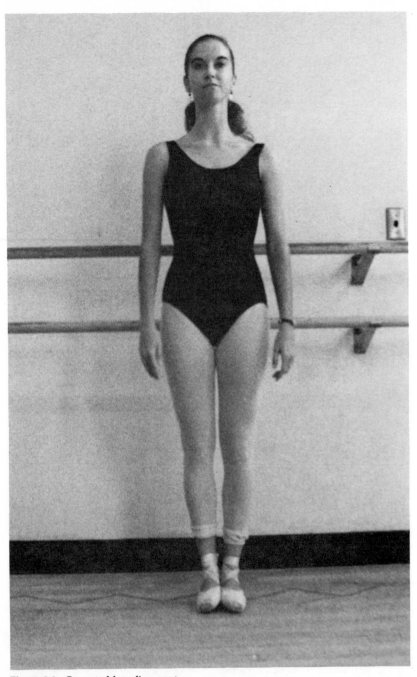

Figure 8.9. Corrected leg alignment

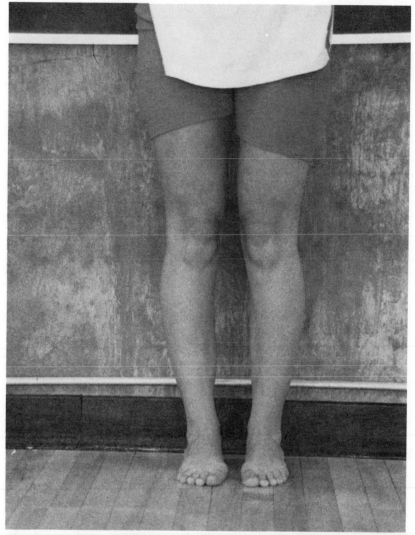

Figure 8.10. "Squinting" kneecaps (internal hip rotation)

Continuing down the body, evaluate the position of the ankles, feet, and toes in parallel position. The ankles should not supinate (roll out, Figures 8.11-8.12) or pronate (roll in, Figure 8.13). From the rear, the Achilles tendon should ascend in a straight line, curving neither to the lateral nor medial sides.

As many forms of dance use both parallel and rotated hip positions, it is important to view the dancer in both stances. After examining the

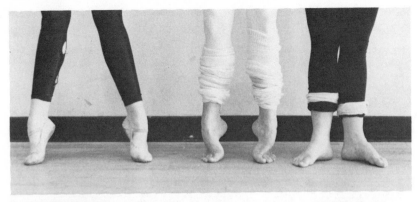

Figure 8.11. Supination (rolling out)

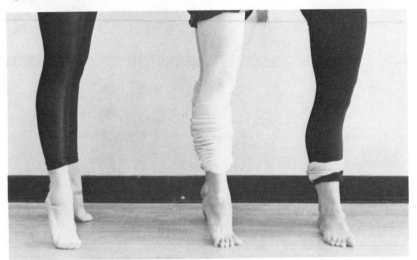

Figure 8.12. Corrected foot and ankle alignment

knees in parallel, have the dancer stand in turn-out. The natural turn-out is easily assessed starting with the feet and continuing upward. The second toe should be in line with the center of the kneecap. The tibia (shinbone) may curve laterally as the evaluator gently glides his/her finger along it toward the center of the patella. The weight of the body should be distributed evenly through the tarsus and forefoot (Figure 8.14). Make sure the dancer understands the correct basic alignment for dance. Careful continuous work can almost always correct and/or adjust lordosis, hyperextended knees, and the pronated or supinated foot. These alignment problems are common in dance,

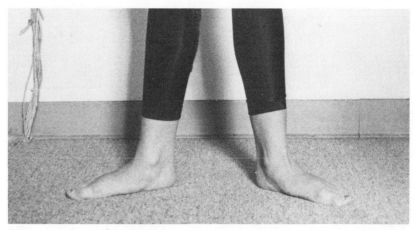

Figure 8.13. Pronation (rolling in)

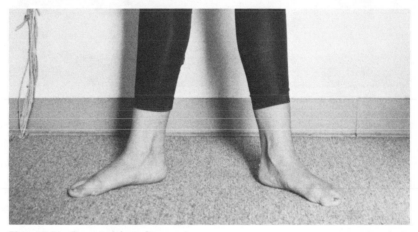

Figure 8.14. Corrected foot alignment

and all this information should be brought to the attention of the dancer verbally and with some hands-on adjustments.

The use of caliper measurements of the foot and of the Podiascope, as designed and used by Barbara Baily Plunk at Irvine, has been extremely helpful in two ways (Figure 8.15).[5] First, although the statistical analysis of the data is not completed at this time, preliminary indications are that the depth of the forefoot at the first metatarsal head as measured by standard calipers is important in the correct fitting of toe shoes. Second, the placement of the bare foot on the Podiascope may show foot placement problems not caught in the visual exam. The negative aspects of the Podiascope are its initial cost,

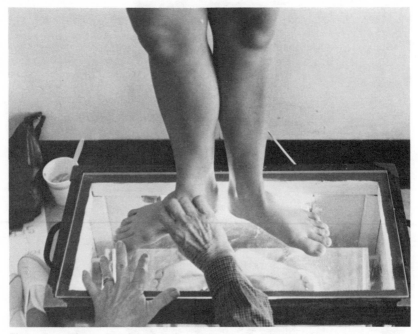

Figure 8.15. The podiascope

and the inordinate amount of time required to examine each foot individually. It is most valuable for examining extreme cases, or to further evaluate those dancers with the most difficult or puzzling problems.

Conclusion

It is important that the dancer is viewed in all of the ways described, the relevant information recorded, and potential problems and appropriate corrective measures brought to his/her attention. Ideally, following the initial screening process, the dancer should be carefully observed while performing any dance movements or positions that are commonly used by the choreographer, school, or company. Particular areas of stress resulting from the demands of the technique on body parts that are not well adapted to them can then be identified. Special exercises might have to be incorporated into or added to the technique class to increase the dancer's strength, flexibility, or endurance, and improve his/her alignment.

References

1. Plastino, J.G. (1988, Jan.-Feb.). [Notes from personal visit to USSR schools, companies and dance medicine facilities]. In possession of Janice Plastino, Dance Department, University of California, Irvine, California.
2. Plastino, J.G. (1988, Nov.). [Interview with Peter Marshall, Physical Therapist, American Ballet Theatre].
3. Vincent, L.M. (1978). *The dancer's book of health.* Kansas City: Sheed, Andrews and McMeel.
4. Plastino, J.G. (1988, Nov.). [Phone interview with Elizabeth Larkam, Dance Medicine Specialist for the Center for Sports Medicine, St Francis Memorial Hospital, San Francisco, CA].
5. Plunk, B.B. (1986-present). *Evaluation of the ballet foot for the fitting of the pointe shoe* [unpublished study]. Irvine, California: University of California.

Recommended Reading

1. Arnheim, D.D. (1980). *Dance injuries: their prevention and care.* 2nd ed. St. Louis: C.V. Mosby.
2. Fitt, S.S. (1988). *Dance kinesiology.* New York: Schirmer Books.
3. Hardaker, W.T., Erickson, L., Meyers, M. (1986). The pathogenesis of dance injury. In: Shell, C.G., ed. *The dancer as athlete.* Champaign, Illinois: Human Kinetics.
4. Plastino, J.G. (1987, May/June). The university dancer: physical screening. *Journal of Physical Education, Recreation, and Dance, 58:*49-50.
5. Stephens, R.E. (1987). The etiology of injuries in ballet. In: Ryan, A.J., Stephens, R.E., eds. *Dance medicine: a comprehensive guide.* Chicago and Minneapolis: Pluribus Press/The Physician and Sportsmedicine.

9

Bartenieff Fundamentals: Early Detection Of Potential Dance Injuries

Sandra Kay Lauffenburger, B.Ed., M.Sc., C.M.A.

Most dance injuries are not sudden or traumatic; they are commonly chronic, stemming from carefully cultivated but inefficient movement patterns developed by the dancer during his/her years of training. These inefficient patterns appear as an unprepared or unaware body tries to cope with technique or choreography. The patterns manifest themselves in improper muscle sequencing, misfiring of unneeded muscles, overuse of certain muscles, and muscle tone imbalance.

In nondancers (or nonathletes) the injury potential resulting from these inefficient movement patterns may not cause concern. However, given the degree of repeated usage required during dance training, rehearsals, and performances, in dancers it deserves serious attention. Inefficient patterns produce muscle misuse or overdependence on inappropriate muscles. As training continues this can lead to overuse of the muscles being engaged, as well as lack of use and subsequent weakening of the more appropriate ones. Finally, muscle imbalance results, and when this is added to excessive stress (repetitive use) and fatigue all the ingredients for injury are present.

The best place to break this potentially destructive chain is at the beginning; the dancer will benefit from early detection of inefficient movement patterns and increased awareness of the functional possibilities. Thus, injury prevention depends greatly on the teacher/trainer's ability to spot incorrect muscle usage and inappropriate motor patterning. Efficient body usage is easiest to observe and correct by looking at simple joint functions. However, given the range and complexity of most dance movement, the teacher/trainer needs a method for organizing, understanding, breaking down and observing movement patterns.

Bartenieff Fundamentals are an effective way of organizing an evaluation of muscle use and motor patterns. The Fundamentals are a series of exercise concepts which are now an integral part of the Laban Movement Analysis System in the United States. These exercise concepts embody the basic internal and external processes that underlie all movement, from athletics to choreography to life-supporting pedestrian tasks. Most of the basic exercises involve simple lifting and lowering, or flexing and extending of limbs or segments of limbs or trunk.

Any aspect of technique or choreography, no matter how complex, can be broken into components that relate directly to one or more specific Fundamentals. A list of the Basic Fundamentals is given in Table 9.1. This chapter will focus on the use of some of these Fundamentals to identify inefficient motor function and the consequent potential for chronic injury. I will illustrate this with one example for the lower body, one for the upper body, and one example for integrated full body movement.

Lower Body Movement Analysis

One of the simplest Fundamentals is the "thigh lift." The exercise procedure is outlined in Figure 9.1. The kinesiologic action is pure flexion and extension at a single hip joint.

TABLE 9.1.
Basic Eight Bartenieff Fundamentals

Fundamental Exercise	Associated Kinesiological Action
Heel Rock	Flexion/Extension of spine Breath support
Thigh Lift	Flexion of hip
Forward Pelvic Shift	Extension of hip
Lateral Pelvic Shift	Abduction/Adduction of hip (minor rotation)
Body Half	Abduction/Adduction/Rotation of proximal joints (and minor spine)
Knee Reach	Rotation of spine and proximal joints
Arm Circles	Rotation/Abduction/Adduction/Flexion/Extension of shoulder joint Protraction/Retraction/Upward and Downward Rotation of scapula Flexion/Extension (small) of other shoulder girdle joints
"X" Rolls	Rotation/Circumduction of proximal joints and spine

Hip flexion and extension are very basic components of dance technique and choreography (*plié, passé,* walking, running, etc.). Through this exercise the teacher/trainer has a chance to observe the dancer's motor pattern and possible muscle imbalances, and to draw the dancer's attention to problems before repetitive use causes chronic pain and the potential for injury. When performed correctly and with awareness, the same exercise can be used to train for a safer and more efficient motor action.

There are three main injury-prone locations related to simple hip flexion and extension: the spine, the hip joint, and the knee joint.

The Spine

The potential for spinal injury can be detected by observing the relationship of the sacrum to the floor as the degree of flexion increases. An anterior tilt of the pelvis (particularly to initiate the movement) or a loss of full sacral contact with the floor (by rolling onto the coccyx or the lumbar spine) should not occur. Either indicates as inability to stabilize the pelvis during hip flexion; thus, true articulation at the hip joint is lost. Often shortening rather than lengthening of the lumbar area is observed, signaling misuse or overuse of the lumbar erector spinae muscles to perform the action, and a concurrent lack of use or weakness in the abdominal muscles (rectus and transversus abdominii, in particular). This shortening not only creates compression on the vertebrae, but the misuse of the erector spinae can lead to hyper-contraction and muscle spasm. These are all symptoms indicating potential low back problems.

The Hip Joint

The hip is a second site to evaluate for injury potential. The action of flexion should involve only the rectus femoris and iliopsoas of the working leg, with the rectus and transversus abdominals stabilizing the pelvis and the balanced usage of the hamstrings and quadriceps stabilizing the knee in its flexed position. However, careful observation of this exercise often reveals overinvolvement of the tensor fascia latae and gluteal muscles. A shortening along the lateral side of the working hip and/or abduction of the thigh are key indicators of this muscular involvement.

Actual hip joint injuries are not so common, but continuance of this rotary tension leads to spinal misalignment. Muscle spasm and pain in the sacral area and hip joint often occurs from hyper-contracted

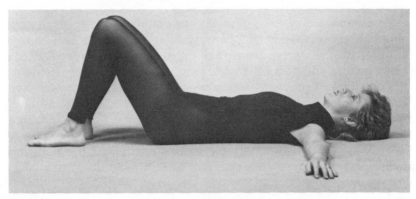

Figure 9.1-A

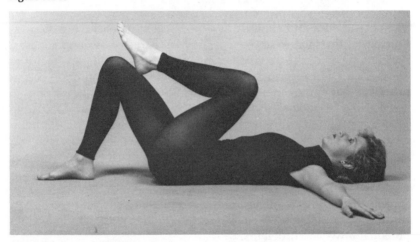

Figure 9.1-B

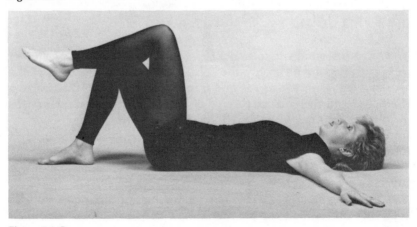

Figure 9.1-C

gluteals. Overused abductors can result in overall thigh muscle imbalance, which is a precursor of knee problems.

The Knee Joint

The potential for knee injury as a result of hip flexion and extension may seem less obvious, but it exists and can be detected by examination of the performance of this exercise. As the knee moves toward the chest it should maintain a constant distance from the body's midline. Deviation toward the midline signals too much adductor and/or gracilis tension; deviation away can indicate abductor (tensor fascia latae, gluteus medius) predominance. Imbalance of the lateral and medial thigh muscles can cause pain and potential for injury by distorting the alignment of the knee. Tight or overactive adductors can cause a medial distortion in alignment and put strain on the medial ligaments and meniscus. Overuse of the abductors leads to lateral distortion in alignment. The knee joint's healthy functioning is greatly dependent on the maintenance of pure tracking in its movement. Strain on ligaments is the first step in weakening or tearing these important support fibers.

Injury potential resulting from muscle imbalance or misuse can be found when performing this action in parallel position. Any inappropriate muscle functioning will be intensified when working in outward rotation, and particularly when bearing weight.

Other Bartenieff Fundamentals also address movement patterns of the lower limbs; however, let us now consider the potential for injury in the upper body. Although dance injuries in this area tend not to be as severe, the potential for problems still exists. This potential may manifest itself in later life as arthritis or limited shoulder mobility, or in relatively benign ways such as unattractive form and line in dance movement.

Figure 9.1. (Opposite Page) Fundamental Exercise: Thigh Lift.

Action: Lie back in a "hook lie" position (9.1-A). Exhale and hollow the abdomen to initiate the movement of leading with the top of the knee to lift the thigh toward the chest (9.1-B). Maintain the same amount of flexion in the knee while returning to the starting position (9.1-C).

Dancer Experience: Lumbar extensor muscles begin to lengthen (i.e., tension diminishes in them). The gluteal muscles gradually relax so the whole sacrum settles on the floor. This allows the iliopsoas to function. The whole process will be experienced as a changing of tension around the greater trochanter. Anchoring of the rest of the body occurs in the opposite (nonworking) leg from ischium to heel, and in the utmost width across the back and front of the chest.

Upper Body Analysis

The upper body is a very complex system of joints, the shoulder joint forming only one small part. The whole shoulder area is a remarkably mobile arrangement of bones connected by a variety of ball and socket joints. The scapular-humeral joint is the major ball and socket joint; however, the sternoclavicular joints, the acromioclavicular joints, as well as the meeting of the ribs with the sternum are all ball and socket joints. Movement in the upper body results from an integrated function of all these joints. Injury potential arises from the fixing, holding, or over-stabilization of one or more joints.

The Bartenieff Fundamental termed "arm circles" addresses the functioning of the upper body. Fixing, holding, and over-stabilization can be evaluated by the "arm circle" exercise (Figure 9.2 explains the basic actions of this exercise). The Laban Movement Analyst (a qualified teacher of Bartenieff Fundamentals) looks primarily for scapula mobility, folding and opening in the sternum, and gradated rotation throughout the arm circle. Each of these items may uncover a potential for injury.

Scapula Mobility

Although shoulder dislocations have been fairly uncommon in dance, the increased popularity of aerobic dance and of athleticism in modern choreography may yield a greater potential for this type of injury. During any arm movement the head of the humerus must stay in its socket, which is located on the lateral edge of the scapula. The range of motion available to the humerus means that the scapula must also have concurrent movement. This synchronized movement, called scapulo-humeral rhythm, must support the humeral movement and provide connection between these two bones. In the arm circle the scapula should float smoothly, with control, on the posterior and lateral surfaces of the torso. Over-stabilization of the scapula, or non-synchronized movement, will begin to weaken the ligaments that keep this joint intact. Continued use of a non-synchronized pattern can also lead to tearing of the small muscles of the rotator cuff that support this joint.

The muscle interaction in scapulo-humeral rhythm is complex. A constant involvement of all three main muscle groups of the shoulder joint (flexor/extensors, abductor/adductors, internal/external rotators) must occur.[1] In performing the arm circle exercise, an unbalanced involvement of these three groups manifests as a lopsided or irregular circle. For example, often a circle that has more height than width indicates an overuse of the upper trapezius and a weakness of the lower trapezius fibers and serratus anterior. The potential for injury begins with neck-shoulder tension and ultimately shifts to lower back and neck problems.

Sternoclavicular Mobility—Chest Folding and Opening

This is a subtle problem because our Western culture generally places a high value on jutting the chest forward and holding it there. Nonetheless, this holding is not functional. It is identified in the dancer by doing the arm circle and looking for discomfort or difficulty when the arm enters the portion of the circle where it crosses the midline of the body to the opposite side. The circle will probably lose width in this portion of the circle, and often the arm appears detached at the shoulder. Kinesiologically, the dancer needs to become aware of the availability of movement in the sternoclavicular joint as well as in the rib-sternum joints. The dancer also must learn to synchronize the actions of the middle trapezius, the rhomboids, and the pectoralis major. The injury potential identified here is related to humeral detachment from the scapula. However, immobility in the chest can also lead to problems with breathing and breath support of movement.

Gradated Rotation

There are circles within circles in the "arm circle" exercise. In addition to the humerus and scapula describing full circular paths during this activity, the head of the humerus must also rotate within the joint. This action is called gradated rotation. If there is no internal rotation, bony and muscular impingements can occur. This is particularly a problem under the coraco-acromial arch. Several tendons (the supraspinatus in particular) and bursa lie in this area. If the head of the humerus does not rotate properly during abduction and/or elevation, several problems can occur. These include: 1. Chronic microtrauma and damage to the tissues under the coraco-acromial arch; 2. Vascular impairment, which in turn can lead to swelling and inflammation; 3. Partial tear of the rotator cuff; and 4. Distortion of the bones or joints.[2]

These problems may not result from simple *port de bras* work, but when heavy hand-held props are used, or active upper body choreography is demanded, the potential for problems exists if gradated rotation is lacking.

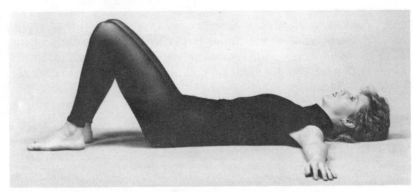

Figure 9.2-A

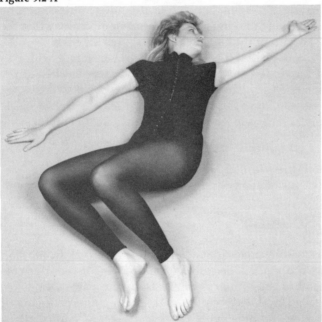

Figure 9.2-B
Figure 9.2. Fundamental Exercise: Arm Circles

Action: Lie on back in "hook lie" position with arms horizontally spread (9.2-A). Let the knees drop to the right side without the feet moving (9.2-B). Allow the left arm to extend itself into the diagonal pull (9.2-C). From there the left arm moves in a large counterclockwise circle. Allow the eyes to follow the hand with a slight movement of the head. When the hand returns to the starting position, rest (9.2-D). Then reverse the direction of circling. (Repeat whole sequence to opposite side.)

Dancer Experience: As soon as the circling movement begins, feel a gradual outward rotation of the arm, noticing how the palm changes the direction it faces. The pelvis must remain anchored. As the arm crosses the body's midline to the opposite side, feel the scapula come "around the side" of the body with the arm. Also, a folding or softening sensation is felt in the sternum area. Thus movement is experienced on the front and back of the body.

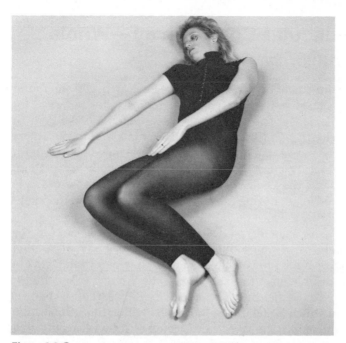

Figure 9.2-C

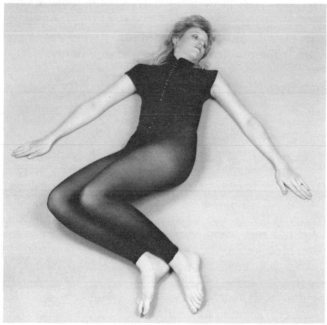

Figure 9.2-D

Neuromuscular Connectivity—Whole Body Analysis

Even if upper and lower body activities have been analyzed and found to utilize acceptable movement patterns, there is still potential for injury when the dancer has to integrate the upper and lower body in full body activity. Again, Bartenieff Fundamentals provide a context for assessing the injury potential in the integrated movement pattern. There are several "exercises" which address full body integration. Here I will discuss the "body half" exercise, and use a case example to show the need for analyzing full body coordination for injury potential.

The "body half" exercise, as described in Figure 9.3, looks at the dancer's awareness of the midline division of the body. It is often important in movement to be able to stabilize one part of the body in order to free up movement of the other side. Among other things, this exercise gives the dancer a clear sense of which part of the body is operating, and which is stabilizing (however, within this stabilization there must not be a holding or nonfunctional muscle activity that inhibits full or needed movement).

This exercise is done primarily in the vertical plane, thus identifying muscle actions that support lateral movement. Any forward-back movement signals the nonfunctional muscle activity which, as I have stated throughout, is the precursor of misuse/overuse injury.

The Case of the "Functionally Inflexible" Dancer

I worked with a client who complained of left hamstring pain and groin tightness, as well as some gluteal spasming. The concern was prevention of both muscle tearing and decreased mobility from sciatica pain. After checking for hamstring flexibility (which was excellent) and hip joint patterning using the "thigh lift" (which was pure and functional), I observed the dancer in rehearsal. I noticed a subtle loss of support on the left side when both the right arm and leg were actively gesturing. I recognized the "body half" exercise as a component of this choreographic movement, and thus examined the dancer doing the "body half" exercise.

In performing the "body half" exercise on the right side (with the left side as "stabilizer") rotation in the right hip joint must occur in order to keep the body in the vertical plane. Rotation must also occur in the anchoring (left) side's hip joint as a counterbalance. However,

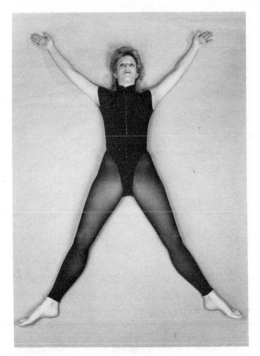

Figure 9.3-A

Figure 9.3. (This page and next) Fundamental Exercise: Body Half

Action: Lie on back in a symmetrical and large "X" position (9.3-A). Exhale as you simultaneously draw the right elbow and right knee toward each other on the floor. The right side of the torso may shorten slightly and the head can tilt to the side (9.3-B). Reverse this action by retracing the original path back to the starting position, leading with the fingers and toes (9.3-C). (Repeat on left side.)

Dancer Experience: Feel the midline of the body separating the major activities of the two sides. The body should stay as flat (in the vertical plane) as possible, thus using primarily the abduction and rotational muscles of the working joints. Opposite (non-moving/stabilizing) side is anchored by a counterbalancing outward rotation in the hip joint, initiated by the deep lateral rotator muscles. The nonmoving side stays open and extended, undisturbed during the movement of the other side.

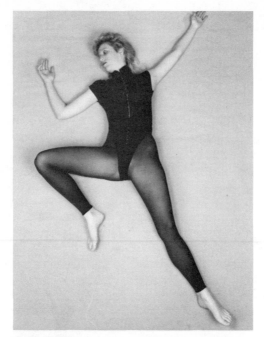

Figure 9.3-B

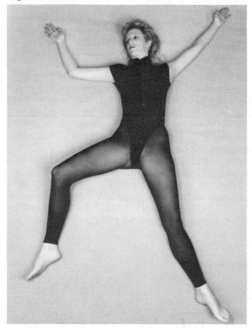

Figure 9.3-C

in this dancer this subtle action of the deep lateral rotators was not activated. Instead, the hamstrings (and gluteals to some extent) contracted to an exaggerated degree, thus signaling the beginning of a nonfunctional "misuse" pattern.

When this action is performed in the standing position, the hip joint serves several functions: the body's weight must be supported, and the above discussed counterbalancing achieved. When the hamstrings and gluteals "grip" too strongly, the beginnings of overuse are set in motion. Ultimately, as in the course of this performer's choreography, the stabilizing side may be called upon to provide stability during locomotor activities. If the hamstrings and gluteals are in a state of frozen contraction, and action at that hip joint is required (i.e., some sort of flexion, either in a *plié* or forward motion), the quadriceps must work against those "frozen" hamstrings/gluteal muscles. The likelihood of microtearing or even major tears exists. I call this type of muscular holding "functional inflexibility" because the muscle is capable of sufficient flexibility in a passive mode; however, when certain neuromuscular patterns are activated this flexibility ceases to exist. In this case the hamstrings lacked the ability to lengthen when called upon to function in the eccentric mode while supporting the body.

By guiding the dancer through a correct performance of the body half exercise on the floor I was able to alert her to the complex and inefficient way she was organizing her body's actions. Once her attention was drawn to what was occurring she was better able to understand a correction. We used the body half exercise in a variety of formats to re-pattern this neuromuscular action.

Summary

Screening for injury potential can be done by using one or more of the Bartenieff Fundamentals. However, Bartenieff Fundamentals assess more than just kinesiological action. They help to organize the body's understanding of efficient movement patterns. They also aid the teacher/trainer in drawing the dancer's attention to an inefficient pattern, "interrupting" it, *and* facilitating the development of functional usage. Knowledgeable, trained usage of the full spectrum of Bartenieff Fundamentals allows the teacher/trainer to work on any movement problem.

Training in Bartenieff Fundamentals is available through the Laban/ Bartenieff Institute for Movement Studies (New York City, Seattle, and several regional extensions), or through individual Certified

Movement Analysts (graduates of the above mentioned training programs).

References

1. Bartenieff, I., Lewis, D. (1980). *Body movement: coping with the environment.* New York: Gordon and Breach.
2. Roy, S., Irvin, R. (1983). *Sports medicine: prevention, evaluation, management and rehabilitation.* Englewood Cliffs, New Jersey: Prentice-Hall.

Photos: Randy Bradley

10

In Search of More Efficient Dance Training

Professor Ruth Solomon

There is an anecdote in Eugene Herrigel's classic *Zen in the Art of Archery* that comes to mind each time I confront a new group of students in technique class. Herrigel recounts how, after several years of frustrating failure to learn the all-important Way to release the string of his Japanese bow, he happened upon a trick which simulated the desired technique and produced adequate results. He could hardly wait to shoot for his Zen Master. When that day arrived, however, and the Master had witnessed just one shot utilizing the bogus technique, he turned away in total disgust and refused even to speak to Herrigel for weeks.

The parallel may not be exact—I don't suppose many of our dance students knowingly deceive us—but surely most dance teachers share with me the impression that many of their students come to them with work habits that are "inappropriate" (I prefer to say "inefficient") in some respects. Even students who have had no previous instruction may, like Herrigel, seek and find ways of shortcutting what we try to achieve with them and thereby fall into faulty movement patterns or bad habits. It has always been my belief that "It is the main business of dance technique classes to eliminate the tendencies which lead to inefficient and deleterious movement, and get the students working in a more effective manner."[1] Like Herrigel's archery instructor, we must help our students get out of their own way.

Fortunately, many of the "tendencies" which lead to movement that is aesthetically unpleasing and, from a medical point of view, potentially harmful are readily apparent because they visibly influence the contour of the body. In fact, it is one of the tenets on which my own approach to teaching technique rests, and which I would like to

191

explore here, that movement is inefficient specifically when it is initiated by the peripheral muscles which lie near the surface of the body (and are therefore highly visible) rather than by those deep in the body, most particularly the psoas system which connects the front of the spine to the thigh. I will present several examples of this type of movement, discuss them especially in terms of their medical ramifications (injury prevention has long been one of my primary concerns), and then describe with the aid of illustrations some exercises I use to try to overcome these tendencies.

Let us look first at the common *plié*, a movement which recommends itself for my purposes because: 1) it is a basic component of virtually every dance technique; 2) it is so central to the achievement of results that are both aesthetically and medically sound; and 3) the key to observing when it is being performed inefficiently, though small, is also very clear. The "key" I have in mind here involves the tibialis anterior, that band of tendon that runs down the lower leg and can be seen quite prominently at the front of the ankle when the muscles of the foot and leg are used in contraction (Figure 10.1). When *plié* is performed efficiently, the weight of the body is held, as we say, "out

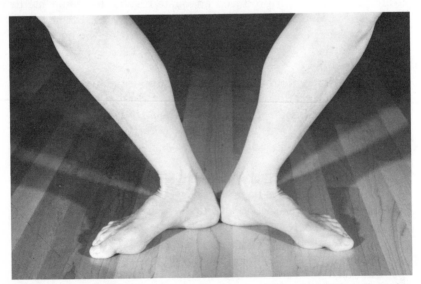

Figure 10.1. Anterior tibialis tendon incorrectly contracted as *demi-plié* is performed in turned-out (first) position.

From Micheli, L.J., Solomon, R. (1987). Training the young dancer. In: Ryan, A.J., Stephens, R.E., eds. *Dance medicine: a comprehensive guide*. Chicago and Minneapolis: Pluribus Press/The Physician and Sportsmedicine, 70. Reprinted by permission.

of the legs" by the psoas system, minimizing tension in the leg muscles and allowing the feet to relax on the floor. The knee and ankle act as simple hinges, there is a strong stretch on the achilles tendon, and *the anterior tib is not prominently protruding* (Figure 10.2). When you see a student's anterior tibialis contract during a *plié* you are keyed into the fact that that student is engaging muscle groups which ought to be released, and this in turn means that they are relying on the legs and feet to do the work rather than using the psoas system to maintain control in the pelvis.

The primary use of *plié* is, of course, to initiate and cushion the landing from jumps. Indeed, the height of a jump or leap, and therefore to some extent its aesthetic appeal, is the direct result of power generated by the preparatory *plié*. Similarly, a soft, weightless landing results from a controlled, well-balanced *plié*. If, conversely, the feet are, as I like to say, "gripping the floor" in order to push off and regain control, the leap will be truncated, and the landing will lack resilience. The reverberation from the impact of such a landing travels up the unnecessarily tense leg and, especially given the number of times a dancer jumps over the course of weeks and months, can contribute to

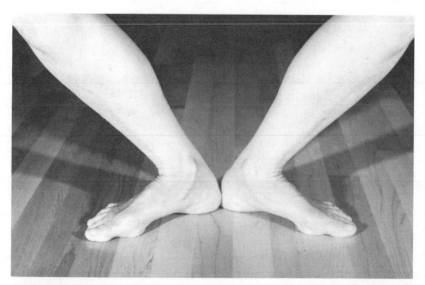

Figure 10.2. *Demi-plié* in turned-out (first) position with anterior tibialis tendon released. Note increased flexion and stretch of achilles tendon.

From Micheli, L.J., Solomon, R. (1987). Training the young dancer. In: Ryan, A.J., Stephens, R.E., eds. *Dance medicine: a comprehensive guide*. Chicago and Minneapolis: Pluribus Press/The Physician and Sportsmedicine, 71. Reprinted by permission.

shin splints and even stress fractures. So, again, keep an eye out for that protruding anterior tibialis. It is only one small factor in the *plié*, but it is significant.

Let us consider now the case of the student who is having trouble achieving full extension: the leg comes up to 90° easily enough, but beyond that whatever extension can be managed is accompanied by obvious tension. Further, if this problem has persisted long enough there may be popping sounds at the site of the hip socket and grinding sensations that may become painful enough in themselves to inhibit the student's ability (or willingness) to raise the leg.

This we readily perceive to be a positioning problem: the extended or "gesturing" leg is not moving in the proper vertical plane relative to the position of the pelvis. Normally we address this problem by simply taking hold of the leg and gently searching out the place where it can be raised without constriction (Figure 10.3). This is fine as far as it goes: a high, graceful, stress-free extension requires proper positioning, and in this respect all the teacher can do is try to help the student experience where that is. I would only add the caveat that as the bony construction of the hip socket and the angle of femoral insertion in the acetabulum differ for every individual, so the "proper" position for extension will vary, however minutely, from one dancer to another. Ultimately the dancer must *feel* right when performing the extension rather than satisfying some externally imposed image of what *is* right.

However, there is another whole aspect of this problem which tends to get short shrift, if it is considered at all. If we look closely at the gesturing leg of the student who is experiencing inhibited extension, we will often see that as the leg passes 90° the quadriceps muscles along the top of the thigh are strongly contracted. In effect, what the student is trying to do is lift the leg by using the muscles of the leg itself. Unfortunately, this effort not only contracts the quadriceps but also the tendons which surround the hip socket. Far from promoting the desired elevation of the leg, this tightening of the tendons actually seems to pull the leg *down*. It is a classic example of how the body can work against itself when inappropriate anatomical means are utilized to accomplish a task.

The quadriceps are, of course, engaged in extension, but their role is secondary to that of the "hip flexor," a lay term for the psoas. Through its attachment to the lesser trochanter at the back of the femur, the psoas provides the primary impetus for raising the leg.[2] The muscles of the leg itself simply respond to this impulse from deeper in the body—as we tend to say, "from the pelvis." Therefore, another correction which should help the student who is having problems with inhibited extension achieve better results (in addition to

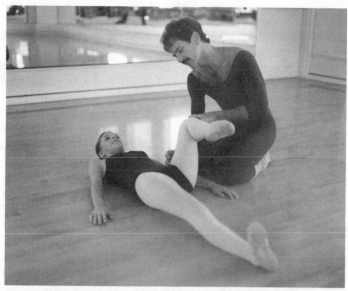

Figure 10.3. Teacher testing for release at the head of the rectus femoris and iliacus.
From Micheli, L.J., Solomon, R. (1987). Training the young dancer. In: Ryan, A.J., Stephens, R.E., eds. *Dance medicine: a comprehensive guide*. Chicago and Minneapolis: Pluribus Press/The Physician and Sportsmedicine, 63. Reprinted by permission.

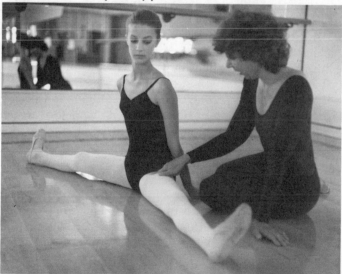

Figure 10.4. Teacher helping student to experience release of the hip socket and quadriceps in second position.
From Micheli, L.J., Solomon, R. (1987). Training the young dancer. In: Ryan, A.J., Stephens, R.E., eds. *Dance medicine: a comprehensive guide*. Chicago and Minneapolis: Pluribus Press/The Physician and Sportsmedicine, 64. Reprinted by permission.

placing the leg in the proper position) is to encourage him/her to *release* the tendons of the hip socket and the quadriceps muscles, especially at initiation of the movement (Figure 10.4).

Nor should those popping sounds at the hip socket be taken lightly. We believe those sounds are produced when contracted rectus femoris or iliopsoas tendons (on the inside of the hip socket) and/or tensor fascia lata (on the outside) slide across the head of the femur. The frequent repetition of this action as the femur is rotated for such movements as *ronde de jambe* and *développé* can progressively irritate the tendons, causing the symptoms associated with tendinitis (iliopsoas tendinitis is a common complaint of dancers). Once the tendons are irritated the dancer becomes reticent to lift the leg because of the pain involved, he or she tends to try to protect the hip socket by holding on even more tightly, and the tendinitis syndrome can become chronic (Figure 10.5).

A final example of movement that is inefficient and ultimately harmful can often be seen in the student who perpetually suffers from back pain, both in the lumbar and thoracic areas. As I watch these students work, one movement trait frequently catches my eye. Probably responding dutifully to an injunction they have received somewhere in their training to "pull up," these students are literally trying to hold themselves up by the rib cage. That entire anatomical structure is thrust forward and up in an attempt similarly to elevate everything below it. Raising the leg in extension, for example, or going into the air are incorrectly thought of as movements to be initiated by this lift of the rib cage.

This is another self-defeating strategy; the student is working very hard, but in the wrong area. Holding the rib cage forward and up creates a conflict of movement in that it contracts the relatively weak peripheral muscles of the back to do work that properly belongs to the large muscles on the front of the spine. What we really want our students to learn to do is *release* the rib cage, thereby enabling them to decontract the back muscles, and in turn bring the psoas fully into play. This placement of the rib cage will be quite apparent to any experienced dance teacher. Affecting the desired realignment in this area will decrease stress in the back and reduce the likelihood of muscle spasms.

This is one manifestation of "tight back." There are others, most notably those associated with lordosis. A lordodic spine may result from a number of different causes; in dance we tend to think it is influenced by the forward tilt of the pelvis that in some dancers accompanies the attempt to increase "turn out." My own feeling is that lordosis signifies a weak or underutilized psoas. However, a

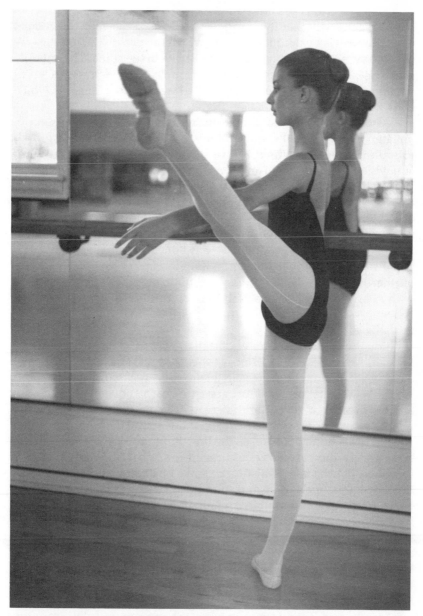

Figure 10.5. Incorrect extension in second position. The gluteus maximus is engaged, causing internal rotation of the extended leg.

From Micheli, L.J., Solomon, R. (1987). Training the young dancer. In: Ryan, A.J., Stephens, R.E., eds. *Dance medicine: a comprehensive guide*. Chicago and Minneapolis: Pluribus Press/The Physician and Sportsmedicine, *60*. Reprinted by permission.

"tight back"—whether it is related to lordosis, a malaligned rib cage, or whatever—is by definition one in which the peripheral muscles are overly contracted, causing a lack of flexibility in the spine. The antidote is exercises that encourage the student to release those muscles which impede movement in the spine and to engage those muscles which enhance it.

As I place so much emphasis on the role of the psoas system in initiating movement, it should come as no surprise that the approach to training dancers which I have developed focuses primarily on strengthening that system and sensitizing the student to its workings. What follows is a description of the sequence of exercises with which the warm-up phase of my technique class normally begins.[3] This is essentially floor work, that is, work done while sitting or lying on the floor. We begin with floor exercises because the support we derive from the floor helps to "unload" the bones and joints we want to articulate and to reduce tension in the muscles which support them. Further, work of this sort tends to minimize most students' concern with balance—and perhaps with the external shape of the movement generally—thus freeing them to concentrate on what is happening anatomically.

Throughout the warm-up vocalization is used as an integral part of virtually every exercise; that is, the students are asked to make sounds—more than just breathing sounds; actual words or vocalized syllables—on the strong effort aspect of each movement. Thus, an audible breath/sound pattern is created: allow the breath in on the release aspect of the movement, breathe (sound) out on the strong effort. This is done because, as the breathing process originates in the same area of the pelvis as does movement (what I call the "center"), the quality of the sound a student makes will emulate the quality of the movement: a clear, strong sound demonstrates that the center is being used in an uninhibited manner; a weak, constricted sound indicates that tension is limiting the movement flow. Students quickly learn to hear and interpret their own sounds and to adjust without the instructor having to make corrections. This holistic approach to breathing-movement has the additional advantage of making the breathing process a conditioned reflex—out on effort, in on release— so that when the dancer comes to perform, he/she will 1) not hold his/ her breath, and 2) be free to express the movement fully, from the center.

The intention here is to present enough of this material not only to indicate how I deal with the kinds of problems discussed above, but to allow anyone who wants to work through it to experience what feels right to them and what is problematic. The next step would

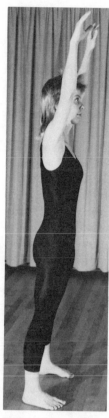

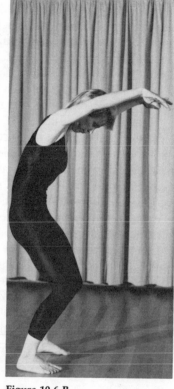

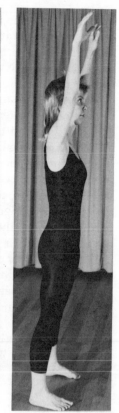

Figure 10.6-B.

Figure 10.6-A.

Figure 10.6-C.

be to utilize these discoveries within the context of already familiar techniques. This is, of course, only one in an infinite number of approaches to training, but it is broad-based enough to be applicable to virtually any other approach.

Standing relaxed, with the feet in parallel position, arms above the head (Figure 10.6-A), we curve the lumbar spine back, keeping the shoulders over the hip sockets and bending the knees as needed to deepen the curve (Figure 10.6-B). This articulation in the lumbar area allows the spine, from lumbar through sacrum and coccyx, to form one continuous curve, the lower end of which, if extended forward in imagination between the legs, would strike the floor at a point well in front of the feet. We are aided in this imaging by the curve of the coccyx which, when viewed in profile, already tilts forward. The lumbar articulation simply deepens and extends that curve. By keeping the shoulders over the hip sockets we cause the dorsal spine to reflect the curve below it; hence, the entire spine, up through the cervical curve, is drawn into one continuous arc. Enhancing the dorsal curve has the additional advantage of releasing the rib cage—indeed, the dorsal spine can't curve if the rib cage is held forward or lifted—in turn relieving tension in the psoas, which is being pulled in the opposite direction to create the lumbar curve.

This effort cycle of the exercise is given three counts and sounded with one continuous word-exhalation, for example "oouut." We then release for three counts, allowing the breath in and returning to the standing position, again making sure that the shoulders remain over the hip sockets (Figure 10.6-C). This simple exercise allows us to focus our attention on the center-of-movement area, to articulate virtually the whole spine in relation to that center, thus beginning to warm it up and align it, and to engage the psoas directly in this process.

Once we have done enough repetitions of this exercise to sense the area in which we are working, we move on to exercise 2. This begins with the same standing lumbar curve (Figure 10.7-A), which is maintained and lowered by bending the knees until the coccyx almost touches the floor (Figure 10.7-B). We hang in this position for three counts and then roll backward on the curve, keeping the knees close

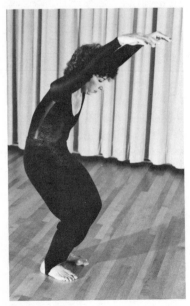

Figure 10.7-A.

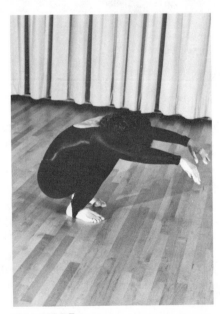

Figure 10.7-B.

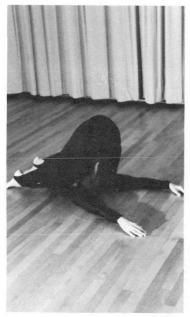

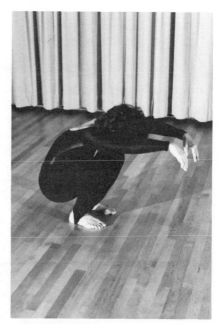

Figure 10.7-C.   Figure 10.7-D.

into the chest to deepen it, touch the floor behind the head with our
toes (three counts, Figure 10.7-C), and roll forward on the curve until
we are back on our feet (three counts, Figure 10.7-D). It is important
that the feet, knees, and thighs remain in parallel, and the knees
should be over the second toe. We again hang in this low parallel
position for three counts and then rise to standing (three counts), as
always making sure that the shoulders are over the hip sockets (Figure
10.7-E). This exercise continues using the same movement sequence
with a more rapid, continuous flow of motion, completing the exercise
in six counts: three counts for rolling down until the toes touch the
floor behind the head, and three counts for rolling forward to stand.
The use of the lumbar curve in this exercise—first establishing it, then
controlling with it as the body's weight is lowered to the floor, then
rolling on it (which we could *not* do smoothly if the spine were not
consistently curved)—provides ample opportunity to experience and
thereby image the spine. Throughout this first part of the warm-up
we want to "think bones."

We end exercise 2 by releasing the spine flat onto the floor instead
of completing the forward roll in the last repetition, and, with bent
knees, allowing the feet to land flat in parallel (Figure 10.8-A). This

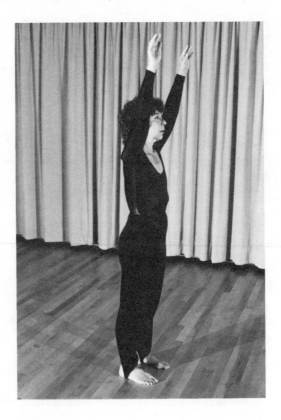

Figure 10.7-E.

places us in position to begin exercise 3, which involves what I call "pelvic rocks." First we roll the lower spine off the floor, starting with the coccyx and continuing as far as the 12th dorsal vertebrae (Figure 10.8-B). This I call an "undercurve"—the equivalent of the "pelvic tilt" in many other techniques (and much physical therapy). The "rock" is completed by reversing this process into an "overcurve" (Figure 10.8-C), which requires a release in the hip socket (rectus femoris and iliacus). This exercise is performed first on two slow counts, then the time is doubled, and doubled again.

Exercise 4 develops on 3 in much the same way 2 did on 1. Starting in the same position, and having established the same undercurve from coccyx through sacrum to 12th dorsal (Figure 10.9-A), we extend the undercurve up the spine until we are resting on the shoulder blades, thus fully involving the dorsal spine in the articulation (Figure

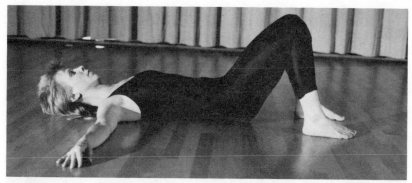

Figure 10.8-A.

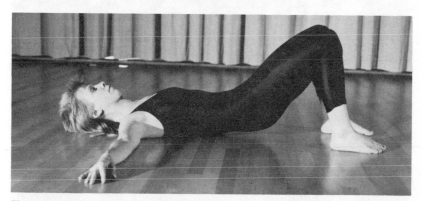

Figure 10.8-B.

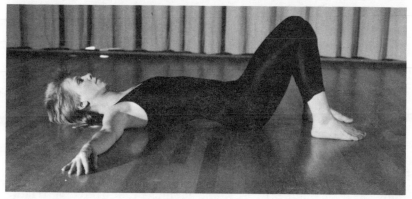

Figure 10.8-C.

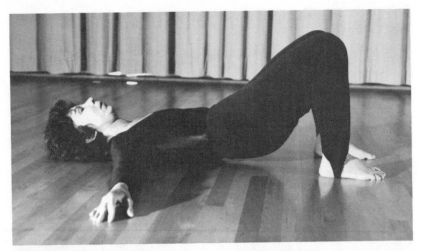

Figure 10.9-A.

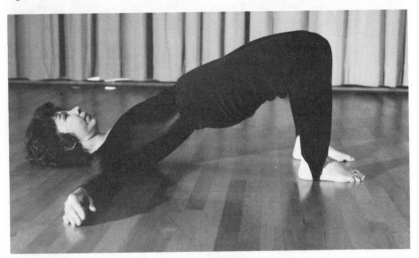

Figure 10.9-B.

10.9-B). Then we start down from the top, cascading the entire spine onto the floor (Figure 10.9-C), and ending in an overcurve (Figure 10.9-D). The breathing is especially important in this exercise and the one that follows as students tend to hold their breath through the strong effort cycles. The movement is designed to combat this tendency; we breathe/sound out for four counts as the pelvis rises, release and allow air in for two counts at the top, breathe/sound out for four

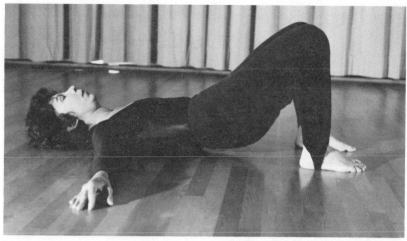

Figure 10.9-C.

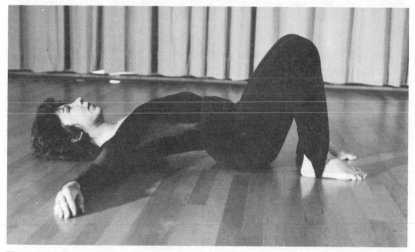

Figure 10.9-D.

counts coming down, and release for air in on two counts in the overcurve. Exercise 5 maintains this same breathing pattern and begins in the same way, but having released for two counts at the top (Figure 10.10-A), we reverse the downward flow of the vertebrae by lowering the coccyx to the floor first (Figure 10.10-B), then the sacrum and dorsal spine (Figure 10.10-C).

As a relief from our focus on the spine, and in order to get some blood flowing through the limbs and joints, in exercise 6 we turn our

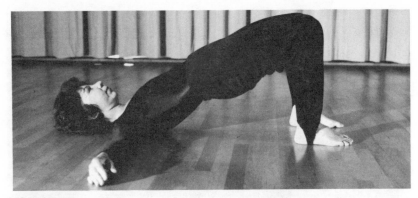

Figure 10.10-A.

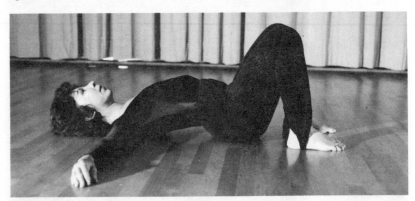

Figure 10.10-B.

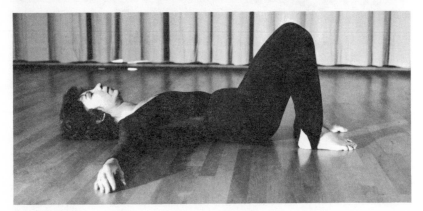

Figure 10.10-C.

attention to the legs and arms. Exercise 5 has left us with spine and feet flat on the floor, knees bent. We now lift the legs above us and shake them loosely for eight counts, letting air in (Figure 10.11-A). Then we flex the feet, bend the knees slightly, and, holding that basic shape, vibrate the legs vigorously, sounding the breath out for eight counts (Figure 10.11-B). We then drop the feet heavily onto the floor in parallel position and repeat essentially the same process with the arms, first shaking them loosely above us (Figure 10.11-C), then shaping them at the elbows and wrists and vibrating for eight counts (Figure 10.11-D).

Exercises 7 and 8 begin as we lift our bent legs above us, knees softly folded, and take hold of the tibia with our hands (Figure 10.12-A). Then, by pressing through the knees into the hands, we drag the head off the floor (Figure 10.12-B), and breathing/sounding out, let it curve sequentially forward (Figure 10.12-C). This simple movement articulates the dorsal and cervical vertebrae, the ones that have been only marginally worked earlier. Then we release the spine back onto the floor, allowing the air in, and repeat. Gradually we begin to rock on the lumbar curve (Figure 10.13-A), rounding it down to a base of support in the sacrum, and (exercise 8) "lever" down through this

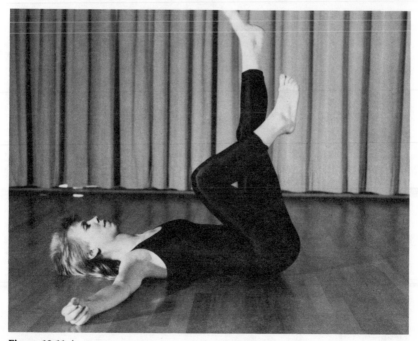

Figure 10.11-A.

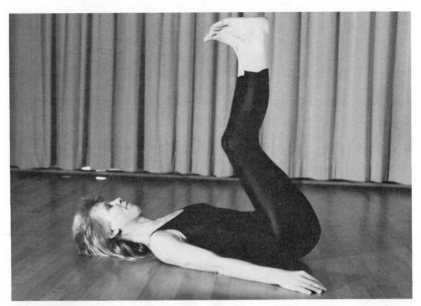

Figure 10.11-B.

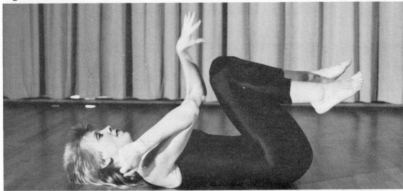

Figure 10.11-C.

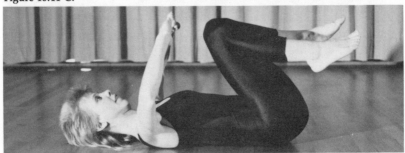

Figure 10.11-D.

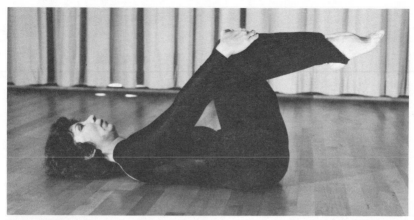

Figure 10.12-A.

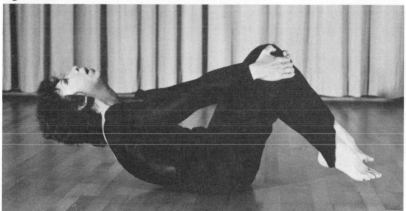

Figure 10.12-B.

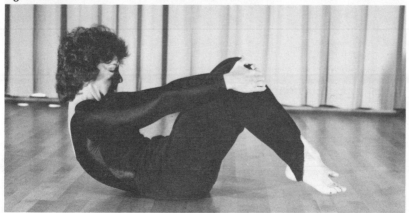

Figure 10.12-C.

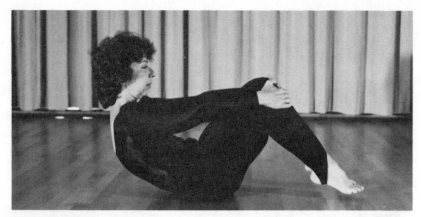

Figure 10.13-A.

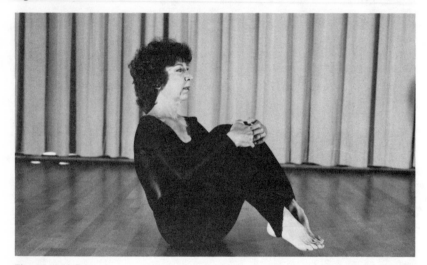

Figure 10.13-B.

base of support to bring ourselves onto a balance point slightly behind the coccyx (Figure 10.13-B).[4] The exact placement differs from one individual to another. Even when we are up on the balance point, the lumbar and dorsal spine remain in an easy curve. It is important not to try to straighten the spine entirely as to do so causes undue strain in the low back, which must then support the weight of the legs. Naturally we breathe/sound out on the levering (effort) action, and release for air in as we curve back down to the starting position.

All of the final exercises in this sequence begin on the balance point. In 9 we circle the head, first to the side (Figure 10.14-A), then forward

(Figure 10.14-B), then side (Figure 10.14-C), and back (Figure 10.14-D), sounding out on the extension back, which is the long arc of the cervical vertebrae. We reverse direction each time, to make sure we are articulating the vertebrae equally on all sides. It is important throughout this exercise to maintain an open throat for easy passage of breath and voice.

In exercise 10 we circle the arms from the shoulders, first one at a time (Figures 10.15-A, 10.15-B), then both together, back to front, then reversing the circle (Figures 10.15-C, 10.15-D, 10.15-E). This not only

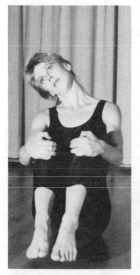
Figure 10.14-A.

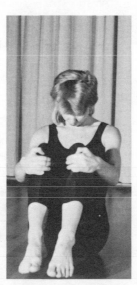
Figure 10.14-B.

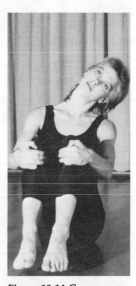
Figure 10.14-C.

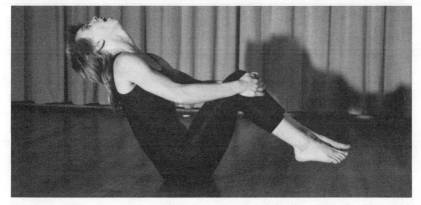
Figure 10.14-D.

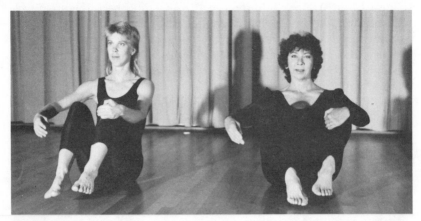

Figure 10.15-A.

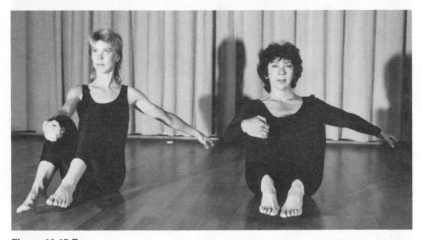

Figure 10.15-B.

lubricates the shoulder joints, but has the added advantage of causing the psoas, which is already engaged in sustaining the body on the balance point, to work even harder to offset the free flow of the arms. The same effect is heightened in 11, where we add the extension of the legs to the work the psoas is doing, extending them in a V shape with the torso, femurs as close to the chest as possible, and tibias articulated to line up with femurs (Figure 10.16-A). Then we alternately fold at the knees (Figure 10.16-B) and straighten the legs, breathing/sounding out as the tibias extend and releasing for breath in as they fold. This exercise also starts to lubricate the knee joints.

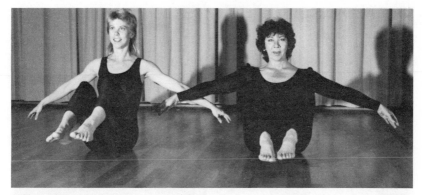

Figure 10.15-C.

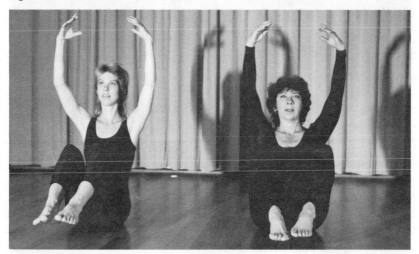

Figure 10.15-D.

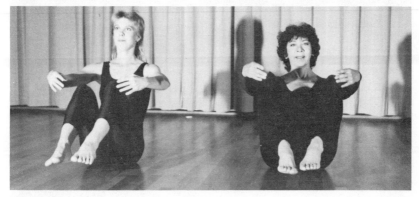

Figure 10.15-E.

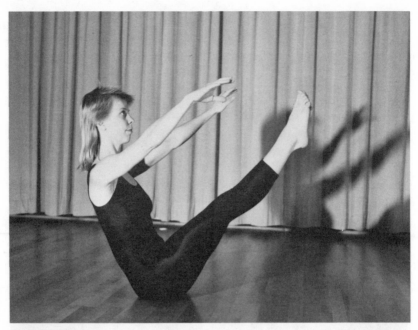

Figure 10.16-A.

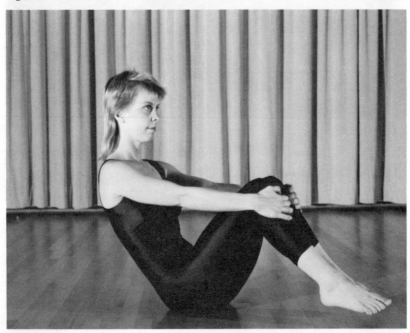

Figure 10.16-B.

Exercise 12 works primarily on lubricating and warming up the hip joints (and strengthening the psoas). From the starting position on the balance point, knees together in parallel and arms extended outside the legs (Figure 10.17-A), we open the knees to the side, bringing the arms inside the legs (Figure 10.17-B). Then we reverse the process—knees in, arms out (Figure 10.17-C). After each set of four repetitions we catch the ankles and allow the weight of the legs to rest in the palms of the hands, releasing the hip sockets. Having performed this exercise several times with bent knees, we straighten the legs and continue, thus increasing the need for control in the pelvis (Figures 10.17-D, 10.17-E, 10.17-F). It should be clear that the strength and

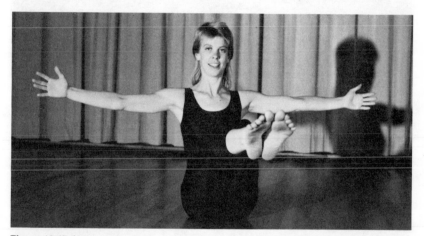

Figure 10.17-A.

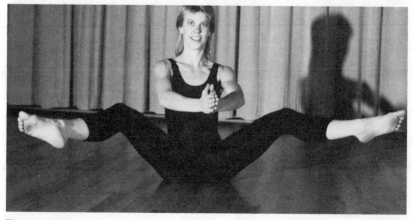

Figure 10.17-B.

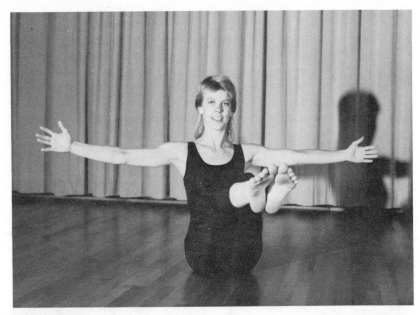

Figure 10.17-C.

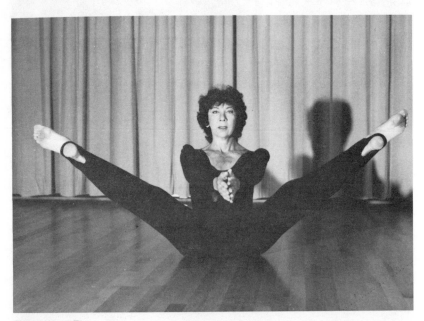

Figure 10.17-D.

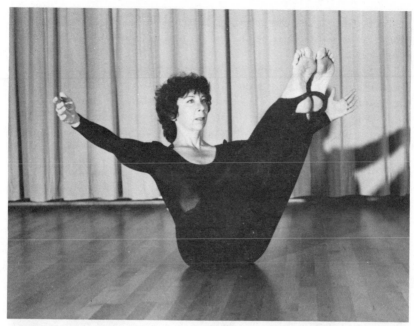

Figure 10.17-E.

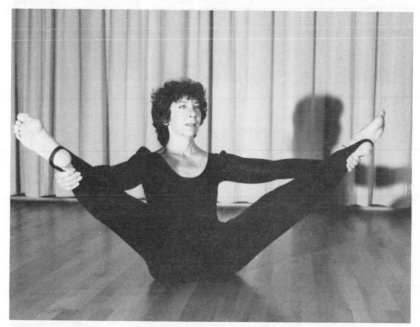

Figure 10.17-F.

facility we are developing throughout these balance-point exercises is exactly what we will use when, in standing position, we work on extension.

The final exercises in this sequence complete the first phase in our preparation for standing work. In 13, still on our balance point with the legs out straight in a raised second position, we take hold of the ankles and fold the knees in (Figure 10.18-A), then return to extended legs in second (Figure 10.18-B). As always, we breathe/sound out on the extension, in on the release. In 14, with the legs together and extended in parallel, we alternately flex and point the feet (Figures

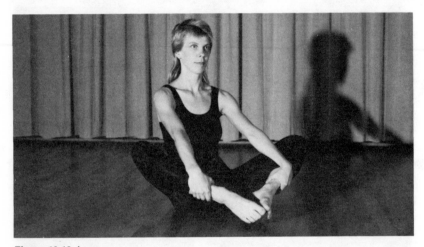

Figure 10.18-A.

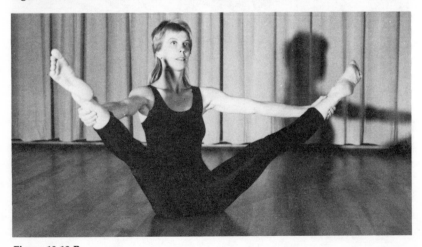

Figure 10.18-B.

10.19-A, 10.19-B). This begins to warm up the ankles and feet. Last (15), we let go with the hands and, while continuing to flex and point the feet and maintaining the lumbar-dorsal curve, lower the legs until the heels are six to eight inches off the floor (Figures 10.20-A, 10.20-B). Then, with the feet flexed, we rotate the legs out from the hip sockets and cross or "beat" the legs as in *entrechat* for at least four sets of eight (Figure 10.20-C). Finally, lowering the legs flat onto the floor, we lever down through the sacrum, bringing the torso up to sitting position and then, releasing in the hip sockets, allow the torso to fold

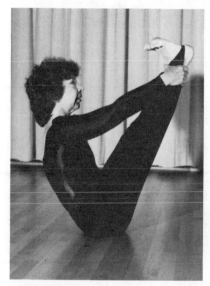

Figure 10.19-A.

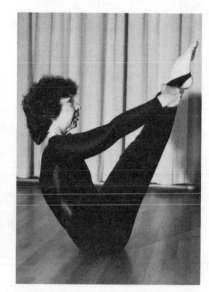

Figure 10.19-B.

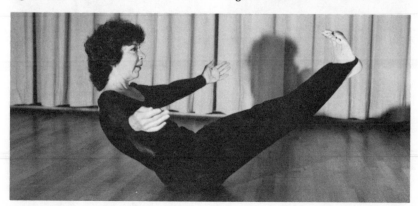

Figure 10.20-A.

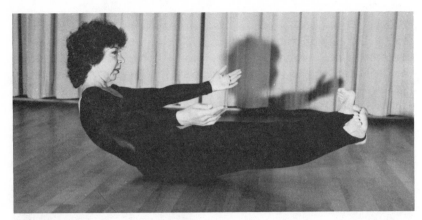

Figure 10.20-B.

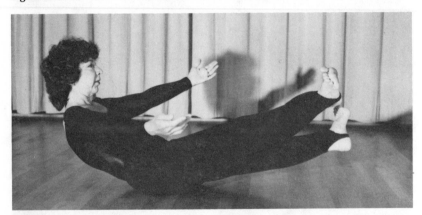

Figure 10.20-C.

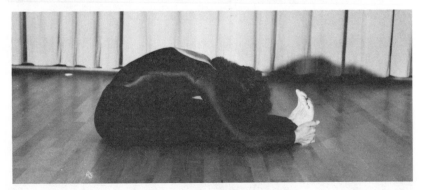

Figure 10.20-D.

over the legs (Figure 10.20-D). It is important in this final phase to make sure that all the muscles around the hip socket—the tensor fascia lata, rectus femoris, and iliacus—are released. The principle throughout exercises 11-15 is to articulate the leg while maintaining a soft hip socket and *not* engaging the quadriceps as the primary motivator of the movements.

The entire sequence described here takes approximately 10 minutes when each exercise is repeated four to six times.

When we see movement performed in a way that evokes our admiration, one of the things we frequently say about it is that it was "effortless." More accurately, what we mean is that it *appeared* effortless because the dancer was able to find the means within his/her body to generate it efficiently. It is the search for the source of this efficiency that has shaped my approach to teaching.

"Talent" is part of the answer; genetic endowment is another part. Some bodies are by nature better equipped to dance than others. Well-formed bones, strong muscles, and pliable connective tissue are not in themselves enough, however; indeed, they can sometimes get in the way of, or be used as a substitute for, the body mechanics that actually do produce "effortless" movement. I am thinking now particularly of the use of peripheral muscles to do the work that really needs to be initiated much deeper in the body—for example, using the quadriceps as the primary motivation to lift the leg in extension, rather than as conveyors of the impulse that has originated in the psoas. Many of our students, even those (or perhaps *especially* those) who seem furthest along technically, have slipped into such habits before they come to us. Fortunately, the results of movement produced in this way are sufficiently different from the effortless results of anatomically efficient movement to be instantly apparent to the trained eye.

I believe it is our primary responsibility as technique teachers to help our students find the most efficient way possible to use their bodies. I emphasize the roles of the psoas, the pelvis, and the spine because the study of anatomy has led me to believe that they are the prime motivators of movement. If the dancer is able to initiate action by the use of these components, all else should follow, and the movement produced will be relatively stress free, efficient, and safe.

References

1. Solomon, R. (1987, May/June). Training dancers: anatomy as a master image. *Journal of Physical Education, Recreation, and Dance, 58*:51-56. (Parts of this chapter are reprinted from that publication.)

2. Ranney, D.A. (1979, Sept). The functional integration of trunk muscles and the psoas. *Kinesiology for Dance*, 9:10-12.
3. *Anatomy as a master image in training dancers* [Video-recording]. Santa Cruz, California: Ruth Solomon [1988]. 1 videocassette; 59 minutes; color; 1/2 inch, VHS or Beta, 3/4 inch, U-matic. (Available from Ruth Solomon, Arts Business Office, Porter College, University of California, Santa Cruz, CA 95064.)
4. Sweigard, L.E. (1974). *Human movement potential*. New York: Dodd, Mead.

Acknowledgements

The author wishes to thank the models in the photographs for this chapter: Sharon Cullem, Martha Curtis, Gregg Lizenbery, and Sativa Saposnek.

Photography: Bruce Berryhill

11

Strengthening and Stretching the Muscles of the Ankle and Tarsus to Prevent Common Dance Injuries

Sally Sevey Fitt, Ed.D.

Introduction

Many surveys of dance injuries indicate that the region of the body with the highest rate of injury is that which includes the lower leg and foot.[1-8] Injuries in this region include traumatic injuries (such as fractures, sprains, and strains) and chronic conditions (such as tendinitis, shin splints, recurring muscle spasms, and persistent muscle soreness). The lower leg and foot are the general regions where the pain is felt. However, because movement occurs only at joints (the articulations of adjacent bones), the focus of this chapter will be the ankle and tarsus joints where the movement actually occurs. The terms lower leg and foot will be used in discussion until the more specific terminology related to the ankle and tarsus joints has been defined.

Traumatic injuries often occur because the musculature lacks the strength to adjust readily to extreme and immediate demands. For example, when one "falls off balance" there is a need for greater strength than normal to pull back to the balanced position. If strength is insufficient, traumatic injuries can result. Likewise, a misaligned landing from a jump or leap requires greater strength than a properly aligned landing. In the ideal world, dancers would never fall off balance, nor would they ever land in a misaligned position, but the fact is they do. For this reason they need more strength in the muscles of the lower leg and foot than is developed in the normal dance class.

Chronic conditions occur because the baseline capabilities of the muscular system (both strength and flexibility) are insufficient to meet the

223

everyday demands. For example, tendinitis is thought to be caused by one of two major training errors. First, asking more from a muscle than it has to give, either in strength or muscular endurance, can temporarily "wear out" the musculotendinous unit (muscles and tendons are not separate entities, but rather different components of the same unit) causing a reaction of the body of the muscle (muscle soreness or spasm) or the tendon of the muscle (tendinitis). Second, tendinitis can be caused by insufficient stretching of a muscle after an intensive exercise bout, leaving the muscle in a state of partial contraction. (It should be noted that the two causes of tendinitis listed above are the hypotheses of this author and have not been systematically studied by her under controlled conditions. However, William Stanish, M.D., supports these hypotheses.)[9] Other chronic conditions also seem to respond positively to conditioning for strength and stretch when exercises are specifically targeted to the exact muscle. The problem for the technique teacher is deciding exactly which muscle needs attention.

Unfortunately, the teachers of dance technique classes seldom have time to study surveys of dance injuries or textbooks and articles on efficient and effective conditioning practices. As a result, the gap between current conditioning theory and actual practice in the dance studio widens. Based on the high occurrence of injuries to the lower leg and foot in dancers, it would seem that the conditioning practices employed in technique classes for this region of the body are, quite simply, inadequate. Dance classes are very valuable for the development of specific dance skills, but strength and mobility conditioning tend to be based more on tradition than on up-to-date theories. Specialized conditioning for dance has four primary objectives: to prevent injuries, to enhance performance, to increase efficiency of action, and to increase the performance longevity of the dancer. No teacher of dance would quarrel with these commonly accepted goals, yet few teachers of dance technique have studied the anatomy and kinesiology of the lower leg and foot intensively. (It should be noted that most dance kinesiologists cannot teach dance technique, either!) The purpose of this chapter is to narrow the gap between conditioning theory and common practices in dance technique classes in order to reduce the rate of dance injury at the foot, ankle, and lower leg. Further, it is hoped that this chapter will not only provide practical solutions to present problems with the ankle and foot, but will also provide the dancer and teachers of dance with principles to use to avoid new problems. For this reason a certain amount of background information is necessary.

This chapter will present information on the conditioning process in four sections: principles of conditioning; anatomical and kinesiological information about the possible actions; evaluation of the present status of conditioning for the lower leg and foot in technique classes (including evaluation of injuries); and description of exercises to increase strength and mobility of the muscles of the ankle and tarsus.

Conditioning for Strength and Elasticity (Flexibility)

There are five fundamental types of conditioning which build the capacities of the human body: (1) muscular strength, (2) muscular elasticity or flexibility, (3) muscular endurance, (4) cardiorespiratory endurance, and (5) neuromuscular coordination.[10] Even though this chapter will focus only on increased strength and elasticity to prevent injury and to speed rehabilitation after injury, it may be helpful to define each of the types of conditioning. *Strength* is defined as the ability to contract a muscle or muscle group against a resistance. *Flexibility* is defined as the ability of a muscle to be stretched to its maximum length. *Muscular endurance* is the ability of a muscle to continue contraction over time. *Cardiorespiratory endurance* is the ability of the cardiovascular and respiratory systems to support, over time, the increased demands caused by exercise. *Neuromuscular coordination* is defined as the establishment of neuromuscular patterns necessary for performance of specific tasks. Strength and elasticity are chosen as the focus of this chapter because they are often neglected in dance classes.

There will certainly be some dancers and teachers of dance who say, "Neglected? That's impossible! Look at all the time we spend on our feet!" However, it must be pointed out that this time is not necessarily spent in exercises that are effective for increasing strength and elasticity. Most exercises conducted in dance technique classes are focused on either neuromuscular coordination or muscular endurance for the foot and lower leg. The principles for building strength are often neglected, and those for increasing elasticity are sometimes misdirected.

Building Strength

The fundamental rule for building strength is to contract the target muscle maximally for 5-10 repetitions. The key word in this statement is "maximally." Maximal contractions require that the muscle be activated to its full potential, which often requires some type of external resistance. Isometric contractions are contractions of the muscle against a nonmovable resistance. When one hears the term maximal contraction, one often thinks of this kind of isometric contraction. However, strength is specific to both the angle of the joint in which the maximal contractions are performed, and to the velocity of the contraction (slow or quick repetitions).[11] For this reason, isometric contractions (with no movement through the range of motion) are less effective than exercises which require maximal contraction throughout the entire range of motion. The most effective exercises for strength are those which are isokinetic; that is, they involve movement against a graded resistance which modulates the resistance depending on the strength of the musculature at the specific joint angle. The major problem with isokinetic exercises is that the highly refined equipment needed to do them is very expensive, and often beyond the budget limitations of dance departments. The second best type of exercise to build strength is isotonic exercise (movement through the range of motion) against an external resistance, performed at both slow and quick tempos.

Increasing Muscular Elasticity

Every dancer knows how to stretch, but not every dancer knows how to stretch effectively. Like strength, flexibility or muscular elasticity is specific to the joint position. This is because the muscles of a given joint have highly specified roles in the production of motion. One must reverse the joint action which is normally produced by a muscle to achieve the most effective stretch position. A muscle that flexes and outward rotates a given joint is most effectively stretched when the joint is placed in a position of extension and inward rotation. While the muscle will also be stretched in a position of extension without rotation, the stretch is not nearly as effective as when all of the actions of the muscle are reversed. Consequently, different muscles will be stretched if a slight shift is made in the joint position. Specific information about the possible joint actions and the musculature which produces those actions is necessary to design effective and efficient stretches.

The process used to stretch muscles is as important to increasing the range of motion as the accurate identification of the joint position for the stretch. Ballistic or bouncing stretches are not effective. Bouncing stretches drive hard into a partially contracted muscle, causing microscopic tearing of the muscle tissue. Therefore, bouncing stretches are to be discouraged. One of the most effective methods for stretching a muscle is the use of reciprocal inhibition to facilitate the stretch.[10] Reciprocal stretches are most effective when the muscle mass of the opposing muscle groups is approximately equal. Unfortunately, the muscle mass of opposing muscle groups is not equal for the ankle and tarsus joints, and this reduces the effectiveness of reciprocal stretches for these muscles. Second in effectiveness to reciprocal stretches are the long, slow, sustained stretches described by DeVries as "static stretches."[12]

A long, sustained stretch involves 1) identifying the joint position which produces the most efficient stretch for the targeted muscle, 2) assuming that position in such a way that gravity can assist in the stretch, 3) maintaining the position while consciously relaxing the target muscle and giving in to gravity to increase the stretch, and 4) continuing the stretch for at least 30 seconds to one minute. Because of the imbalance of muscle mass of opposing muscle groups in the ankle and tarsus, the long, sustained stretch is most effective for stretching in that region. Some people find that a gentle, repetitive pulsing action is effective for increasing stretch. The problem with the pulsing stretches is that it is quite easy to increase their tempo and force, thereby slipping into a bouncing stretch. However, if care is taken to avoid bouncing, the pulsing stretches may be effective.

Stretching has a number of different objectives. One has already been mentioned; to increase the range of motion of a joint. Other objectives of stretching include: warm up of the musculature before class; cool down of the musculature after class; reducing the level of residual contraction in a muscle after a heavy exercise bout to reduce subsequent muscle soreness; general relaxation; and correcting muscular imbalances. The nature of stretching shifts somewhat according to the objective of the stretch. The pulsing stretch may be effective for warm-up, but the long, sustained stretch is thought to be most effective for all other objectives at the ankle and tarsus. The stretches described in this chapter are primarily for the purposes of increasing range of motion, and stretching muscles after heavy exercise bouts. Therefore, the long, sustained stretch is recommended.

The Ankle and Tarsus Joints and Possible Actions

The foot is a miraculous architectural structure. Just imagine: you walk, run, jump, and leap off of and on to some of the smallest bones of the body! When one considers the pounding we give them, it is truly amazing that feet last a lifetime! The reason they do last is that they incorporate the strongest of architectural structures, the arch. Moreover, there are many joints in the foot to disperse the force of landings.

The toes are made up of two or three small bones (phalanges) with joints between the bones (the interphalangeal joints). The proximal phalanges articulate with the metatarsal bones at the phalangeal-metatarsal joints. The proximal* ends of the metatarsal bones articulate with the distal tarsal bones, forming the metatarsal-tarsal joints. There are seven bones in the tarsus region (cuboid, three cuneiforms, navicular, talus, and calcaneus) which articulate with each other and cumulatively provide the actions of the tarsus. The talus, of the tarsus region, articulates with the tibia and fibula (bones of the lower leg) to form the ankle joint. The potential for motion is increased by the number of joints in the foot. This makes the foot resilient to the stresses of locomotion, but it also makes the foot susceptible to injury.

The ligaments (inelastic, connective tissue which connects bone to bone) of the foot and ankle stabilize the joints and provide for protection against hypermobility of joints which, in turn, produces injuries. However, strength in the muscles of the ankle and tarsus is also needed as support against the extreme demands that dancers place on their feet. In addition, these muscles must be elastic to meet the dancer's need for mobile feet.

The ankle and tarsus joints are crucial to all locomotion. The ankle joint has two possible actions: plantar flexion (pointing the foot), and dorsiflexion (flexing the foot). The tarsus joint (actually a series of joints) also has two possible actions: pronation (a combination of abduction and outward rotation) and supination (a combination of adduction and inward rotation). The ankle and tarsus and the actions allowed for in those two joints are the focus of this chapter. The ankle and tarsus work synergistically to produce the familiar motion of what is normally called the ankle, but what is actually the combination of ankle and tarsus.

The "Feel" of Dorsiflexion, Plantarflexion, Supination, and Pronation

Dancers seem to learn best when the kinesthetic sense is used to fortify the definition of terms. Hence, this section has been added to clarify,

---

*Proximal and distal are terms used to describe relative positions: proximal means closer to the "center" of the body, and distal means farther from the center of the body.

in motion, the action-definitions of the movements possible at the ankle and tarsus.

Dorsiflexion of the Ankle

Sit on the floor with the legs stretched out straight in front of you (the "long sit" position) and with no rotation at the hip (have the kneecaps pointing straight at the ceiling). Push the heels down on the floor, causing the toes to point straight up toward the ceiling without moving the heels on the floor, and without turning the feet outward or inward. Some people call this a flexed foot, but in truth it is dorsiflexion of the ankle joint. Often dorsiflexion of the ankle is accompanied by extension of the toes (pulling the toes up toward the body).

Plantar Flexion of the Ankle

In the same "long sit" position as you used to feel dorsiflexion, press the feet down toward the floor, attempting to touch the toes and/or the balls of the feet to the floor. Make sure the feet are in alignment for pure plantar flexion—i.e., that there is no pronation or supination of the tarsus. Plantar flexion of the ankle is often accompanied by flexion of the metatarsal phalangeal joint (gripping of the toes).

Supination of the Tarsus

Sit on a table with the thighs on the table, the knees bent, and the lower legs hanging off the table in a relaxed fashion. Turn the soles of your feet toward each other as if you were going to clap them together. There is both inward rotation and adduction (movement of each foot toward the midline between the feet) of the tarsus or foot. In dance classes the action of supination of the tarsus is often called a "sickled foot." With the legs dangling from the table, and with both tarsal joints supinated, the appearance of the lower leg and foot is like a closed parentheses ().

Pronation of the Tarsus

Still sitting on the table with the legs dangling off the table from the knee down, turn the soles of the feet away from each other, out toward the sides. There is both outward rotation and abduction (movement away from the midline) of the tarsus in this action. In dance classes the action of pronation of the tarsus is often called a "beveled foot."

With the legs dangling and both tarsal joints pronated, the appearance of the lower leg and foot is like an open set of parentheses)(.

Neutral Position of the Tarsus

In addition to the actions of pronation and supination, it is important to point out that a tarsus that is neither pronated nor supinated is considered a neutral tarsus. In the neutral position of the tarsus, the second toe is approximately aligned with the true center of the ankle joint. This position of the tarsus places the least stress on the lateral and medial ligaments and muscles of the ankle and tarsus, particularly in weight-bearing positions or in locomotion.

Combined Actions of the Ankle and Tarsus

In the demonstrations described above, you were asked to focus your attention on the actions at either the ankle or tarsus joints. Now we will combine the actions at the two joints.

Dorsiflex both ankles and supinate both tarsal joints (soles of the feet together). Next, still maintaining dorsiflexion of the ankles, pronate both tarsal joints (turn the soles of both feet out and away from each other). You have been holding dorsiflexion of the ankle joint constant while moving at the tarsal joints in actions of supination and pronation.

Plantar flex both ankles and supinate both tarsal joints. Then try plantar flexion and pronation. For many dancers this action is quite difficult to find. This is indeed unfortunate because it is the muscles that plantar flex and pronate that stabilize the outside of the foot in *relevé* or *pointe* position. Without strength in these muscles, the likelihood of sprains of the tarsus (often called ankle sprains) is greatly increased.

Now that you have kinetically examined all of the possible motions of the ankle and tarsus region, do some "ankle circles" and observe how the ankle and tarsus work in a close partnership to allow all of the possible actions of what is normally called the ankle. On the chart below, enter key words that describe, for you, the feel of the combined actions listed.

Combined Actions of the Ankle and Tarsus		
Actions of the Tarsus	Actions of the Ankle	
	Plantar Flexion	Dorsiflexion
Pronation		
Supination		

Muscle Groups that Perform the Actions of the Ankle and Tarsus

Muscles are generally grouped and identified by the actions which they perform on the joints they cross. It is the joint that determines what actions are possible, and it is the muscles that produce the force for the actual movement. Joint actions are bipolar opposites, such as plantar flexion and dorsiflexion, or pronation and supination. Likewise, the muscles follow this pattern, with muscle groups having opposite actions. Agonist muscles perform a given action at a particular joint, while the antagonists perform the opposite action at that joint. For example, the plantar flexor muscles are agonistic for the action of plantar flexion and antagonistic for the action of dorsiflexion. However, because the ankle and tarsus joints operate in such close synergy, one must often consider paired actions to determine the antagonistic muscles. Only three of the muscles which cross the ankle joint have action only at the ankle joint (the gastrocnemius, the soleus, and the plantaris). All of the other muscles which act upon the ankle joint also act upon the tarsus. These are two-joint muscles, and the combined actions at the two joints must be considered when strength and stretching exercises are designed for these muscles. There are some muscles which cross the ankle and tarsal joints and also cross the toe joints (flexor hallucis longus, extensor hallucis longus, extensor digitorum longus, and flexor digitorum longus). For these three-joint muscles, in addition to considering the actions at the tarsus and ankle one must take into account the agonistic actions produced at the toes when designing strengthening exercises, and the antagonistic actions for the toes when designing stretching exercises.

This all sounds unnecessarily complex. Simply put, the principles described above are as follows: 1) to strengthen a muscle, do all of the joint actions performed by that muscle against a resistance, and do them through the full range of motion; 2) to stretch a muscle, reverse all of the joint actions performed by the muscle and do a long, sustained stretch in that position. The list below gives the specific muscles that perform the isolated joint action. The muscles indicated in italics are those that have only that action. All the other muscles have actions at more than one joint.

Muscles by Joint Action

Plantar Flexion (Ankle Joint):
  Gastrocnemius, Soleus, Plantaris, Tibialis Posterior, Peroneus Longus, Peroneus Brevis, Flexor Digitorum Longus, Flexor Hallucis Longus
Dorsiflexion (Ankle Joint):
  Tibialis Anterior, Peroneus Tertius, Extensor Hallucis Longus, Extensor Digitorum Longus
Pronation (Tarsus Joints):
  Peroneus Longus, Peroneus Brevis, Peroneus Tertius, Extensor Digitorum Longus
Supination (Tarsus Joints):
  Tibialis Anterior, Tibialis Posterior, Flexor Digitorum Longus (slight action of supination by the Flexor Hallucis Longus and the Extensor Hallucis Longus)

Note: Intrinsic muscles are those muscles which do not cross the ankle joint; they have both proximal and distal attachments on the bones of the foot. None of the intrinsic muscles of the foot are included in the list above. However, there is one exercise given for these muscles in the exercise section.

While the listing of muscles and single-joint actions gives the reader a sense of which muscles do what, the more important information for the purpose of designing exercises combines the actions of the ankle and tarsus.

Ankle/Tarsus Muscles Listed by Combined Actions

Pronators and Plantarflexors: Peroneus Longus, Peroneus Brevis
Pronators and Dorsiflexors: Peroneus Tertius, Extensor Digitorum Longus
Supinators and Dorsiflexors: Tibialis Anterior, Extensor Hallucis Longus
Supinators and Plantar Flexors: Tibialis Posterior, Flexor Hallucis Longus, Flexor Digitorum Longus

Note: The gastrocnemius and soleus are not listed because they do not have an action at the tarsus, since they do not cross that joint.

All of these lists of specific muscles are included for those who wish to refer to anatomy books for illustrations of the specific muscles. The names of the individual muscles are not really necessary for the development of strengthening and stretching exercises. Actually, all that is needed to design exercises is to know the four combined actions of the ankle and tarsus, and to have done a systematic evaluation of strength and elasticity of the relevant muscle groups.

Common Conditioning Practices in Dance Classes

Strength conditioning of the lower leg and foot in dance technique classes is commonly minimal in that no progressive resistance exercises are used to increase the strength of the musculature. *Relevés* on one foot approach maximal contractions for the plantar flexors, but no maximal contractions are done for dorsiflexors, pronators, or supinators in dance classes.*

Conditioning for muscular endurance does receive some attention in technique classes due to the repetitive nature of *tendues*, *pliés*, and *relevés*, but even this conditioning is insufficient when one considers that time constraints limit the number of repetitions that are necessary to achieve the desired results.

Conditioning for muscular elasticity of the muscles of the lower leg and foot is usually limited to stretches of the dorsiflexors of the ankle to increase the *pointe* of the foot, with an occasional "token" stretch of the gastrocnemius (calf muscle and Achilles tendon). Generally speaking, the stretches given in class are based more on tradition than on the structure of the muscular system or the particular needs of the students in the class.

Use of *warm-ups* is fairly common in dance classes, but the focus is often on comfortable exercises rather than what is needed to prepare the body to dance. Also, it is rare to find dancers spending much time in *cool-down* exercises, or stretching out overworked muscles at the end of class.

For much too long, teachers of dance have depended on tradition to determine the content and structure of the classes they teach. In certain components of any dance class, tradition—and adherence to it—is quite appropriate. However, ignoring the principles of conditioning which have been shown to be effective in building strength and muscular elasticity is, quite simply, foolish. Recent research has clearly demonstrated an unusually high incidence of injuries to the lower leg and foot. It should therefore follow that dance educators need to reevaluate the conditioning practices which are commonly used.

---

*I have in mind throughout this discussion the basic *ballet* technique class. Some modern techniques provide a wider range of conditioning for the foot and ankle—significant contractions of the dorsiflexors, for example—though none, I believe, systematically use weights or maximal contractions for strength training.

Identification of Gaps between Principles of Conditioning and Actual Practices in Dance Classes

A number of gaps are immediately obvious when one compares conditioning theories and common conditioning practices in dance classes. It is clear that dance classes do not employ the *overload principle* (contracting the muscle or muscle group maximally against a resistance). Occasionally one might find a maximal contraction in a dance class when a dancer is about to fall off a balance, or when all of the body weight is on one foot, but the systematic use of overload to build strength is notably absent. There is *lack of specificity* in conditioning the musculature of the ankle and tarsus to increase either strength or stretch. Whatever strength or muscular elasticity is built in the technique class is seldom intentionally directed at specific muscle groups. Conditioning is most often based on habit instead of need—on what has always been done rather than on the specific requirements of the students. Often the needs of the individual take a back seat to the needs of the group as a whole. Moreover, what is taught frequently encourages marked muscular imbalances of strength and/or elasticity of opposing muscle groups.

These comments may seem excessively harsh, but the intention here is not to make technique teachers feel guilty. There is no need for that, since in most cases technique teachers do a wonderful job of conditioning for neuromuscular coordination. They are simply unaware of the inefficiency of traditional training practices. Clearly, those traditions have been somewhat effective; after all, the teachers themselves learned to dance with those traditional teaching techniques. However, it must be emphasized that the frequency of injuries to the lower leg and foot is high enough to necessitate a critical review of how we are training our young dancers. It would seem wise to integrate the principles of efficient conditioning into dance classes, not to replace traditional teaching, but to augment it.

Dancer's Specific Demands on the Ankle/Tarsus Joints

In a normal standing position, gravity is a dorsiflexor of the ankle joint and a pronator of the tarsus. Therefore, maintaining a simple standing position requires counteraction of the effect of gravity by the plantar flexors of the ankle and the supinators of the tarsus. In a "half-toe" position, gravity most commonly will supinate the tarsus and dorsiflex the ankle. Thus, the pronators and plantar flexors are the key muscles to counteract gravity in the half-toe position. It should be noted that the muscle groups shift as the position (relation to gravity) changes. The examples given (normal standing and half-toe balances) are only two examples of the possible demands on these joints. As the dancer moves through a complex combination, many different demands are placed upon the musculature of the ankle and tarsus to counteract the ever-changing effect of gravity on those joints. In all locomotion, including all but the most stylized of walks, runs, jumps, leaps, and hops, the plantar flexors of the ankle are the key muscles for opposing gravity. If a dancer has excessive range of motion in plantar flexion, as many dancers do, strength in the dorsiflexors of the ankle is necessary to stabilize the ankle joint in half-toe or *pointe* position. Functionally, the optimal position of the tarsus is neutral: neither pronated nor supinated. Neutral alignment of the tarsus allows for direct transference of weight from one segment of the foot to another, and it produces less stress on the ligaments and tendons. A balance of strength between pronators and supinators is therefore necessary to maintain a neutral position of the tarsus.

Results of Insufficient Conditioning

Lack of strength in the muscles of the ankle/tarsus region severely reduces the capacity to stabilize the joint, a factor which is critical in the demanding balances executed by dancers. In the worst scenario, lack of strength in these muscles can lead to debilitating strains, sprains, or fractures. In less traumatic instances, lack of strength can be a contributing factor in the occurrence of tendinitis or shin splints when demands exceed the capabilities of specific muscles or muscle groups.

Lack of muscular endurance ultimately has the same effect as lack of strength in that the demands placed on the musculature can no longer be met. The need for muscular endurance is most pronounced in rehearsals where the dancer is required to perform the same combinations over and over. Without sufficient muscular endurance, injuries can be the result.

Lack of muscular elasticity (flexibility) can cause tearing of muscles when the joint is moved beyond its normal range of motion. These tears can be severe, as in the case of a ruptured achilles tendon, or relatively mild, as in the case of a minor strain. Lack of muscular elasticity is also an important factor in the everyday aches and pains the dancer experiences. These minor strains are one cause of aches and pains, but another cause is excessive demands in standard dance movements. When one muscle group is inelastic, the opposing muscle group must work harder to accomplish motion than if the inelastic muscle group were stretched out. Thus, increasing muscular elasticity makes motion easier and less stressful than working with limited mobility. A prime example of this principle is stretching the hip extensors (specifically the hamstrings) to make dance "extension" (flexion of the hip joint) more efficient.

Specific stretching of a muscle group immediately following a demanding exercise bout with that muscle group can reduce the level of muscular stress that eventually might lead to tendinitis or other chronic conditions if ignored. For example, a regular "cool-down" procedure after *pointe* class—or any class which emphasizes plantar flexion of the ankle (such as *relevé*, jumps, or leaps)—should include specific stretching of both the gastrocnemius and the soleus muscles (see exercise section of this chapter). Clearly, stretching to increase muscular elasticity is a critical factor for all phases of a dance class, rehearsal, or performance.

Evaluation of Pain and Identification of Injuries

Dancers have a keen kinesthetic awareness. Even if they don't know the names of the muscles or the joint actions, they still can begin to identify a particular pain and deal with it effectively. They need to identify *where, when,* and *how* the pain occurs. This information will be valuable whether or not it is necessary to see a physician for precise diagnosis and treatment. While the following guidelines for analyzing pain are written for the ankle and tarsus region, the same principles can be generally applied to other regions of the body.

Where do you hurt (localization of the pain)?
- Is the pain anterior or posterior (front or back)?
- Is the pain on the medial or lateral side of the lower leg (inside or outside)?
- If the pain radiates, what is its path?
- Is the pain isolated in the foot? Where in the foot?

When do you hurt (functional analysis)?
- When performing the possible combinations of actions of the ankle and tarsus, which action makes it hurt?
- Does it hurt differently when performing different actions (see How do you hurt?)?

- Which actions in technique class (or everyday activities) cause the most pain? What kind of pain (how it hurts)? Is it different for different activities?

How do you hurt (the nature of the pain itself)?

- What does the pain feel like? Try to find words that describe the "feel" of the pain. Some words that are often used are: sharp, shooting, isolated, diffuse, prickly, burning, jabbing, crunching, grating, deep, superficial, and grabbing.
- Is the pain related to stretching the muscle (hot, prickly, pulling, or lengthening), or is it contraction pain (shortening, gripping, or cramping)?

After you have analyzed the pain in this way, you have an information base for identifying different types of injury. The most common injuries to the ankle and tarsus are tendinitis, shin splints, muscle spasms, sprains, strains, and fractures. A brief description of each of these common conditions is given here to assist the dancer who is evaluating an injury.

Common Injuries to the Ankle and Tarsus

Tendinitis is inflammation of the tendon (the attachment of muscle tissue to bone tissue). It most often occurs when the strength of a muscle is inadequate to meet the demands being made on it, or when muscles are not stretched out following intense exercise bouts. The location of the tendinitis follows the location of the muscle and the path of the tendon. In order to determine which tendon is inflamed, the dancer can go through the possible combined actions of the ankle, tarsus, and toes (both contracting the muscle against resistance and stretching the muscle) and identify which actions cause stretching pain and which actions cause contracting pain. Knowing the joint actions which cause pain can help in determining what activities to avoid in the acute stages of tendinitis. Gentle stretches should be done using the joint actions opposite to the contraction pain. Once the pain is gone, the muscle groups causing the pain should be strengthened. Home remedies for tendinitis include icing, rest, and gentle stretching of the muscle. In addition, aspirin can be taken as an anti-inflammatory drug, with dosages of two with each meal and two before bedtime (eight per day). If a tendinitis persists even after the home remedies, it is essential to see a physician.

The term *shin splints* once had a very specific meaning: it referred to the microscopic pulling of muscle fibers away from the bone where the belly of the muscle attached directly to the bone. Over the years, shin splints has become a general term which includes anything that hurts from the knee down.[13] True shin splints can only occur in those muscles which have no tendonous attachment on one end. Functionally, true shin splints are like a tendinitis where there is no tendon. The cause of shin splints is similar to the cause of tendinitis: asking more from the muscle than it has to give. Like tendinitis, the treatment for shin splints follows the pattern of rest, icing, and gentle stretching. To determine how to stretch for shin splints, one can use the same technique as is used for tendinitis: run through the possible combinations of joint actions and identify which actions produce stretch pain and which produce contraction pain. Gentle stretches should be done using the joint actions opposite to the contraction pain. Once the pain is gone, the muscle groups causing the pain should be strengthened. If shin splints persist for more than a week or two, one should examine the possibility that the injury is not really a shin splint, but perhaps is a stress fracture. The "feel" of shin splints and stress fractures is quite similar, and can therefore be easily confused.

Sprains are injuries to both soft tissue (muscle, nerve) and connective tissue (ligaments, joint capsules, tendons, and other connective tissue) which are caused by overmovement of a joint. The most common sites of sprains are on the lateral side of the tarsus (overmovement in the direction of supination usually caused by landing on an improperly aligned tarsus) and in the toes (caused by stubbing). It is prudent to always have a sprain examined by a physician to rule out the possibility of a fracture. General treatment of a sprain includes icing, compression, elevation, and rest. It should be noted that sprains, which almost always include injuries to the ligamentous structure, often take as long as 18 months to heal completely. Even then there is often some residual loss of range of motion from a sprain. Following the period of recuperation, muscles around the sprain should be strengthened and stretched to prevent reinjury and to regain lost capacities.

Strains are, like sprains, injuries caused by overmovement of a joint. However, in strains the injury is limited to the soft tissue, and does not include connective tissue. The same general treatments as are used for sprains can be used for the treatment of strains. Reconditioning the muscles after recovery from a strain is essential, or the injury will likely recur. Without rehabilitative exercises, the muscles are even weaker than they were when the original injury took place.

Fractures fall into a number of categories, including simple, compound, green stick, and stress fractures. All fractures exhibit some kind of loss of integrity of the bone structure: a break, a crack, a chip, or a shattering of a bone. The belief that if one can move a body part it is not broken is simply not true. Therefore, one should not depend upon one's own judgment in assessing a potential fracture. Treatment for fractures should always be directed by a physician.

Any discussion of pain would be incomplete without mentioning the value of pain. Pain is truly an ally; without pain, it would be impossible to identify and treat an injury. Pain tells us when movement activities are asking too much of the body, and when to stop— *if we will listen.*

Self-assessment of Strength and Range of Motion

The first step in actually using this information to guide conditioning is the assessment of capabilities. The two features of conditioning which must be assessed are strength and elasticity (or range of motion).

There are many technical tools for measuring strength, but the easiest is manual strength testing. This technique involves manually resisting the joint action while contracting against the resistance. For example, testing the strength of the plantar flexors and pronators involves manually pushing the foot toward dorsiflexion and supination while muscularly trying to pronate and plantar flex. Manual testing is far from the most precise measurement of muscular strength, but it is practical because no special equipment is necessary. The person doing the testing can, with relative ease, identify the contraction as "strong," "average," or "weak."

In range-of-motion testing of the ankle and tarsus, the subject relaxes the foot and lower leg while the tester manipulates the foot into the different positions. Similar to the rough but informative assessment of strength, manual testing of range of motion can be grossly identified as "marked," "average," or "limited." Below is an assessment sheet for recording the results of strength and range-of-motion testing.

Assessment of Strength and Range of Motion

Strength	Strong	Average	Weak
Plantar flexors (neutral tarsus)			
Dorsiflexors (neutral tarsus)			
Plantar flexors/Pronators			
Plantar flexors/Supinators			
Dorsiflexors/Pronators			
Dorsiflexors/Supinators			

Range of Motion	Marked	Average	Limited
Plantar flexion (neutral tarsus)			
Dorsiflexion (neutral tarsus)			
Plantar flexion/Pronation			
Plantar flexion/Supinator			
Dorsiflexion/Pronation			
Dorsiflexion/Supinator			

Once completed, this chart becomes a guide for the tested dancer's conditioning program. Weak muscles should be strengthened and inelastic muscles stretched.

Guidelines for Increasing Strength

Maximal Contractions

Exercises for building strength require maximal contractions that move through the full range of motion. In the initial phases of some of the exercises described below, the weight of the body alone, or the simple movement of a joint through an unfamiliar action, is sufficient to achieve a state of maximal contraction. That is because the muscles in the first phases of conditioning are not yet very strong. However, as strength increases it becomes necessary to find a way to add resistance to the performance of the exercise in order to continue to build strength.

Increasing Resistance

Certain systems of increasing resistance are more effective than others for this area of the body. Free weights are difficult to use because they do not attach readily to the foot. Elastic bands can serve this purpose, and they come in many different forms. For example, wide sewing elastic, wrapped around the foot in such a way as to resist the action being performed, can be used in the first phase of the conditioning program. As strength increases, one might first double the layer of elastic, then move to the use of surgical tubing (available at any medical supply house) which provides greater resistance than the elastic, and finally to cross-sections of inner tubing (cutting an automobile inner tube across the tube in about two-inch selections, forming a circle of rubber), which is quite inelastic.

These forms of resistance are most effective for strengthening the muscles of the tarsus (both pronators and supinators) and the dorsi-flexors of the ankle. For the muscles which exclusively plantar flex the ankle joint (those that are already quite strong in most dancers), other systems which add greater resistance are appropriate. One very simple method for building strength in the plantar flexors is to shift the weight to one foot in performing normal dance exercises such as *pliés* and *relevés*. This action actually doubles the load on the muscles.

Match the Weak to the Strong

The specific nature of the exercises that are needed is determined by the manual assessment of strength done previously. If there is a major muscular imbalance between opposing muscle groups in the ankle and tarsus, the first step should be to bring the strength of those muscles more closely in balance. Thus, the first strengthening exercises should be those for the weakest muscles. In doing the exercises to build strength, one may also identify a difference in strength between opposing muscle groups or between the same muscle group of the right foot and the left foot. This information is valuable; remember, one of the goals of any conditioning program is to achieve balance of muscular capacity. When an imbalance of muscular strength is discovered, the general rule is to do a few extra repetitions with the weak muscles or muscle group to work toward more balanced strength. If the action is hard to do, do more—within reason.

Condition by Muscle Groups

While it might be helpful to know the specific muscles in each muscle group, this knowledge is not essential to the conditioning process. It is sufficient to approach conditioning by muscle groups, starting with those that control the joint actions of the ankle and tarsus (plantar flexors, dorsiflexors, pronators, and supinators), and then isolating the combined actions of the ankle and tarsus (plantar flexors and pronators, plantar flexors and supinators, dorsiflexors and pronators, and dorsiflexors and supinators). The exercises described below are designed to build strength according to muscle groups.

Five Past the "Burn"

In doing any exercise to build strength, one must be aware of how much is enough, and how much is too much. One must go beyond existing capacities to build strength, but going too far can lead to excessive muscle soreness, or even injury. One rule of thumb involves the burn. Whenever one is doing exercises for strength, a point is inevitably reached when the muscle or muscle group starts, as we say, "to burn." To build strength beyond existing levels it is necessary to go beyond this point, but not so far as to induce injury. About five repetitions past the burn is usually demanding and safe.

Stretch Out After Strengthening

Maximal contractions are extraordinarily beneficial and build strength with amazing speed, but one must be careful always to stretch out after a strength-building exercise bout. Without stretches, the residual neuromuscular tension remains, and tends to increase the normal level of muscle soreness. In addition, stretching the active muscle group after an intense exercise bout seems to reduce the build-up of excessive muscle bulk.[14] The general principle for stretching out is to reverse the combined joint actions used in the strengthening exercises and do a long, sustained stretch. Specific positions for stretching the different muscle groups are identified in the stretching section of this chapter.

Vary the Tempo of Strength Exercises

Increased strength is specific to the angle of the joint and the velocity of the contraction used in conditioning. Therefore, it is necessary to do the exercises for strength at both slow and fast tempos for the maximum benefit.

Specific Exercises to Increase Strength

The Ankle/Tarsus Series (for strengthening all combined actions of ankle and tarsus)

This series can be done in a long-sit position or lying on one's back. Dorsiflex the ankle joint. Press the soles of the feet out to the sides (pronate), without rotating at the hip joint and without lessening the degree of dorsiflexion. Then press the soles of the feet inward (supinate), isolating the action to the tarsus. Alternate the in-and-out action and repeat at least five repetitions past the burn. Repeat the same sequence with the ankle joint in a position of plantar flexion. As strength increases, add more repetitions until about 40 or 50 can be done easily. Then go on to the advanced ankle/tarsus series.

The Advanced Ankle/Tarsus Series (for strengthening all combined actions of the ankle and tarsus)

Add resistance to the previous series in the form of elastic, surgical tubing, or inner tube cross-sections. The elastic is placed around the balls of the feet, and the exercises are performed against the resistance. In the action of pronation (both in plantar flexion and dorsiflexion—Figures 11.1-A and 11.1-B respectively), the feet readily press out against the elastic. However, when doing supination it is necessary to cross the legs below the knee in order to achieve resistance when a circle of elastic is used. When using surgical tubing, crossing of the legs is not required, as illustrated in Figures 11.1-C and 11.1-D.

The "Mouth" (for strengthening the dorsiflexors of the ankle)

In the long-sit position, place the right heel on top of the left ankle joint. Place an elastic resistance device around the toes of both feet (Figure 11.2). Holding the elastic in place with the left foot, pull straight up against the resistance with the toes and foot on the right side. Repeat the exercise with the left foot on top, dorsiflexing it against the resistance. If one foot (ankle) is stronger than the other, one or two extra repetitions should be done on the weak ankle to begin the process of equalizing strength.

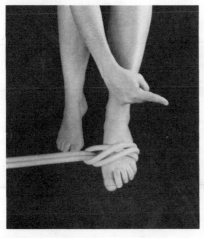
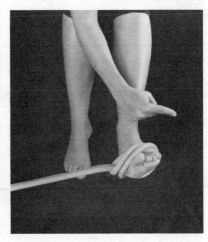

Figure 11.1-A.   Figure 11.1-B.

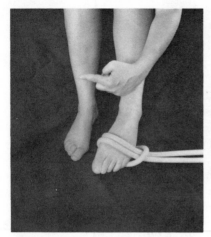

Figure 11.1-C.

Figure 11.1-D.

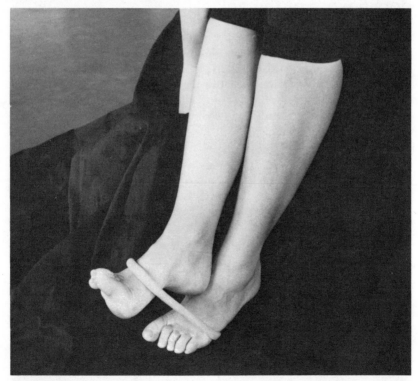

Figure 11.2.

Toe Gripper (for strengthening the intrinsic muscles of the foot)

In a long-sit position, flex the knees slightly, dorsiflex the ankle, and grip the toes as hard as possible (Figure 11.3). Simultaneously grip the hands into a tight fist (this fortifies the contraction of the foot muscles by activating the flexor reflex). Hold the contraction about 15 to 20 seconds, but not to the point of cramping the muscles of the foot. Release, stretch, and wiggle the toes. Repeat the whole exercise, including the stretch.

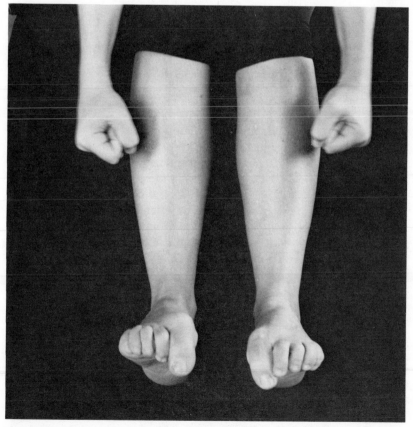

Figure 11.3.

Stair-step Full Relevés (to strengthen plantar flexors of the ankle and increase awareness of a properly aligned tarsus during action of the ankle)

Stand on a stair-step with the balls of the feet on the edge of the step, the heels unsupported (Figure 11.4-A). Allow the heels slowly to descend as far as possible, while keeping the tarsus in a neutral position (Figure 11.4-B). Then rise through the normal standing position and, maintaining neutral alignment of the tarsus, go on to full *relevé* or half-toe (Figure 11.4-C). Lower the heels to the starting position. Repeat this exercise five times past the burn. When your strength has developed to the point that it is easy to do 30 repetitions, try this exercise with all your weight on one foot. Reduce the number of repetitions accordingly.

Weighted Pliés/Relevés (to strengthen the plantar flexors of the ankle as well as all of the muscles involved in plié and relevé)

Do a complete *plié/relevé* sequence in all positions with weight added to the normal body weight. A scuba diver's weight belt can be used, or free weights, or even a dance bag held in the hands with the arms hanging at the sides (Figure 11.5). As strength increases, do more repetitions or add more weight. With even more strength, reduce the amount of weight and repetitions and do the sequence on one foot at a time. Again increase weight or repetitions as strength increases. *Note:* Pay careful attention to alignment in both the torso and legs as you would in an unweighted *plié* series.

How Much Strength Is Enough?

Clearly, there comes a point when the dancer says "This is enough"; otherwise, strength conditioning could continue *ad nauseum*. There is no pat answer to the question of how much is enough. Each dancer must review the demands he or she makes on the ankles and feet. Those demands serve as a guide for strength conditioning, but it is important to remember that one should always have a reserve of extra strength so that the body can accommodate to unusual demands.

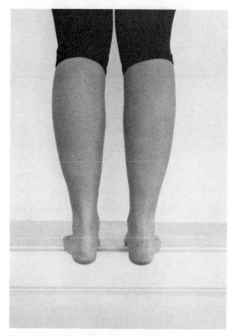

Figure 11.4-A.

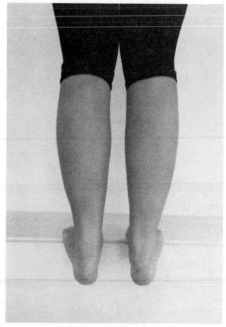

Figure 11.4-B.

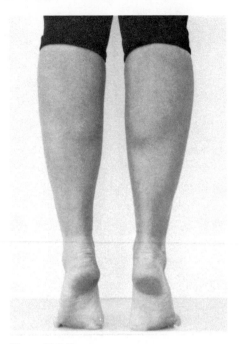

Figure 11.4-C.

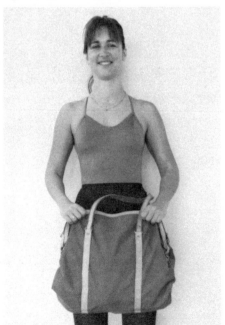

Figure 11.5.

Guidelines for Increasing Elasticity

Use of the Long, Sustained Stretch

The use of the long, sustained stretch for the muscles of the ankle and tarsus has been recommended earlier in this chapter. The rationale is based on the fact that the ankle and tarsus do not have a balance of muscle mass between agonists and antagonists. The long, sustained stretch is therefore most effective in this region.

Balance the Elasticity of Opposing Muscle Groups

Imbalance in the muscular elasticity of opposing muscle groups at the ankle and tarsus has just as serious consequences as does an imbalance of strength. Having more range of motion in one direction than another (for example, more supination than pronation) means that the agonists are inelastic (in this case, the supinators) and the antagonists (the pronators) are quite elastic. In motion, this means that the tarsus will take a neutral muscular position somewhere between the extreme possibility of supination and the limited possibility of pronation. This is a muscular neutral, not the neutral position of the tarsus joint, which is considered the ideal. It means that the foot will fall into a position of supination whenever it is not bearing weight. Landing on a supinated tarsus greatly increases the likelihood of sprains and strains of the tarsus, commonly called ankle sprains.

Stretch by Joint Action

The most effective and efficient way to stretch any muscle is to reverse all of its joint actions. It is possible to stretch effectively by performing all of the combinations of actions possible at the relevant joints. Thus, stretching of the ankle and tarsus muscles requires stretching in the following combinations of actions: pronation and plantar flexion; pronation and dorsiflexion; supination and dorsiflexion; and supination and plantar flexion. Because there are four muscles which cross the ankle, tarsus, and also the toe joints, the addition of flexion and extension of the toes as another feature of the stretch ensures that one has stretched all of the muscles of the ankle and tarsus.

Stretch Past the Comfort Zone

It is not unusual to find dancers doing what I call "token stretches"—stretches of very short duration that stay within the comfort zone, never going past the point of pain. For a stretch to be effective—that is, to increase the elasticity of the muscle—it is necessary to go beyond the existing capacities of the muscle to stretch. Therefore, stretching is not simply "hanging out" in the comfort zone, but rather going beyond comfort to increase capacities. In addition, the familiar, well-worn stretches are often not the stretches that are most needed. For example, most dancers don't really need to stretch while sitting in second position; they can already put their chests on the floor, or at least come close. Those "oldies but goodies" feel good because they are easy to do, but that means we really don't need to do them. The stretches that are least comfortable to do are the ones that are needed the most.

Use Gravity or Other External Forces to Increase the Stretch

The long, sustained stretch is most effective if the target muscles are in a passive state (i.e., not contracted at all). For this reason, it is helpful to place the joint in a position where gravity will increase the stretch on the target muscles. For example, if the plantar flexors are the target muscles, a joint position should be taken that allows gravity to assist in the dorsiflexion of the ankle joint. If it is difficult to use gravity in this way (and it is for some of the combined actions of the ankle and tarsus), other sources of external force can be used to increase the stretch, as long as the person experiencing the stretch has control over them. One easy way to provide external assistance for a stretch is by manually pushing the joint into the stretch position. Doing this for oneself is the safest technique for using manual stretches. With another person doing the pushing it is difficult to control the pressure, and an injury might result. For this reason I do not recommend "partner stretching."

How Long is Long Enough?

Holding a stretch for less than 20 to 30 seconds is a "token" stretch. There is really not enough time in short-duration stretches for the connective tissue of the muscle to be stretched. One should hold a stretch for at least one minute, particularly when the muscles have been inelastic for sometime. Moreover, each stretch should be repeated at least three or four times during the day to reinforce the sense of stretch in the muscles and the new position of the joint allowed for by the stretch.

Relax and Reassemble After a Stretch

A period of relaxation and reassembly is critical after a long, sustained stretch. This is particularly true of stretches that are new to the dancer, and are focused on muscles that have not been intensively stretched in the past. The body needs time to adjust to the new information given to it by a long, sustained stretch. It is important to allow that time by relaxing and paying conscious attention to the changes that have occurred. The period of relaxation should be followed by imaginary movements of the joint, and then gentle movements of the joint to reawaken the muscles around it to the demands of contraction.

Specific Stretching Exercises

Gastrocnemius and Soleus (Achilles Tendon)

Assume a parallel lunge position with the right leg forward and the hands reaching out to rest against a wall. Keeping the left knee straight and the left heel on the floor, press forward through the hips onto the right leg, taking more weight on the hands. Hold this position for 30 seconds to one minute (Figure 11.6-A). Then slowly bend the left knee, still keeping the left heel on the floor, and hold this stretch position for 30 seconds to one minute (Figure 11.6-B). Come out of the stretch of the left ankle slowly, taking time to assess the changes and process the new information. Repeat the exercise on the other side, with the left foot forward and the right ankle the focus of the stretch.

Note: Always do this stretch in both positions of the knee, as different muscles are stretched when the knee is straight and bent.

Stretch for Pronators and Plantar Flexors

Sitting in a chair with the right lower leg resting on top of the left thigh, assume a position of dorsiflexion and supination of the right ankle and tarsus. Place the right hand on the inside of the right ankle joint and take hold of the foot with the left hand (Figure 11.7). Pull with the left hand and push with the right, thereby applying an external force to increase the stretch in the direction of dorsiflexion

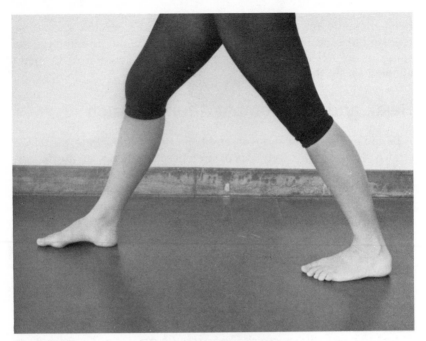

Figure 11.6-A.

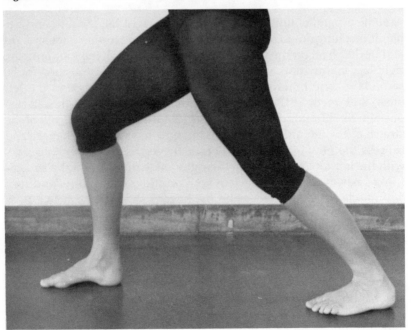

Figure 11.6-B.

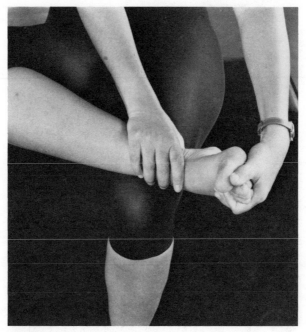

Figure 11.7.

and supination. Hold the stretch for 30 seconds to one minute. Relax for a moment before repeating the exercise on the other side.

Stretch for Pronators and Dorsiflexors

Sitting in a chair with the right lower leg resting on top of the left thigh, assume a position of plantar flexion and supination of the right ankle and tarsus. Place the right hand on the inside of the right ankle joint and take hold of the foot with the left hand (Figure 11.8). Push with the right hand and pull with the left hand to increase the joint actions of supination and plantar flexion. Relax for a moment before repeating the exercise on the other side.

Adding the Toe Muscles

While doing this stretch, add powerful gripping of the toes, or manually pull the toes into flexion (Figure 11.9).

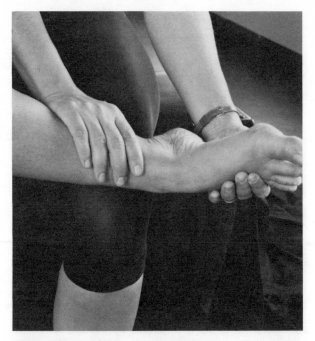

Figure 11.8.

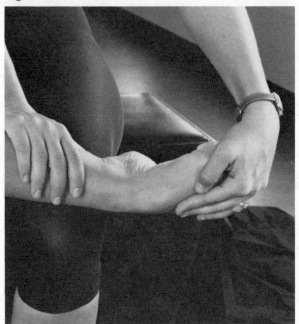

Figure 11.9.

Stretch for Supinators and Plantar Flexors

Sitting either in a chair or on the floor, draw the right knee up to the chest and take hold of the right foot with the right hand on the little-toe side of the foot (Figure 11.10). With the hand, pull the foot up (into dorsiflexion) and to the outside (into pronation). Hold the stretch for 30 seconds to one minute and relax for a moment before repeating the exercise on the left side.

Adding the Toe Muscles

To include the muscles of the toes in this stretch, while maintaining dorsiflexion and pronation with the right hand pull the toes up into a position of extension with the left hand. Add stretch of the toe muscles to the left side of the stretch as well.

Stretch for Supinators and Dorsiflexors

Sitting in a chair with the right lower leg resting on top of the left thigh, assume a position of plantar flexion of the ankle and pronation of the tarsus with the right foot. Hold the right ankle with the right hand, the thumb toward your chest and the fingers on the outside of the ankle. Place the heel of the left hand on the most medial aspect (toward the middle) of the ball of the foot (not shown). Press with the left hand and pull with the right hand while maintaining a plantar-flexed position of the right ankle. Hold the stretch for 30 seconds to one minute and then relax for a moment before repeating the stretch on the other side.

Other Helpful Exercises for the Ankle and Tarsus

Anterior Shin Splint Stretch

Kneel and sit back on the heels with the ankles plantar flexed. Place the hands on the floor on either side of the knees. Lift the knees off the floor, taking the weight of the body on the hands and on the tops of the feet while keeping the buttocks close to the heels (Figure 11.11). Allow gravity and the weight of the body to increase to plantar flexion of the ankle joints. Keep the tarsus in a neutral position (neither supinated nor pronated) throughout this exercise. Hold the position

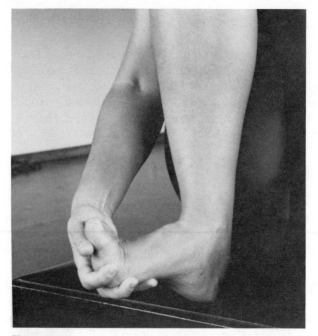

Figure 11.10.

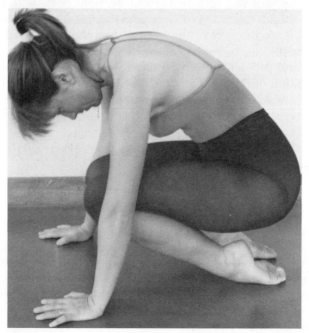

Figure 11.11.

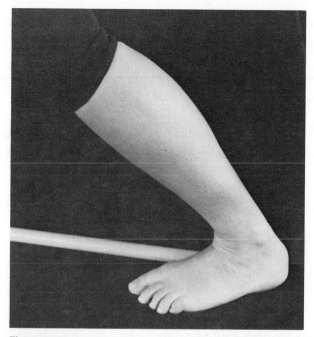

Figure 11.12.

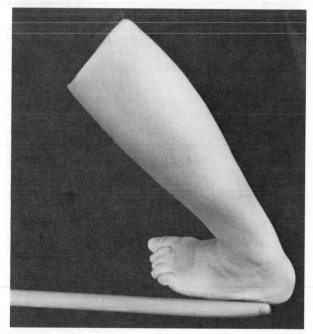

Figure 11.13.

for 30 seconds to one minute. Relax and do some easy ankle circles on completion of the exercise.

Stretch for Shin Splints on the Posterior and Medial Aspect of the Lower Leg

Do the bent-knee portion of the gastrocnemius and soleus stretch described above with the back foot turned out (Figure 11.12). As usual, hold the stretch for at least 30 seconds to one minute, and relax for a moment before doing the second side. Then do the soleus stretch with the back foot turned in (Figure 11.13).

Conclusion

The primary rationale for this chapter is that dance classes do not sufficiently focus on building strength and elasticity in the foot and lower leg to prevent injuries to that region. Efficient and effective conditioning practices are often ignored, and the injury rate in this region, for dancers, is inordinately high. A simple system for increasing strength and elasticity of the muscles of the ankle and tarsus is presented. The general steps of the system include: 1) identification of areas of weakness, inelasticity, or injury; 2) identification of joint actions in those areas; 3) identification of key muscle groups; 4) analysis of present conditioning practices and special demands on those areas; 5) assessment of strength and range of motion; and 6) using the principles of conditioning to design exercises to balance strength and mobility of agonist and antagonist of the right and left sides.

I realize that all of the analysis involved in the process outlined above could transform a passionate dance technique class into a sterile class with no fire to it. That is certainly not my intention. I sincerely believe that effective strengthening and stretching exercises can be incorporated into technique classes in such a way as to continue to work toward the central goal: *to dance*. Indeed, that is the creative challenge offered to teachers and dancers: to develop capacities through a fusion of art and science.

References

1. Shaw, J.L.H. (1977). The nature, frequency, and patterns of dance injuries: a survey of college dance students [Thesis]. Salt Lake City: University of Utah.

2. Fuller, P.E. (1975). An identification of common injuries sustained in ballet and modern dance activities [Dissertation]. Denton, Texas: Texas Women's University.

3. Miller, E.H., Schneider, H.J., Bronson, J.L., McLain, D. (1975, Sept.). A new consideration in athletic injuries: The classical ballet dancer. *Clinical Orthopaedics and Related Research, 111,* 181-191.

4. Ryan, A.J., Gilbert, R.S., Schuster, R., Subotnick, S.I. (1976, Nov.). Ballet dancers' injuries pose sportsmedicine challenge. *The Physician and Sportsmedicine, 4,* 44-57.

5. Schneider, H.J., King, A.Y., Bronson, J.L., Miller, E.H. (1974, Dec.). Stress injuries and developmental change of lower extremities in ballet dancers. *Diagnostic Radiology, 113,* 627-632.

6. Bachrach, R.M. (1988, Oct.). The relationship of low back/pelvic somatic dysfunctions to dance injuries. *Orthopaedic Review, 17,* 1037-1043.

7. Nagrin, D. (1988). *How to dance forever.* New York: Morrow.

8. Washington, E.L. (1978). Musculoskeletal injuries in theatrical dancers: site, frequency, and severity. *American Journal of Sports Medicine, 6*(2), 75-98.

9. Stanish, W. (1984). *Tendinitis: its etiology and treatment.* Lexington, Massachusetts: The Collamore Press, D.C. Heath and Co.

10. Fitt, S.S. (1988). *Dance kinesiology.* New York: Schirmer Books.

11. Fleck, S.J., Kraemer, W.J. (1987). *Designing resistance training programs.* Champaign, Illinois: Human Kinetics.

12. DeVries, H.A. (1966). *Physiology of exercise for physical education and athletics.* Dubuque, Iowa: W.C. Brown.

13. Gans, A. (1985, Aug.). The relationship of heel contact in ascent and descent from jumps to the incidence of shin splints in ballet dancers. *Physical Therapy, 65,* 1192-1196.

14. Fitt, S.S. (1981-82). Conditioning for dancers: investigating some assumptions. *Dance Research Journal, 14*(1 and 2), 32-38.

Photography: Rosalind Newmark

12

A Biomechanical Approach To Aerobic Dance Injuries

Stephen P. Baitch, P.T.

Since its inception, sports medicine has focused on treating the athlete's injuries in order that he or she may return to athletic participation as quickly as possible. Initially, the emphasis of treatment was centered on alleviation of symptoms of injury, followed by an aggressive rehabilitation program. Presently, due to the emergence of high technology and in-depth experimentation in the field of biomechanics, the focus is shifting from the treatment of injury to dealing with causes. This shift has been applied to injuries in all sports, including aerobic dance. This article will discuss the mechanisms of aerobic dance injuries, and the biomechanical make-up of the body as it affects movement in aerobic dance.

The increasing popularity of aerobic dance has brought with it an alarming incidence of injury. According to a study performed on aerobic dancers in February 1985, 75.9% of aerobic dance instructors and 43.3% of students reported injuries.[1] Aerobic dance injuries have specific characteristics with regard to location and frequency. In a study conducted with 61 aerobic dancers at the Union Memorial Hospital Sports Medicine Center in Baltimore, 82% of the injuries reported involved the lower extremities.[2] The most common site of injury was the heel (spur syndrome or plantar fasciitis). The second most common site was the inner portion of the shins (shin splints). The present author's experience supports these findings.

Several predisposing factors of injury were observed. Of primary concern was the number of classes taken per week: the difference between the average for students (3.3) and for instructors (4.7) showed a significantly increased incidence of injury. A concrete floor covered with carpet also yielded a high injury rate (50%). (It is interesting to note, however, that a soft resilient floor did not always reduce the risk of injury; in fact, a wood-over-air-space floor covered with padded carpet had the second highest injury rate.) Shoewear was another component which was analyzed. Barefoot dancers had a 65% injury rate as compared with 49% for dancers wearing shoes. Although this speaks well for using some form of footwear, it also suggests that more work needs to be done on the construction of aerobic dance shoes. Several studies have indicated that excessive cushioning in shoes allows extraneous motion to occur in the foot and leg, thereby increasing the incidence of injury.[3, 4] Training techniques were considered to be another contributing factor in aerobic dance injuries. Many aerobic dancers who were injured revealed that they did not stretch adequately before and after exercise. Some injuries could also be attributed to a too rapid increase in the number of classes taken over a given period of time. This was found to be equally true in runners who increased their weekly mileage too rapidly.

In several studies it has been noted that repetitive movement combined with a hard surface definitely yielded a higher rate of injury.[1, 2, 5] It was hypothesized that an inability to dissipate shock might be the underlying cause for most aerobic dance injuries. However, shock reduction as a form of treatment was not always effective; nor had it proven efficacious in runners with complaints similar to those found in aerobic dancers. More recently the emphasis of treatment has been geared toward increasing control and stability of the foot while running. There is much literature to support the concept that realignment of the foot is extremely successful in treating various problems in runners.[6, 7, 8, 9] We are now beginning to apply the same theories of realignment to aerobic dancers.

An examination of the biomechanics of the aerobic dancer's lower extremities has become crucial in our treatment approach. Characteristics such as excessive rotation of the femur and malalignment of the patella, for example, have been proven to be highly correlative with knee pain (this same finding was noted previously in runners). Also observed was a correlation of tibial varum (bowed legs) and excessive foot pronation (rolling in) with symptoms of heel and shin pain as well as metatarsalgia (pain in the ball of the foot). The abnormal alignment of the foot has been known to cause problems as proximal as the hip and low back.

Many movements in aerobic dance demand the support of the entire body weight on one foot for a short period of time. The muscles of the foot, ankle and leg contract both concentrically (shortening) and eccentrically (lengthening) in order to control the ascent and descent of the movement. At the same time, the joints of the foot and ankle must lock and unlock at precise moments to provide stability and mobility. A structural malalignment of the foot can cause excessive strain on the muscles, as well as abnormal rotation of the lower extremity. Aerobic dancers (or runners) with excessive pronation, for example, must overuse the posterior medial muscle groups of the shin in order to control the rate of ascent and descent during exercise.[10] Static evaluation reveals that when a dancer with this condition is viewed from the rear, the heel is in an everted position relative to the floor, the arch is dropped, and the tibia demonstrates bowing and rotation.

With the recent advances in high technology we are able to enhance the static evaluation with a dynamic analysis utilizing a high speed video camera system. The slow motion and frame by frame capability of this system can record abnormal movement of the foot and lower extremity. The results are given in the form of a computer printout which provides angular measurements of the foot and lower leg.

Once the static and dynamic results are obtained, a treatment plan is implemented. If it is determined that the dancer's symptoms are occurring as a result of abnormal foot mechanics, a balanced orthotic (shoe insert) might be used to re-align the foot. By placing the foot in a neutral position with the orthotic, problems of the heel, shin, and knee can be eliminated.

It might be argued that the orthosis simply acts in this case as a shock absorber. Interestingly, however, as indicated earlier, aerobic dancers and runners have used a significant amount of cushioning in their shoes to self-treat injuries without success. In contrast, we have used a semi-rigid polypropylene orthosis with minimal shock absorption capability to correct alignment of the foot. A specific case study will illustrate the efficacy of this treatment.

A forty-one year old female aerobic dancer presented with a complaint of chronic right heel pain which had developed over the past six months, apparently as a result of her participation in high-impact aerobic classes. She said that the heel pain began after she increased the frequency of her dance classes from two to three per week. The onset of the pain was gradual, and initially was noticed only after dancing. By the time she came to our clinic the pain was present during and after dance classes, but was most intense when she got up in the morning. Other relevant facts were that the patient had tried different types of aerobic shoes in an attempt to alleviate the heel pain, but without success; she had been dancing on wood floors covered with carpet at the time of the injury; she wore high heels frequently during the day, due to her job requirements; and prior treatment for her heel problem with anti-inflammatories and a cortisone injection had given minimal relief.

The patient's history is extremely valuable in these cases because it helps to formulate a course of treatment based on the underlying mechanism of injury. This particular history allowed the clinician to determine that the right heel pain was secondary to a gradual onset resulting from small repeated stresses after the dancer increased her activity from two to three classes a week.

Once a history is taken, a thorough static biomechanical examination is performed. The evaluation searches for any limitation or excessive joint motion in the foot or lower extremity that may be the cause of a malalignment problem. The results in the case reported here indicated that in the nonweight bearing position, subtalar joint inversion and eversion range of motion measurements were within normal limits. The subtalar joint neutral position was 2 degrees varus, bilaterally. The forefoot to rearfoot relationship indicated a 4 degree varus on the right symptomatic foot and a perpendicular relationship on the left foot. Ankle dorsiflexion was measured to be 5 degrees with the knee extended and 15 degrees with the knee flexed, bilaterally. In the standing position, tibial varum (bowing) was noted to be 5 degrees bilaterally. The relaxed calcaneal stance measurement indicated a 4 degree everted position on the right and a 2 degree everted position on the left foot.

To confirm these findings a high speed video analysis was performed during a simulated aerobic dance routine. The patient was instructed to do a series of aerobic dance movements similar to those used in her normal aerobic dance workout. Points of reference placed on the bisection of the lower legs and heel counters of both shoes were digitized and then analyzed frame by frame with the use of a computer. It was found that in the standing position the medial side of the forefoot was actually being raised in relationship to the ground when the subtalar joint was in the neutral position (Figure 12.1). However, in order to bring the forefoot to the ground, the subtalar joint had to pronate as a compensatory mechanism, causing an everted position of the calcaneus (Figure 12.2). The high speed video analysis not only verified that the abnormal pronation occurred, but it demonstrated that the dynamic pronation angle on the symptomatic right foot (9 degrees) exceeded the static pronation angle (4 degrees).

From a biomechanical standpoint it was determined that the excessive pronation had caused unlocking of the subtalar and mid-tarsal joint of the foot and subsequent eversion of the heel, producing hypermobility of the foot. In turn, this unlocking effect was creating an excessive strain on a band of tissue which has its attachment on the posterior medial surface of the heel (plantar fascia), thus causing heel pain. It was also noted that this dancer had limited ankle dorsiflexion,

RIGHT FOOT
(ANTERIOR VIEW)

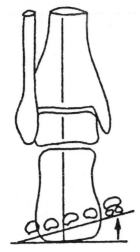

FOREFOOT VARUS

(UNCOMPENSATED)

Figure 12.1. The medial side of the forefoot is elevated in relation to the ground with the subtalar joint in neutral, indicating a forefoot varus

bilaterally. This condition, also known as an equinus deformity, prevents the ankle from moving adequately in the upward direction in a nonweight-bearing situation (Figures 12.3-A, 12.3-B). During weight-bearing activity it prevents the tibia from moving forward on the foot. In order to compensate for this problem the mid-tarsal joint of the foot must unlock and pronate so that adequate dorsiflexion can occur at the ankle joint, thus allowing the tibia to move forward over the foot.

Dancers with limited ankle dorsiflexion (5 degrees or less) are not unusual. These same dancers often report that they frequently wear high-heeled shoes during working hours. In theory, wearing a high heel may place the gastroc-soleus muscle, located in the posterior calf, in a shortened position for a prolonged period of time (Figure 12.4-A). Conversely, an aerobic dance shoe, which has minimal elevation in the heel, can be a drastic transition from wearing a two-inch high heel (Figure 12.4-B). The aerobic dance shoe, with its relatively lower inclination angle, places an undue strain on the already compromised length of the gastroc-soleus muscle during exercise. As the heel makes contact with the ground, increased mid-tarsal joint pronation may

RIGHT FOOT
(POSTERIOR VIEW)

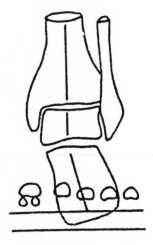

FOREFOOT VARUS
(COMPENSATED)

Figure 12.2. The calcaneus everts past perpendicular in order to bring the medial side of the forefoot to the ground, causing excessive pronation

occur, allowing the tibia to move forward over its base of support (the foot), due to the inadequate amount of ankle dorsiflexion available.

Initially, the treatment prescribed for the patient described above with plantar fasciitis consisted of ice massage to the right heel and stretching exercises for the gastroc-soleus muscles, bilaterally. This regimen was performed before and after her aerobic dance routine. She was also instructed to reduce her classes from three to two a week. The patient was then casted for semi-rigid orthotic devices, which were made of high density subortholin material. These orthotics were designed to control the abnormal subtalar and mid-tarsal joint pronation, in an attempt to minimalize the strain placed on the plantar fascia.

The patient gradually broke in the orthotics until she was able to wear them for her entire dance routine. After wearing them for six weeks she reported that her right heel pain had disappeared, and she had returned to her pre-injury level of three classes per week. A post-treatment evaluation was performed using the high speed video analysis system. The results indicated that initial maximum pronation

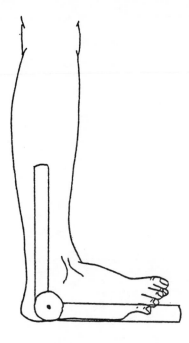

Figure 12.3-A. Abnormal amount of ankle dorsiflexion indicating an equinous deformity of the ankle

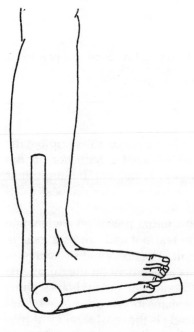

Figure 12.3-B. Normal amount of ankle dorsiflexion needed for adequate ambulation is 10-15 degrees

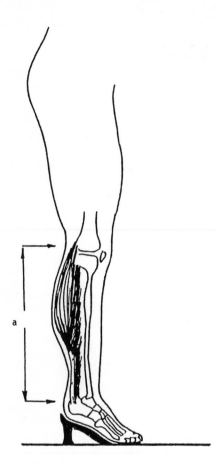

Figure 12.4-A. Shortened position of the gastroc-soleus muscle when foot is in high-heeled shoe

angles were reduced from 9 degrees to 5 degrees on the symptomatic right foot. The asymptomatic left foot showed a reduction in the maximum pronation angle from 4 degrees to 2 degrees. It is important to note that the dancer was wearing her orthotics for the post-treatment evaluation.

Theoretically, the decrease in the maximum pronation angle while wearing orthotic devices stabilizes the rearfoot and causes a locking effect of the mid-tarsal joint during gait. The abnormal stretching of the plantar fascial tissue, which has its attachment on the calcaneus, is prevented by limiting the amount the subtalar and mid-tarsal joints can pronate. However, the literature remains inconclusive on whether decreasing the maximum pronation angle is the most significant contribution of orthotic devices. It must be kept in mind that the pronation

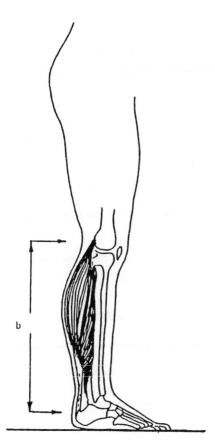

Figure 12.4-B. Length of gastroc-soleus muscle when foot is in aerobic dance shoe

angle is only one, parameter now being studied as a correlative factor in the cause-effect relationship between injuries of the lower extremity and orthotic devices.

This article demonstrates the systematic approach that is being implemented in order to evaluate and effectively treat lower extremity problems. The study of biomechanics has already had a tremendous impact on training regimens, as well as floor, shoe, and equipment design. There are still many questions to be answered regarding the role that abnormal biomechanics plays in the cause of injury. However, by shifting the focus of treatment toward the biomechanical causes of injury, we anticipate being able to return many injured dancers (and athletes) to a relatively high level of activity.

References

1. Richie, D.H., Kelso, S.F., Bellucci, P.A. (1985, Feb.). Aerobic dance injuries: a retrospective study of instructors and participants. *The Physician and Sportsmedicine, 13,* 130-140.
2. Vetter, W.L., Helfet, D.L., Spear, K., Matthews, L. (1985, Feb.). Aerobic dance injuries. *The Physician and Sportsmedicine, 13,* 114-120.
3. Cavanagh, P. (1982). The shoe-ground interface in running. In: Mack, R.P., ed. compilation of *The American Academy of Orthopaedic Surgeons symposium on the foot and leg in running sports.* St. Louis: C.V. Mosby, 30-44.
4. Nigg, B.M. (1986). *Biomechanics of running shoes.* Champaign, Illinois: Human Kinetics.
5. Francis, L.L., Francis, P.R., Welshons-Smith, K. (1985, Feb.). Aerobic dance injuries: a survey of instructors. *The Physician and Sportsmedicine, 13,* 105-111.
6. Bates, B.T., Osternig, L.R., Mason, B., James, L.S. (1979). Foot orthotic devices to modify selected aspects of lower extremity mechanics. *American Journal of Sports Medicine, 7,* 338-342.
7. Botte, R.R. (1981). An interpretation of the pronation syndrome and foot types of patients with low back pains. *Journal of American Podiatric Medical Association, 71,* 243-253.
8. Brody, D.M. (1980). *Running injuries.* CIBA Clinical Symposia Annual, 32(4).
9. Subotnick, S.I. (1976, Jan.). The shin splints syndrome of the lower extremity. *Journal of American Podiatric Medical Association, 66,* 43-45.
10. Viitasalo, J.T., Kvist, M. (1983). Some biomechanical aspects of the foot and ankle in athletes with and without shin splints. *American Journal of Sports Medicine, 11*(3), 125-130.

Illustrations: David Petrie

13

The Neuroanatomical and Biomechanical Basis of Flexibility Exercises in Dance

Robert E. Stephens, Ph.D.

Flexibility is a critical factor in the overall fitness of a dancer. Although dancers are generally quite limber, many have limited range of motion due to tight muscles in specific areas. Therefore, it is important that dancers and dance teachers know and understand the basics of safe and effective stretching techniques. This chapter will discuss the importance of flexibility exercises, central and peripheral factors in flexibility, eight guidelines for safe and effective stretching, and four of the best flexiblity exercises for dancers.

The Purpose of Flexibility Exercises

Although warming up prior to stretching may not improve the permanent elongation of the target muscle, it certainly feels good, and it decreases the risk of small tears in the connective tissue of the muscle. Warming up also increases blood flow and tissue metabolism. Therefore, an adequate warm-up should precede stretching.

The proper performance of any dance technique requires maximum range of motion of the joints of the spine and extremities and extremely supple, flexible muscles. Unfortunately, professional dancers frequently develop specific muscle imbalances as a result of their dance training. The most common areas are the rotator muscles of the hips and the triceps surae (gastrocnemius and soleus muscles). This tendency to muscle imbalance should be addressed through flexibility exercises, which in turn should be *training specific* for dancers; that is, they should prepare the dancer to perform the specific movements which are characteristic of better or safer dancing. Proprioception, or position-sense exercises, should be regularly incorporated into a flexibility program. The circumduction movement involved in *rond de jambe à terre* (both *en dedans* and *en dehors*), for example, is an excellent proprioceptive training exercise for the deep musculature of the hip joint.

If a dancer has been injured, it is very important that he/she maintains strength and flexibility during the rehabilitation period. This is also an optimal time to reeducate the body for returning to dance and preventing further injuries. Hence, flexibility exercises serve a therapeutic function.

Having a trained dancer visualize a mental image or images of the correct sequence of a motor movement pattern will facilitate proper performance of the movement. Intense visualization of the elements of complex movement patterns during relaxation apparently results in a sequential firing of gamma motor neurons in preparation for performance of the movement. This gamma motor activity controls proprioception sensitivity and muscle tone and, therefore, has a direct positive influence upon the accuracy and quality of the potential subsequent muscle contraction. By intensely visualizing the basic components of a combination of dance steps, for example, it is possible to have a "rehearsal" effect upon the efficient sequential firing of the gamma motor system. Performance can be enhanced through this mechanism. Therefore, visualization/relaxation techniques should be incorporated into the flexibility regimen.

Motor Activity and Muscle Flexibility

The motor system portion of the nervous system is a complex intermingling of subsystems which initiate, modify, control, and coordinate all motor movement patterns, from those that are simply postural to precise movements of the limbs. The motor system also controls *muscle tone*, which is defined as the resistance a muscle provides to passive movement or stretching of its associated limb.

Muscle flexibility is definitely affected by muscle tone. Likewise, muscle tone is the substrate for muscle flexibility and movement. For example, individuals who have had a stroke in the motor region of the cerebral cortex may exhibit spasticity of postural or limb musculature. Spasticity is the increased resistance of muscles to passive movement in one direction. The person may have chronically contracted flexors of the upper extremity (e.g., biceps brachii, and forearm flexors) and extensors of the lower extremity (e.g., the psoas, quadriceps femoris, and triceps surae). The increased muscle tone (hypertonia) or "tightness" of these muscle groups would demonstrate a drastic reduction in muscle flexibility. There would be increased resistance to passive extension of the upper extremity and flexion of the lower extremity.

However, the motor system is not the only factor that controls or determines muscle flexibility. There are a number of central and peripheral factors which contribute to muscle flexibility (Table 13.1). Effective stretching techniques may utilize one or more of these central and peripheral factors in order to increase muscle flexibility. The three major mechanisms of improving flexibility involve: altering the

TABLE 13.1.
Flexibility Factors

CENTRAL FACTORS
- **Limbic System and Cerebral Cortex**
  Emotional and behavioral input from the limbic system and the prefrontal lobes of the cerebral cortex affects muscle tone via the reticular formation.
- **Motor Systems**
  Descending pathways from the Reticular Formation, Vestibular, Extrapyramidal, and Pyramidal Systems influence muscle tone and movement.
- **Sensory Pathways**
  Proprioception
    Information from receptors in the muscles as well as specialized input from the visual and vestibular systems provide essential cues as to the position of the body and limbs in space.
  Tactile
    Various types of receptors in the skin for general and discriminative touch supply information about weight distribution over the supporting body part, and physical contact between body parts and with other dancers.
- **Spinal Cord Reflex Pathways**
  Myotatic Reflex
  Autogenic Inhibition Reflex
  Reciprocal Inhibition Reflex
  Gamma Efferent Pathway
PERIPHERAL FACTORS
- **Sensory Receptors**
  Neuromuscular Spindles in the Muscles
    These receptors detect tonic (static) and phasic (changing) stretching of the muscle. The sensitivity of the NMS is controlled by the gamma efferent system.
  Golgi Tendon Organs
    GTO's are specialized receptors in tendons that detect tension. They are part of a protective circuit to prevent injury to the musculo-tendinous unit due to excessive amounts of tension.
- **Biomechanical**
  Mechanical limits to Range of Motion
    Osseous, muscular, articular (joints), scar tissue
  Connective Tissue Mechanics
    Elastic (non-permanent) Stretch
    Plastic (permanent) Stretch

descending influences from the reticular formation in the brain through the use of relaxation/visualization techniques; utilizing spinal reflexes such as the autogenic inhibition, reciprocal inhibition, and gamma reflex pathways; and emphasizing biomechanical factors that elongate the plastic (permanent) elements of the connective tissue surrounding the muscle fibers. Each of these mechanisms is based upon the proper utilization of the central and peripheral factors that control muscle flexibility.

The Limbic System and Cerebral Cortex

Muscle tone and, to a certain degree, flexibility are controlled primarily by intricate complex neuroanatomical and neurophysiological mechanisms. Probably the most sophisticated of these—and certainly the least appreciated by dancers in terms of their contribution—are the extensive influences of the cerebral cortex and the limbic system. The prefrontal lobe of the cerebrum has a potentially powerful affect upon the initiation and modification of emotional behavior, while the limbic system tends to set the basic or primal emotional "tone" of a particular behavioral response.

Both of these areas of the brain can have an obvious affect on muscle tone, relaxation, and, ultimately, flexibility, because of their strong input into the reticular formation, which controls muscle tone. For example, when you are feeling very anxious about a particular situation, your muscle tone often increases. Remember the anxiety and nervousness of your first performances or auditions. Your muscles felt tense or tight, especially in the areas of the neck, shoulders, or lower back. Your movements were stiff, awkward, or robotic. Your timing was off. The slightest noise could cause you to nearly jump through the ceiling. This is a good example of how a psychological state (fear or anxiety) can directly influence muscle tone and physical performance. On the other hand, relaxation techniques can produce a reduction in muscle tone and a corresponding increase in flexibility (Figure 13.1). These techniques link deep breathing, positive visualization, and gentle stretching with the process of learning to "turn off" extraneous, tension-producing messages from the prefrontal and limbic cortices.

Effective stretching exercises require the use of relaxation and breathing techniques. When stretching, you should close your eyes, isolate the particular target muscle group, remove any anxiety associated with the exercise, relax and breath slowly and deeply, and try to visualize the correct performance of the exercise. Appropriate relaxing

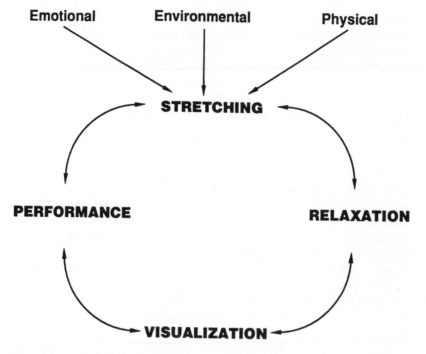

Figure 13.1. The Cycle of Stretching

or soothing music can help create a meditative ambience and aid in the slow progressive pacing of the exercises during a session.

The Motor System

Since muscle tone and, to a certain degree, muscle flexibility are controlled by the motor system, it is important for us to have a rudimentary conceptualization of how the motor system generates the complex motor movement patterns that form the basis of dance technique. The motor system may be conceptualized into six functionally interrelated parts: ideation, initiation, modification, modulation, transmission, and refinement of motor movement patterns (Table 13.2).

All areas of the cerebral cortex contribute to the initial formation of the impulse or "idea" to move. How a simple "idea" or intent to move (e.g., "I want to do an *assemblé* ") is transformed from a memory into a complex firing of neuronal impulses is a fascinating and little understood phenomenon. Once the "idea" is created, it is the job of the basal ganglia in the core of the brain to initiate a motor movement

TABLE 13.2.
Neurological Analogues of Motor Movement Patterns

CONCEPTUAL COMPONENTS		NEUROANATOMICAL LOCATION
Ideation	———	Cerebral Cortex
Initiation	———	Basal Ganglia
Modification	———	Cerebellum
Modulation	———	Motor Cortex
Transmission	———	Descending Motor Tracts
Refining	———	Primary Sensory & Reflex Circuits

pattern which will eventually activate those muscles involved in the *assemblé*. The cerebellum will then modify the motor movement pattern by coordinating and synchronizing the action of each of the muscles involved in the *assemblé*. The cerebellum relays this information back to the motor cortex for final modulation prior to sending impulses down the spinal cord. When these descending impulses reach a specific level of the spinal cord, they undergo a final "refining" process by incoming information from the spinal nerves before leaving the spinal cord to innervate the appropriate muscle groups necessary for performing an *assemblé*.

Motor movement patterns receive contributions and influences from five levels of the brain, and these specific patterns are subsequently superimposed upon a preexisting framework of muscle tone, which is largely under the control of spinal cord reflexes. Each system is located at successively higher levels of the brainstem and cerebrum. Generally, the higher the level, the more sophisticated or specialized the particular system. The five systems that contribute to the motor system are located at three general levels of the brain (Table 13.3). The

TABLE 13.3.
Components of the Motor System*

Medulla
   Vestibular System: Equilibrium stimuli affecting the axial muscles of the torso

Midbrain
   Tectum: Reflex responses from visual and auditory stimuli
   Reticular formation: Muscle tone via the gamma efferent system

Cerebrum
   Basal ganglia: Associative movements of the axial and proximal limb musculature
   Cerebral cortex: Movements of the distal limb musculature

*Listed from inferior to superior

systems at each of these levels can affect muscle tone and, therefore, via descending pathways, muscle flexibility.

The descending pathways from the motor system—along with the constant flow of incoming somatic sensory information—cause the continuous alterations in reflex activity which are integral to all motor movement activities. The most important of the descending motor pathways relative to muscle flexibility are the *Reticulospinal Tracts* from the reticular formation. These tracts or pathways play a vital role in controlling muscle tone—and, therefore, flexibility—via the gamma efferent pathway. Gamma efferent neurons control the sensitivity of the neuromuscular spindles in the muscles. These receptors detect stretch and provide the nervous system with critical information as to the position of the body and limbs (proprioception). There is an intimate relationship between proprioception and performance, and muscle tone and flexibility.

Sensory Pathways

The primary source of sensory information essential for motor activity is *proprioception*. Proprioceptive information is derived from the visual and vestibular systems, and receptors located in the muscle and tendons. All motor movement activity, whether crude or precise, requires accurate proprioceptive information to the brain and spinal cord.

Tactile information from the skin also plays a significant role in the successful performance of many motor activities. For example, precise tactile information from the ball of the foot is a critical factor in learning to get your weight over the supporting foot during *pirouettes*. All of these motor and sensory neurological factors that control muscle tone, flexibility, and proprioception merge at the level of the spinal cord and assert their influence upon the numerous intrinsic spinal cord reflex pathways.

Spinal Cord Reflexes

Spinal cord reflexes form the fundamental framework for all motor movement activity, in addition to controlling muscle tone. In fact, motor activity may be thought of as a modification of basic spinal reflexes by supraspinal systems. In computer terms, the spinal cord reflexes are the "hardware," and the brain, or supraspinal systems, are the "software." In this analogy the "hardwired" reflex pathways are constantly modified by new "software programs" developed from incoming somatic sensory information, and descending influences from supraspinal pathways.

COMPUTER	NEUROLOGICAL ANALOGUE
Software (Programs & Input)	Brain & Sensory Systems
Hardware (Circuit Boards)	Spinal Cord Reflexes

All effective flexibility exercises are based upon spinal cord reflexes. There are four fundamental reflex pathways—myotatic, autogenic inhibition, reciprocal inhibition, and gamma efferent—involved in muscle flexibility and stretching exercises. All are based, more or less, upon the basic reflex pathway. There are five components to the basic reflex pathway (Figure 13.2). The components of a basic reflex arc or pathway include both sensory (afferent) and motor (efferent) neurons, along with a highly versatile interneuron.

The key element in this circuit is the *interneuron*. It is the interneuron that determines the fundamental response pattern of the reflex arc. The interneuron may be either excitatory or inhibitory in terms of its neurophysiological function. Neuroanatomically, it may disperse the response to a stimulus to other neurons in that same segment of the spinal cord, or to other levels of the spinal cord, or to the opposite side of the spinal cord. An interneuron may also have extensive connections with the *reticular formation*, which plays a critically important

The Basic Reflex Arc

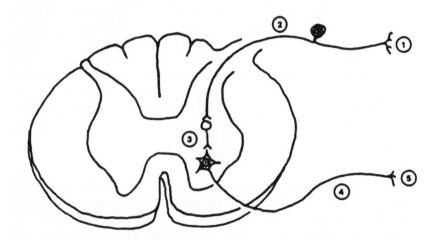

Figure 13.2. The Basic Reflex Pathway
    1. Receptor: detects stretch or tension
    2. Afferent (Sensory) Neuron
    3. Interneuron (excitatory or inhibitory)
    4. Efferent (Motor) Neuron
    5. Effector (Motor End Plate): Muscle

role in conditioned reflex patterns (i.e., patterned motor reflex responses). The reticular formation, along with several other descending motor pathways, has a fundamental role in basic movement patterns and the control of muscle tone.

Myotatic Reflex

The myotatic reflex is a two-neuron pathway involving a sensory afferent neuron (Ia) and an Alpha motor efferent neuron (Figure 13.3). There is no interneuron in this circuit. The sensory fiber conveys information originating from neuromuscular spindles (NMS) embedded in the muscles. These receptors detect tonic and phasic stretching of the muscle. Information from the neuromuscular spindles courses in spinal nerves to the spinal cord, where the type Ia sensory fibers will synapse upon Alpha motor neurons. Alpha motor neurons will, in turn, stimulate the muscle that contained the activated NMS to contract.

The myotatic reflex arc is strongly activated by rapid stretch of a muscle. Rapid stretching of the neuromuscular spindles in a muscle

Myotatic Reflex

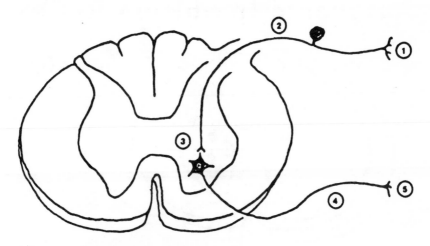

Figure 13.3. Myotatic Reflex
   1. Receptor: Neuromuscular Spindles
   2. Sensory Neuron: Ia Afferent
   3. Interneuron: None
   4. Motor Neuron: Alpha Motor
   5. Effector: Extrafusal Muscle Fibers
      Net Effect: stretch/contract

will cause that muscle to contract. For example, when your physician strikes the patellar tendon below your kneecap, the sudden stretch of the quadriceps muscle results in its contraction and the extension of the leg (Knee-Jerk Reflex).

In a similar way, ballistic or bouncy stretching techniques may elicit contraction of the target muscle group. These exercises activate the myotatic or stretch/contract reflex arc and increase the tightness of the target muscle. Ballistic stretches may also cause microscopic tears in the connective tissue surrounding the muscle cells. Slow, progressive static stretches for 30-60 seconds are more effective and relaxing and should be used for most muscle groups.

Autogenic Inhibition Reflex. The autogenic inhibition reflex is more typical of a basic three-neuron pathway involving a sensory (afferent) neuron, an inhibitory interneuron, and an Alpha motor efferent neuron (Figure 13.4). A sensory fiber (type Ib) conveys information originating from Golgi Tendon Organs (GTO) located in the tendons of muscles. These receptors detect excessive amounts of tension or physical stress in the muscle. Information from the GTO's travels in the spinal nerves to the spinal cord, where the type Ib sensory fibers will synapse upon small inhibitory interneurons. These interneurons will

Autogenic Inhibition Reflex

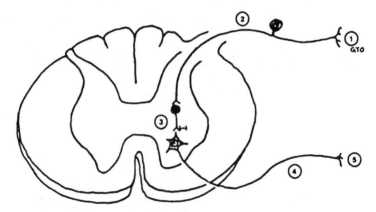

Figure 13.4. Autogenic Inhibition Reflex
1. Receptor: Golgi Tendon Organs
2. Sensory Neuron: Ib Afferent
3. Interneuron: Inhibitory
4. Motor Neuron: Alpha Motor
5. Effector: Extrafusal Muscle Fibers
   Net Effect: tension/relax

inhibit the function of the Alpha motor neurons. The decreased influence of Alpha motor neurons on the associated muscle will cause the muscle to relax. Excessive amounts of tension transmitted to the tendon by muscular contraction tend to cause neurophysiological inhibition of that same muscle. There are specific minimum thresholds for activation and central engagement of this reflex arc.

Autogenic inhibition protects the muscle from being injured by excessive amounts of tension. This tension/relax circuit can be utilized quite effectively in certain stretching techniques. In the specialized exercises at the end of this chapter autogenic inhibition is intentionally activated in order to induce muscle relaxation. During the contraction phase of the Proprioceptive Neuromuscular Facilitation (PNF) stretching technique, the autogenic inhibition (tension/relax) reflex is activated in the working muscle.

Reciprocal Inhibition Reflex.   Reciprocal inhibition is also representative of a basic three-neuron pathway involving a sensory (afferent) neuron, an inhibitory interneuron, and an Alpha motor efferent neuron (Figure 13.5). A type Ia sensory fiber conveys information originating from neuromuscular spindles (NMS) located in the muscles. Information

Reciprocal Inhibition Reflex

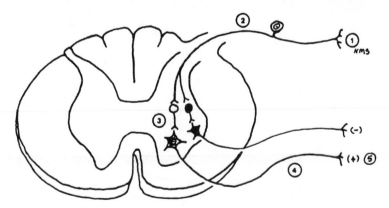

Figure 13.5. Reciprocal Inhibition Reflex
    1. Receptor: Neuromuscular Spindles
    2. Sensory Neuron: Ia Afferent
    3. Interneurons to Agonist (+) and Antagonist (−)
    4. Motor Neuron: Alpha Motor
    5. Effector: Extrafusal Muscle Fibers
       Net Effect: Contraction of agonist muscle,
              relaxation of antagonist muscle

from the neuromuscular spindles in a contracting muscle (agonist) travels in the spinal nerves to the spinal cord, where the type Ia sensory fibers will synapse upon small inhibitory interneurons. These interneurons will *inhibit* the function of the Alpha motor neurons to the antagonistic muscles. The decrease in Alpha motor neuron activity to the antagonistic muscle will cause the muscle to relax.

Contraction of a particular muscle, such as the quadriceps on the front of the thigh, will activate the reciprocal inhibition reflex and induce relaxation of antagonist muscle, in this case the hamstring. While you are performing certain flexibility exercises, you should concentrate upon contracting the muscle group which is antagonistic to the stretching muscle. This technique should provide an additional amount of relaxation of that muscle. Reciprocal inhibition is used naturally in dance when, for example, during the *demi-plié* the anterior tibialis muscle on the front of the legs is contracted in order to stretch the gastrocnemius and soleus muscles, resulting in a deeper *demi-plié*.

Gamma Efferent Pathway.   Muscle tone and proprioception is controlled by the gamma efferent pathway. The key neuron in this circuit is the gamma motor neuron located in the spinal cord (Figure 13.6).

Gamma Efferent Pathway

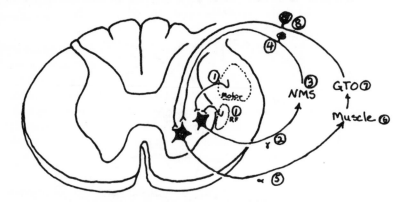

Figure 13.6. Gamma Efferent Pathway
    1. Descending Motor Pathways (corticospinal, reticulospinal tracts)
    2. Gamma Motor Neuron
    3. Intrafusal Muscle Fiber in NMS
    4. Ia Afferent Neuron
    5. Alpha Motor Neuron
    6. Extrafusal Muscle Fiber
    7. Golgi Tendon Organ
    8. Ib Afferent Neuron
       Net Effect: Changes in Muscle Tone

Gamma motor neurons are directly influenced by descending information from the reticular formation (reticulospinal tracts, RetST), in addition to receiving input from the basal ganglia (rubrospinal tracts, RST) and cerebral cortex (corticospinal tracts, CST). Output from the gamma motor neuron leaves the spinal cord, courses in a spinal nerve, and finally terminates in the specialized muscle fibers (intrafusal) which are encapsulated in the neuromuscular spindles.

Intrafusal muscle cells control the amount of tension and, therefore, sensitivity of the neuromuscular spindles. In other words, "tighter" spindles are more sensitive to being stretched. Information from the spindles is conveyed to the spinal cord via type Ia sensory fibers in the spinal nerves. Inside the spinal cord these fibers participate in a myotatic reflex, which will result in the contraction of some of the regular (extrafusal) muscle cells in the originating muscle, thus providing the muscle with tone.

The net result of the gamma efferent pathway is an alteration in muscle tone and the maintenance of accurate proprioceptive (position-sense) output from the neuromuscular spindles. Increased gamma motor activity causes a corresponding increase in muscle tone, or hypertonia. Decreased gamma motor activity results in a reduction of muscle tone, or hypotonia. Both hypertonia and hypotonia result in a decrease in the degree and accuracy of movement performed by an affected muscle. Optimal muscle tone, a dynamic balance between the two, is essential to the proper performance of the precise movements characteristic of dance technique.

However, while performing flexibility exercises it is possible and, indeed, preferable to induce some degree of hypotonia in order to enhance the stretching of the muscle. Since gamma motor activity is controlled by the brain—primarily through the reticular formation—it is possible to decrease muscle tone by incorporating the relaxation, visualization, and breathing techniques mentioned earlier. The gamma efferent pathway, along with the previously mentioned reflexes, form the neuroanatomical basis of the highly effective stretching technique of proprioceptive neuromuscular facilitation (PNF).

PNF, or contract/relax stretching techniques, involves three phases: 1) passive stretch for 20 seconds; 2) an 8 second isometric contraction; and 3) an increase in the amount of passive stretch. Contract/relax stretching exercises take advantage of the decreased muscle tension (hypotonia) that immediately follows an isometric contraction of a stretched muscle (phase 2). During this hypotonic phase, the muscle can be stretched even more (phase 3). PNF techniques are very effective for stretching larger muscle groups, such as the hamstrings, groin muscles, quadriceps femoris, and triceps surae (gastroc-soleus).

PNF is based upon four basic neuroscientific principles: resistance, reflex, irradiation, and successive induction. Voluntary isometric contraction of the passively stretched muscle, along with adjacent muscle groups, activates the Golgi tendon organs and the autogenic inhibition reflex. The subsequent inhibition of the contracted muscle is overridden by the powerful descending influences from the brain, which are causing the contraction. Stretching adjacent muscle groups (irradiation), voluntary concentric activation of antagonistic muscles, and alternating agonist muscle groups against antagonist groups on both sides of the body will induce increased inhibition of the stretched muscle after the voluntary contraction is complete. During the passive stretch phase of the exercise it is important to utilize mental relaxation and deep-breathing techniques in order to decrease gamma efferent activity and its effect upon muscle tone. PNF techniques for the hamstrings, groin adductor muscles, quadriceps, and gastroc-soleus muscles are described in the exercise description section of this chapter.

Biomechanical Factors in Flexibility

There may also be mechanical limits to range of motion, such as osseous, muscular, or articular structures. Osseous (bony) or scar tissue limitation may affect flexibility by physically restricting or impeding the movement of a joint. Muscles that are excessively tight from training, or as a result of neurological factors, may also limit flexibility. Finally, the type of joint may limit range of motion according to its function and structure.

Connective Tissue Mechanics.   When stretched, connective tissue surrounding the muscle cells (endomysium) exhibits both permanent (plastic) and non-permanent (elastic) elongation. Under normal conditions, when the stretch is removed the elastic elongation recovers, but the plastic elongation remains. When connective tissue is stretched, the relative proportion of elastic and plastic elongation within a particular muscle can vary widely, depending upon how, and under what conditions, the stretch is performed. The principal factors that influence the proportion of elastic/plastic elongation are the amount of applied force, duration of applied force, and the temperature of the tissue.

Elastic elongation response is affected by high-force, short-duration stretching, and normal or colder tissue temperatures. Ballistic or bouncy stretching techniques without warming up the muscle are representative of conditions that affect elastic elongation. These conditions also activate the myotatic (stretch/contract) reflex, and may cause microscopic tears in the tissue. Furthermore, they do not result in permanent elongation of the target muscle.

Plastic deformation is enhanced by low-force, long-duration stretching at elevated temperatures (113° F), with cooling taking place before release of the tension. Sustained gentle stretching of a muscle in a whirlpool, followed immediately by icing while the muscle is still stretched, produces permanent elongation of the muscle. This method of stretching also greatly reduces the risk of tissue trauma.

Guidelines for Flexibility Programs

1. Keep your program simple, painless, and soothing. Develop a fixed routine—including a set sequence of stretches—and stick with it.
2. Warm up for 5-10 minutes before starting your flexibility training. Ride a stationary bike, go for a brisk walk, or perhaps just take a nice hot bath or whirlpool before stretching. The resultant elevation in body temperature will make stretching more effective and comfortable, and reduce the possibility of injury.
3. Use static (30-60 sec.) stretches for most muscle groups, and PNF for hamstrings, adductors, and the triceps surae. Alternate stretching agonist-antagonist muscle groups. Your program should integrate gentle progressive exercises with slow, deep breathing and a relaxed mental state.
4. Perform these exercises in a quiet, warm, and comfortable environment. Limit the possibility of interruptions. The morning is usually the optimal time for flexibility and proprioceptive training. Therapeutic exercises are also best performed in the morning because generally a person concentrates better in the morning and has a decreased sensitivity to physical discomfort or mild pain.
5. Concentrate on correct form and alignment of the body. The benefits of any exercise are greatly diminished when it is performed improperly, and the risks of injury are significantly increased.
6. Keep your eyes closed, breathe slowly and quietly, and concentrate on relaxation and isolation of the mind and body. Learn to "turn off" extraneous gamma efferent activity from the spinal cord by removing the elements of anxiety and forceful determination from the exercises. Let the exercises work for you; relax and enjoy the sensation of stretching your muscles.
7. The exercises that follow are for serious dancers; they are not recommended for the general public, who have no need or preparation for the extreme flexibility demanded by high- performance

dance training. If one of these exercises is too difficult or uncomfortable to perform, you should check with an expert to find an alternative exercise or modification.

8. Use common sense when doing these exercises; *if it hurts, don't do it*. Ask yourself why it hurts (are you performing the exercise incorrectly, or is there a structural/functional problem?), and, if necessary, seek the advice of a qualified health professional.

Selected Flexibility Exercises

The flexibility of the groin, hamstring, and calf muscles is important to all dancers. Tightness of any one of these muscle groups will hamper the development of proper dance technique, and seriously predispose the dancer to injury. The following four exercises demonstrate the utilization of basic spinal cord reflexes and the fundamental principles of flexibility training that were discussed in this chapter. A more detailed and complete program of stretching and strengthening exercises for dancers may be found in *The Dancer's Complete Guide to Healthcare and a Long Career.**

1. Partnered Diamond Stretch (Adductors)

The partnered diamond exercise is an *advanced* stretching exercise which uses the contract/relax technique. Your groin (adductor) muscles should be warmed up prior to performing this exercise. You and your partner should be very cautious and aware of the possibility of overstretching. The adductor muscles are very sensitive to excessive tension and stretch; be careful and go slowly.

While you are in the Diamond position, a partner blocks your feet with his or her knees, and *gently and carefully* presses down on your knees until your groin (adductor) muscles are mildly stretched (Figure 13.7). After 20 seconds of static stretch (do not increase the stretch during this phase), very slowly start to push your knees against the resistance of your partner's hands. Gradually increase the intensity of the contraction for six seconds, sustain a maximal contraction for about two seconds, and then relax. Your partner then presses gently to increase the stretch. This initial passive stretch (phase 1), your isometric contraction (phase 2), and the relaxation and final stretch (phase 3), comprise one set of this exercise.

*A.J. Ryan and R.E. Stephens. (1988). *The Dancer's Complete Guide to Healthcare and a Long Career*. Chicago, Bonus, 165-196.

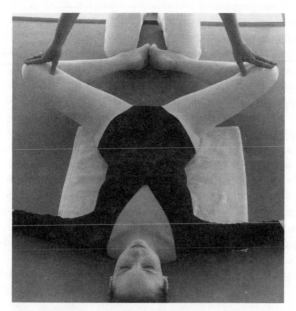

Figure 13.7. Partnered Diamond Stretch (adductors)

Your partner must be ready for the relaxation that initiates phase 3 and avoid applying excessive tension on your knees. A mild stretch is sufficient in this exercise, and both your partner and you need to be very aware of excessive amounts of tension in the groin muscles. If performed properly, you should not experience pain or discomfort. If you do, stop immediately. The abdominal muscles must maintain the proper tilt of the pelvis and alignment of the lower spine during this exercise.

After 20 seconds of relaxation the contraction can be repeated, and a total of three sets can be performed in a continuous series. Your partner should be aware that during the third set the extremely stretched groin muscle will be able to generate little force, and he or she should be very careful not to overstretch. It is best to do three or four sets at lesser intensities than one or two sets at maximal tensions. At the end of this exercise your knees are slowly brought back together by your partner.

2. Contract/Relax Hamstring Stretches

Contract/relax techniques are safe and effective methods for stretching the hamstrings. You may use a partner or perform this exercise on your own. The partnered hamstring stretch is most effective when your hamstrings are warmed up and you have a very trustworthy, responsible partner. As with all partnered exercises you should be very cautious and aware of the possibility of overstretching during this exercise.

While you are lying on your back, a partner supports your right leg with his or her right shoulder. Your partner *gently and carefully* applies pressure to your leg in order to stretch the hamstring muscles on the back of the thigh (Figure 13.8). After 20 seconds of static stretch (do not increase the stretch during this phase), very slowly start to push your right leg against the resistance of your partner's shoulder. Gradually increase the intensity of the contraction for six seconds, sustain a maximal contraction of the hamstring muscles for about two seconds, and then relax while your partner gently applies pressure to increase the stretch. During the contraction phase, both the agonist (hamstring and gluteals) and antagonist (quadriceps) muscle groups of both extremities should be activated.

As in the previous exercise, your partner must be ready for the relaxation and avoid applying excessive tension on your hamstrings (maintaining a staggered stance is important for the partner's balance).

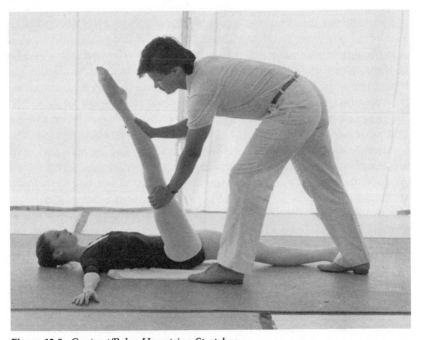

Figure 13.8. Contract/Relax Hamstring Stretches

A moderate stretch is sufficient in this exercise, and both your partner and you need to be very aware of excessive amounts of tension on the hamstrings.

Your partner's initial passive stretch, followed by your isometric contraction, relaxation, and the final stretch, comprise one set of this exercise. Three continuous sets are usually performed without releasing the stretch. By the third set the hamstrings will be so stretched that they will not be able to generate very much force; therefore, your partner should be very careful not to overstretch. It is best to do more sets at a lower intensity than one or two sets at maximal tension. At the end of this exercise the dancer's leg is slowly returned to the floor by the partner.

As an alternative to partnered hamstring stretches you can perform the same type of stretching technique by using a modified contraction/relaxation exercise. Lying on your back, bring the right leg up to hip level and support it by holding the back of the thigh with both hands (make sure you have a good grip). If your hamstrings are too tight to reach comfortably, use a towel to sling around the thigh. Stretch the hamstrings by gently pulling the right thigh towards the chest, keeping the knee straight. The left leg should not lift off of the floor and the left knee should be straight. Maintain a moderate stretch for about 20 seconds. Perform an isometric contraction by pushing against your hands (or towel) for 6-8 seconds. After the contraction, continue to gently stretch the hamstrings. Repeat the sequence two more times, and change sides. If the tension is too much at any point in the exercise, you can either reduce the stretch or bend the knee.

3. Modified Contract/Relax Standing Superficial Calf Stretch for the Gastrocnemius

In order to stretch the superficial calf muscle (gastrocnemius) simply lean toward the *barre* in a lunge, keeping the heel of the straight leg on the floor (Figure 13.9). Continue leaning forward until the heel begins to lift off the floor, and then press the heel down by using the tibialis anterior muscle and pushing against the *barre* with your hands. Hold the stretch for about 20 seconds, slowly rise to *demi-pointe* position against resistance, then slowly lower from the *demi-pointe* position while resisting this action. The *resistance* to *relevé* , produced by using one set of muscles to offset the action of another, is the key factor in inducing muscle stretch in this exercise. Repeat the sequence two more times.

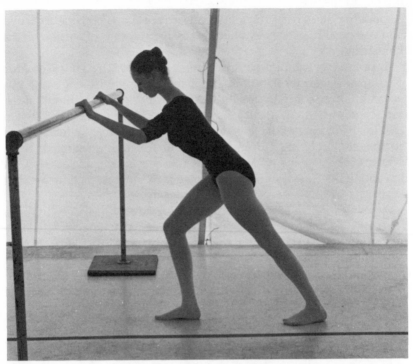

Figure 13.9. Modified Contract/Relax Standing Superficial Calf Stretch for the Gastroc-nemius

4. Modified Contract/Relax Standing Deep Calf Stretch for the Soleus

Continue your calf stretches by slowly bending the right knee of the back leg, while leaning forward and keeping the heel on the floor (Figure 13.10). Lean forward until the heel barely begins to lift off the floor and then press the heel down using the tibialis anterior muscle and by pushing against the *barre* with your hands. Hold the stretch for about 20 seconds, slowly rise to *demi-pointe* position against resistance, and slowly lower from the *demi-pointe* position while resisting this action. Once again, the resistance to *relevé* is the key factor in inducing muscle stretch in this exercise. Repeat this sequence two more times. After working one side, repeat the calf stretches on the other side.

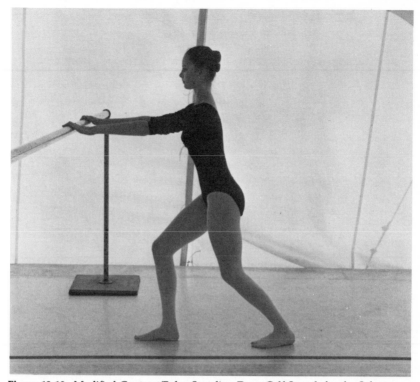

Figure 13.10. Modified Contract/Relax Standing Deep Calf Stretch for the Soleus

Sources

Carpenter, M.B., Sutin, J. (1983). *Human neuroanatomy.* 8th ed. Baltimore: Williams and Wilkins.

Gowitzke, B.A., Milner, M. (1988). *Understanding the scientific bases of human movement.* 3rd ed. Baltimore: Williams and Wilkins.

Noback, C.R., Demarest, R.J. (1981). *The human nervous system: basic principles of neurobiology.* 3rd ed. New York: McGraw-Hill.

Pansky, B., Allen, D.J., Budd, G.C. (1988). *Review of neuro-science.* 2nd ed. New York: Macmillan.

Ryan, A.J., Stephens, R.E. (1988). *The dancer's complete guide to healthcare and a long career.* Chicago: Bonus Books.

Ryan, A.J., Stephens, R.E., eds. (1987). *Dance medicine: a comprehensive guide.* Chicago and Minneapolis: Pluribus Press/The Physician and Sportsmedicine.

Sapega, A.A., Quedenfeld, T.C., Moyer, R.A., Butler, R.A. (1981, Dec.). Biophysical factors in range-of-motion exercise. *The Physician and Sportsmedicine, 9:*57-65.

Stephens, R.E. (1989). *Clinical neuroanatomy: a case history approach.* 5th ed. Kansas City: University of Health Sciences.

Acknowledgements: Photos by the author. Photo model, Jessica Stulik.

14

Stress, Performance, and Dance Injuries: Suggestions for Prevention and Coping

Raymond W. Novaco, Ph.D.

To a much greater extent than is true of other artistic performers, the dancer's training and performance regimens present risk for incapacitating injury. Gelsey Kirkland, for example, in her recent *Dancing on My Grave*,[1] poignantly describes the toll taken on her body by the need to meet choreographers' demands. Enduring perpetual inflammation and traumatic injuries, as well as Ballanchine's and Robbins' insensitivity to such matters, stretched her physical and psychological resources beyond the limit.

One suspects that nothing could have helped Ms. Kirkland—hers is clearly the extreme case—but generally speaking stress coping skills can both help to prevent injuries and facilitate recovery from them. They can also contribute to performance enhancement. These skills, which are based on psychological techniques which have been corroborated by a good deal of research, are being widely used in the field of sports psychology. This chapter will explore some of the potential applications of stress reduction to dance. First, however, some basic ideas about the nature of stress and how we are affected by it need to be discussed.

Stress, Arousal, and Emotion

Stress is something of a two-sided coin: in one sense we feel oppressed and victimized by it; in another, it is a red badge of courage that has become fashionable to wear. Stress-management in fact became a hot business some years ago, with an exponential growth of programs offering ways of boosting productivity while lowering stress.[2] One wonders with reason whether the contemporary sensitivity to stress is not just another form of the narcissistic concern with well-being and tendency to blame external circumstances for psychological states that are endemic in our society. Yet the fact remains that there is considerable research in the health and behavioral sciences that has linked stressful circumstances to health impairments, psychological disorders, and decrements in performance.

In everyday usage, stress refers to forces and feelings "out there" that put pressure on us, and also to something "in here" that is akin to a nervous disorder. This dual point of reference creates some ambiguity in how we envision and discuss the subject. Scientific views of stress are not without ambiguities either, but they generally represent it as a condition inherent in the organism or system, stimulated by exposure to environmental demands, and resulting in impairments to health and performance. Simply put, stress is a condition of imbalance between perceived demands and our resources for coping with them.[3,4,5] The demand/resource imbalance, abstract though it seems, is manifested in concrete physiological and mental disruptions. These conditions can have long-term adverse consequences; when prolonged, they can magnify into recurrent emotional distress, performance failures, and self-destructive behavior. There may also be impairments to physical health, such as ulcers, headaches, and cardiovascular disorders.

The casual incorporation of "stress" into common parlance, in part through the marketing of stress management techniques, has led to such linguistic nonsense as a distinction between "positive" and "negative" stress. Selye[6] inadvertently promoted this distinction by introducing the term "eustress" (as opposed to "distress") to describe those external conditions—such as work pressures, life challenges, performance demands, and even some kinds of crises—that can on occasion motivate one to exceptional levels of achievement. Despite its appeal to management consultants, no one has ever substantially developed the concept of "eustress." Quick and Quick,[7] for example, advocate the dual concept ("eustress/distress"), but throughout their book use the term "stress" to refer almost exclusively to adverse conditions and consequences. The principal effect of this way of thinking has been to confuse stress with coping (i.e., the skills we acquire to produce beneficial outcomes in the struggle with adversity), and especially with arousal.

Arousal is very much a part of stress (although many things that produce arousal are not stressful), and the level of arousal has a great deal to do with health. The ability to regulate arousal, especially that associated with emotional reactions, is a central part of stress management, and bears heavily on such matters as the rehabilitation of injuries. Tension, frustration, and demoralization are common reactions to injury that inevitably impair the recovery process.

Stress research often has involved measures of physiological arousal, and it is routinely assumed that physiological disturbances underlie illness. Scientific interest in the physiology of stress was sparked by Cannon,[8] who called attention to the connection between bodily states associated with emotional arousal and those produced by such extreme physical conditions as cold, lack of oxygen, and blood loss. Since Cannon, the autonomic nervous system (ANS) generally is recognized as central to stress responses. This system regulates the heart and smooth muscles of the body, the digestive system, sweat glands, and certain endocrine functions. While the sympathetic system component of the ANS is activated to mobilize the body's resources in response to threat, the parasympathetic component also is important because of its relevance to digestion, recuperation, and relaxation.

The significance of physiological arousal with regard to stress is threefold. First, pronounced physiological activation constitutes a disturbance of homeostatic balance. The continued onset of arousal and its prolongation are thought to be related to disease processes that affect the heart, gastrointestinal system, kidneys, and pancreas, as well as pain and discomfort in the skeletal musculature. For example, acute psychophysiologic reactivity has been linked to the occurrence of cardiovascular disease.[9] "Hot responders," those who react to threat or challenge with large increases in arousal, are at greater risk for coronary problems.

Second, heightened physiological arousal can have a detrimental effect on performance. If arousal is too high, performance suffers, just as it does when arousal is too low. In the stress literature and in sports psychology this is represented as an "inverted U function" for the relationship between arousal and performance. This concept originated with Duffy[10,11] and Hebb,[12] and was later adopted in research on anxiety. While Duffy focused on the relationship between muscle tension and performance, Hebb discussed the arousal function in terms of information processing. In this regard, Easterbrook[13] explained the arousal-caused impairment of performance in terms of "cue utilization"; arousal narrows the range of cues a person can use in doing a task. The more complex the task, the more cues are involved, and the more disruptive become the effects of high arousal. Therefore, the idea of maintaining an "optimum level of arousal" appears. This implies that the level of arousal needs to fit the task and its performance requirements.

When a task has many mental components, or if there are precise movements to be performed (as there characteristically are in dance), the importance of moderating arousal is greatest. If arousal is too low, there is little effort and no intensity. If arousal is too high, there is decreased concentration and poor execution. The way in which a particular level of arousal will affect performance very much depends on the requirements of the task and the skill level of the performer. High arousal should be less disruptive to gross motor movements that have become automatic in the performer's repertoire.

A third aspect of the significance of physiological arousal as a component of stress is its intrinsic role in the disruptive emotions. Arousal is closely associated with such emotions as fear, anger, and disappointment, and it is in the realm of our thinking about this association that we have come furthest in defining our beliefs about the activation and control of stress. Prior to the eighteenth century emotions were understood as passions by which we are "gripped," "seized," or "torn."[14] This view suggests that emotional reactions are strictly the result of things that happen to us. However, more recently we have come to see ourselves as architects of our experiences, and only rarely as their victims. We construct our experience, and much of that construction takes place in the head, while the rest is produced by our own behavior. This belief in human volition is a major theme of stress reduction interventions. Cognitive control techniques are widely used for stress management and in the regulation of pain. Knowing how to use the power of the mind as a coping skill is partly dependent on recognizing dysfunctional thought processes for what they are.

The Importance of What Goes On in Our Heads

Performance anxiety can be understood as that condition in which we are alarmed about the consequences of performing inadequately. Preoccupation with perceived personal inadequacy has consistently been found to impair performance. Such dysfunctional cognitions not only elicit and heighten anxiety, but they also interfere with task-relevant activity. Sarason aptly described this process: a situation is seen as difficult and threatening; anticipating that situation, we view ourselves as inadequate to the task, focusing on the undesirable consequences of the perceived inadequacy; strong self-deprecatory preoccupations interfere with mental functioning, and the anticipation of failure and loss of regard from others. In this vicious cycle of anxiety-engendering occurrences, a self-fulfilling prophesy is indeed realized.[15]

Among the early pioneers of sports psychology was Timothy Gallwey,[16] who also recognized the importance of what goes on in our head with regard to successful performance. In Gallwey's analysis, performance anxiety springs from self-doubt. The lack of trust in one's ability to perform to full capacity leads to anxiety and to physiological "tightening." Otherwise smooth, efficient movements become halting and self-conscious. Furthermore, the relationship between self-doubt, anxiety, and performance is a vicious cycle, or as system theorists would say, a "deviation-amplification" process: self-doubt produces anxiety, which leads to performance errors, which create further self-doubt, and so on. Sensations of weakness in bodily joints, light-headedness, and general loss of muscle tone can be symptoms of self-doubt. Quite commonly, people in this state compensate by trying too hard.

Stage fright is an amplification of normal anxiety reactions which have escalated to debilitating levels. It is normal to be nervous before performing in front of an audience, but if the performer gives undue attention to anxiety symptoms (e.g., butterflies, dizziness, rapid breathing, excess perspiration, trembling, etc.) nervousness can escalate into panic. The dancer may fear losing control, become hypercritical, and dwell on expectations of failure.

Being on stage, of course, means being the center of attention with few places, if any, to hide. "Dancing in front of an audience involves risk—a slip, misstep, gesture offbeat, forgetting what is supposed to be done. Fear of failure is most troubling. Dreadful apprehension may also occur when the theme of the dance threatens to become real, that is, the roles the dancers enact are too close to the performers' immediate personal life experiences."[17] To be sure, some accomplished dancers experience stage fright throughout their careers, but they are able to focus on the performance, preventing the anxiety from becoming debilitating. This is an application of the idea of being task-oriented, which psychological research has shown to be a fundamental coping skill in controlling disruptive emotions.[18]

In addition to producing certain emotional episodes like stage fright, our cognitions play an important role in the experience of pain. The perception and tolerance of pain are psychologically mediated processes. As Melzack and Wall theorized, pain is a multidimensional phenomenon involving sensory, motivational, and cognitive-evaluative components.[19] Because of intense desires to excel and the pressures of competition, dancers may ignore pain signals from their bodies that warn against continued exertion. Kirkland gives numerous examples of subjecting herself to chronic strain. In describing the compulsory regimens for turn-out, she recalls: "There was no regard for the knees or hips, which in my case were distorted to the breaking point."[1] Despite advice from an orthopedic surgeon regarding her feet which had turned purple from inflammation, she "danced through the pain and compensated." As perhaps in this instance, a dancer's attitude toward physical injury may sometimes involve a touch of self-destructiveness, or be a way to cover career disappointments.[20]

The influence of mind on body has been recognized at least since the Greek and Roman Stoic philosophers. Hence, one can say with some certainty that such mental processes as attention, expectation, appraisal, and reflection have a significant bearing on stress responses. The allocation of attention, our expectations of self and others, the appraisal or interpretation of events and circumstances, and our reflection, reconstruction, and rehearsal of experiences are important determinants of stress and coping.

Stress Interventions

In the past decade, considerable work in the area of cognitive-behavior therapy has spearheaded progress on stress intervention techniques, which have been extended to the field of sports psychology, as well as to behavioral medicine and health psychology.[21,22] Across the now vast body of clinical research, stress reduction interventions can be understood in terms of remediation procedures, regulatory techniques, and preventive strategies. *Remediation procedures* are interventions implemented to curtail and treat stress reactions. Various psychological and medical procedures are available for such therapeutic action. *Regulatory techniques* are psychological coping tactics utilized to counteract precursors or elements of stress reactions, particularly with regard to tension, emotion, and cognition predisposing to stress. Behavior patterns linked with recurrent stress episodes might also be modified in a self-regulatory effort. *Preventive strategies* involve proactive personal and organizational action designed to reduce exposure to stressors, to develop skills for dealing with environmental demands, and to augment environmental and social resources that promote well-being.

The full scope of stress interventions obviously cannot be described here, but two central procedures—arousal reduction and cognitive restructuring—will be briefly discussed. The associated techniques would seem to have utility for dance performance.

Arousal Reduction

Procedures designed to reduce arousal are commonly part of stress management programs. Both mental and physical relaxation are emphasized to control and regulate tension. The first structured approach in the medical and psychological literature was Jacobson's progressive relaxation method of systematically tensing and then relaxing sequential sets of skeletal muscles.[23] Programs of this sort share roots in such ancient Eastern practices as yoga and Tai Chi, but it was not until the emergence of Transcendental Meditation cults in the 1960s and 70s that Eastern ideas about relaxation gained widespread recognition. Basically, in TM technique the person sits comfortably in a quiet place with eyes closed, focuses on breathing, and repeats a mantra silently for 10 to 20 minutes, once or twice daily. Highly significant degrees of arousal reduction across many physiological channels have been found to be associated with TM practice.

Another relaxation induction procedure is autogenic training, developed by Schultz and Luthe. Autogenic training was conceived by Schultz, a German psychiatrist, as a form of self-hypnosis that could be used to create mental resolve for behavior change, as well as to modify physiological conditions in specific organ areas. The technique emphasizes smooth, rhythmic breathing, self instructions of calmness, and the use of suggestions of "heaviness" and "warmth" for body regions, especially limbs.

In addition to these self-administered techniques of arousal reduction, other more technical procedures, such as biofeedback and hypnosis, have demonstrated utility. The goal of each method is to teach the subject to control troublesome internal states. Having the capability to regulate arousal and tension, it has been found, improves the likelihood of optimum performance.

Cognitive Restructuring

Various procedures are being used extensively in clinical work to modify cognitive dimensions of stress disorders. Changing belief systems, modifying perceptions, altering the focus of attention, eliminating intrusive thoughts, and adjusting expectation are among the tactics utilized to help clients restructure how they view the world and themselves. The treatment efficacy of such procedures has been documented.[24,25] Problems involving anxiety disorder, depression, assertiveness, pain, eating disorders, anger, alcoholism, and smoking have all been successfully treated with cognitively based behavioral programs.

With regard to stress, the process of coping effectively entails the ability to ascertain the nature of problems, think of alternative solutions, identify steps to solution, anticipate obstacles, and utilize feedback from coping efforts. These elements all correspond to the necessities of injury rehabilitation. However, not all sources of stress are amenable to mastery. Natural disasters, aging, serious injury, disease, and the death of loved ones are examples of such conditions. Hence, the concept of coping acknowledges that there may well be constraints on possible outcomes and the availability of means. The severity of an injury (e.g., a joint sprain vs. a total rupture of a major tendon) may indeed limit the dancer's ability to regain pre-injury proficiency.

One promising cognitive technique that is getting extensive use in the area of sport psychology is visuo-motor behavioral rehearsal (VMBR). This technique involves relaxation, visualization of performance, and performance in a simulated stressful situation. It is important that the subject have an accurate mental image of optimum performance and be able to visualize the details of the behavioral sequence. Suinn[26] developed this technique as a way of removing emotional obstacles to performance, and has used it effectively with Olympic skiers. Other investigators have tried it with tennis players and karate competitors in tournament situations.[27,28] Although results across dependent measures are not always significant, there is some evidence for performance enhancement. Studies of basketball players also showed positive results.[29,30]

Regarding many kinds of stress arising from economic and occupational experiences, the most effective forms of coping involve the modification of goals and values. Goal setting is a cognitive-behavioral skill that has been incorporated into many stress reduction programs and other approaches to performance enhancement. It involves an assessment of personal values, and a clear specification of short-term goals. A timetable with realistic expectation is a useful tool.

The dancer who may be experiencing stress from competitive pressures, along with the intense desire to perform to perfection, can be helped by a goal setting strategy. The success of this hinges on an accurate knowledge of the performance requirements and a realistic assessment of the dancer's capabilities. In conjunction with this analysis, training procedures can be designed to improve diet, strength, flexibility, and conditioning. The visualization of goals, to be achieved through practice, can be a useful adjunct.

Work stress is often generated by unrealistically high expectations of personal capacity. Trying to accomplish too much in a short time creates overload, which is highly stressful; therefore, time management is an important stress coping skill. Intense, unpredictable, and uncontrollable stressors disturb concentration, so the first step is overload avoidance. Learning to avoid excessive obligations can be difficult for high achievers, but peak performance is more likely to occur through relaxed concentration than frenzied strain. Concentration on the here and now requires quietude of mind, undistracted by preoccupations. A lapse in concentration because of worries or fatigue detracts from proper technique, which raises the probability of injury.

Dance Injuries and Stress Coping Skills

Conditions of stress present risk for injury. A dancer who is preoccupied with worries, frustrations, disappointments, or antagonisms is distracted and tense. Chronic discontent with one's achievement, especially if coupled with fatigue, "sets the stage for carelessness."[20] When competitive pressures and the demands of choreographers raise stress levels, the mind must be focused and the body relaxed to avoid injury.

Kirkland recalls a rehearsal when she had misgivings about a choreographer's insistence on a particular lift and slide, which then had tragic consequences:

> My new partner, John, picked me up and put me down as Jerry (Robbins) instructed. I had the helpless feeling that I was falling from a ten-story building. My foot jammed into the floor with a crunch loud enough to tell me that I was in deep trouble. My foot was broken. Clenching my teeth, I managed to walk off the stage without making a sound. Then I howled, my head full of tears.[1]

Although the injury is construed by Kirkland as resulting from the choreographer's foolishness, what she reveals about her state of mind preceding the incident and her rage reaction afterwards suggests that stress was not irrelevant.

Injury itself becomes a major stressor. As Kirkland states, at the moment of injury the question "Will I ever dance again?" shoots through the brain of every dancer. Mazo gives multiple examples of the "Damn-the-pain-the-show-must-go-on" mentality that permeated the New York City Ballet, leaving the company at times well suited for a hospital ward.[31] However, there is an important difference between enduring discomfort in the spirit of commitment and risking serious injury because of fear that one will be summarily replaced.

The motivating quality of commitment is evident in life-sustaining contexts, enabling the person to withstand severely adverse conditions—physiological ones, such as chemotherapy, or environmental ones, such as concentration camps. The strength of commitment enforces the pursuit of goals in the face of obstacles and thereby blunts the pain experience. The committed person is impelled toward coping with stress and is more apt to sustain the coping efforts.[32] However, although commitment is central to psychological well-being, it also renders the person vulnerable to threat. The dancer who is deeply committed to a distinguished career is more threatened by an injury than one who has less lofty ambitions. Hence, commitment is a two-sided factor with regard to injuries; the difference is between conditions of motivation/determination and those of anxiety/insecurity. It is one thing to endure discomfort, but it is quite another to cause greater tissue or structural damage by ignoring bodily signals.

Although denial of injury is a normal way of coping among intense persons who are dedicated to achievement, the persistence of pain dictates taking the longer view of injury, sacrificing ego for recuperation and rehabilitation. Stress coping skills are useful in dealing with the frustration and demoralization that can ensue. We are affected emotionally by what we pay attention to and how it is appraised or interpreted. Cognitive restructuring combined with a sensible goal-setting strategy, including the visualization of renewed performance strength, can be an effective combination. Having an image of a long-term goal (as, for example, Roger Bannister had an image of breaking the four-minute mile) is one way to start, but the goal should be realistic. Then imagery can be used to envision step-by-step the achievement of that goal, including the overcoming of obstacles anticipated along the way. Because the recovery from injury is often complicated by set-backs of either a physical or psychological nature, visualization can facilitate coping. In visualizing dance performance itself, kinetic, tactile, auditory, and scenic images can be utilized.

Among the most important stress-mitigating factors is the availability and utilization of supportive social relationships. While social relations can have negative as well as positive effects on psychological well-being,[33] it has often been found that social support has a "buffering" effect on stressful life experiences. Supportive relationships can enhance coping with stressful events and perhaps also reduce exposure to such events; it may even directly benefit physical and psychological health. Although the psychological mechanisms remain to be understood, social support protects us from otherwise debilitating forces associated with life crises and daily hassles. When faced with a serious injury, friends and colleagues can provide the best antidote to demoralization and prolonged distress. Using those valued relationships will help to maintain self-esteem and provide encouragement during rehabilitation.

Stress has been neglected as a subject relevant to dance performance and dance injuries. This chapter has pointed to several areas of stress involvement, including arousal functions, disruptive emotions, cognitive interference, and coping with injury itself. There are a number of stress regulatory interventions, shown to be efficacious by clinical research, that hold promise for enhancing dance performance and promoting well-being among dancers. It is the author's hope that the new field of dance medicine will incorporate research on stress and coping.

References

1. Kirkland, G (1986). *Dancing on my grave*. New York: Doubleday.
2. Guenther, R. (1982, Sept.). Stress-management plans abound, but not all programs are run well. *Wall Street Journal, 30,* 33 (sec 2, col 4-6).
3. Cox, T. (1978). *Stress*. Baltimore: University Park Press.
4. Lazarus, R.S. (1966). *Psychological stress and the coping process*. New York: McGraw-Hill.
5. McGrath, J.E., ed. (1970). *Social and psychological factors in stress*. New York: Holt, Rinehart and Winston.
6. Selye, H. (1976). *The stress of life*. New York: McGraw-Hill.
7. Quick, J.C., Quick, J.D. (1984). *Organizational stress and preventative management*. New York: McGraw-Hill.
8. Cannon, W.B. (1929). *Bodily changes in pain, hunger, fear and rage*. 2nd ed. New York: D. Appleton.
9. Krantz, D.S., Manuck, S.B. (1984). Acute psychophysiologic reactivity and risk of cardiovascular disease: a review and methodological critique. *Psychological Bulletin, 96,* 435-464.
10. Duffy, E. (1932). The relation between muscular tension and quality of performance. *American Journal of Psychology, 44,* 535-546.
11. Duffy, E. (1957). The psychological significance of the concept of "arousal" or "activation." *Psychological Review, 64,* 265-275.
12. Hebb, D.O. (1955). Drives and the c.n.s. (conceptual nervous system). *Psychological Review, 62,* 243-254.
13. Easterbrook, J.A. (1959). The effect of emotion on cue utilization and the organization of behavior. *Psychological Review, 66,* 183-201.
14. Averill, J.R. (1974, Oct.). An analysis of psychophysiological symbolism and its influence on theories of emotion. *Journal for the Theory of Social Behavior, 4,* 147-190.
15. Sarason, I.G. (1978). The test anxiety scale: concept and research. In: Spielberger, C.D., Sarason, I.G., eds. *Stress and anxiety, 5.* New York: John Wiley.
16. Gallwey, W.T. (1974). *The inner game of tennis*. New York: Bantam Books.
17. Hanna, J.L. (1988). *Dance and stress: resistance, reduction and euphoria*. New York: AMS Press.
18. Novaco, R.W. (1985). Anger and its therapeutic regulation. In: Chesney, M.A., Rosenman, R.H., eds. *Anger and hostility in cardiovascular and behavioral disorders*. Washington: Hemisphere.
19. Melzack, R., Wall, P. (1965). Pain mechanisms: a new theory. *Science, 150*:971-979.
20. Horosko, M., Kupersmith, J.R.F. (1987). *The dancer's survival manual*. New York: Harper and Row.

21. Meichenbaum, D. (1977). *Cognitive behavior modification: an integrative approach.* New York: Plenum Press.
22. Meichenbaum, D., Jaremko, M.E., eds. (1983). *Stress reduction and prevention.* New York: Plenum Press..
23. Jacobson, E. (1929). *Progressive relaxation.* Chicago: University of Chicago.
24. Kendall, P.C., Hollon, S.D., eds. (1979). *Cognitive-behavioral interventions: theory, research and procedures.* New York: Academic Press.
25. Kendall, P. (1982). *Advances in cognitive-behavioral research and therapy.* New York: Academic Press.
26. Suinn, R. (1972). Removing emotional obstacles to learning and performance by visuo-motor behavior rehearsal. *Behavior Therapy,* 3:308-310.
27. Noel, R.C. (1980). The effect of visuo-motor behavior rehearsal on tennis performance. *Journal of Sport Psychology,* 2:221-226.
28. Weinberg, R.S., Seabourne, T.G., Jackson, A. (1981). Effects of visuo-motor behavior rehearsal, relaxation, and imagery on karate performance. *Journal of Sport Psychology,* 3:228-238.
29. Hall, E.G., Erffmeyer, E.S. (1983). The effect of visuo-motor behavior rehearsal with videotaped modeling on free throw accuracy of intercollegiate female basketball players. *Journal of Sport Psychology,* 5:343-346.
30. DeWitt, D.J. (1980). Cognitive and biofeedback training for stress reduction with university athletes. *Journal of Sport Psychology,* 2:288-294.
31. Mazo, J.H. (1974). *Dance is a contact sport.* New York: Saturday Review Press.
32. Lazarus, R.S., Folkman, S. (1984). *Stress, appraisal, and coping.* New York: Springer.
33. Rook, K.S. (1984). The negative side of social interaction: impact on psychological well-being. *Journal of Personality and Social Psychology,* 46:1097-1108.

Recommended Reading

1. Benson, H. (1975). *The relaxation response.* New York: Morrow.
2. Charlesworth, E.A., Nathan, R.G. (1982). *Stress management.* New York: Ballantine Books.
3. Garfield, C.A. (1984). *Peak performance: mental training techniques of the world's greatest athletes.* Los Angeles: JP Tarcher.
4. Mason, J.W. (1975, Mar. and June). A historical view of the stress field. *Journal of Human Stress,*1,6-12, 22-36.
5. Solway, D. (1986, June). In a dancer's world, the inexorable foe is time. *New York Times,* 8:1 (sec 2, col 1).

PART IV:

Practical Concerns

15

Finding the Right Physician

Allan J. Ryan, M.D.

Should I See a Doctor?

Let's face it, from a health standpoint dance is a hazardous line of work. One statistical study after another indicates that if you dance long enough you *will* have injuries. Some of these will be severe and obviously require medical attention, others will appear at least to be minor, while most will fall in the gray area between. Because your ability to pursue your chosen occupation depends so heavily on maintaining the health of your body, it is crucial that you handle these situations properly.

I would like to suggest that if there is any question in your mind about whether or not to consult a physician regarding an injury you encounter as a dancer, you *should* do it. "Of course," you say to yourself, "that's a doctor speaking. They all think they (and only they) have the answers to all things, and besides, they need to drum up business." Also, probably, this advice runs against your grain; you are concerned about the expense and fearful of being told to stop dancing. You know that there is plenty of sympathetic help closer at hand; other dancers, directors, or choreographers always seem to have been through something like what you are experiencing, and can therefore tell you what to do and who to see for treatment.

The problem is that diagnosing injuries is often anything but a simple matter, and proper diagnosis is crucial to getting injuries quickly under control. There are plenty of "therapists" in virtually any community who can administer a wide variety of treatments— some entirely valid, others less so—but none of these people is certifiably qualified to do *diagnosis*. That is the exclusive province of MDs, who have not only extensive training in this area to draw upon, but also an arsenal of super-sensitive technologies at their disposal. The therapists to whom one might go, including those who are being drawn increasingly into the offices and clinics of dance/sports medicine doctors, can often do wonderful things toward restoring ailing bodies to health, but, again, they are not qualified to determine what is wrong. It is for this reason that in most states today physical therapists can see patients only on the referral of a doctor. The understanding implicit in that law is that doctors will diagnose and therapists will treat.

Choosing the Right Physician

Now let us consider what kind of doctor you should see. Like professional sports teams, some of the larger dance companies today have formed affiliations with their own physician(s). If you are fortunate enough to belong to one of these companies, the business of choosing a physician has been done for you; the company's doctor will deal with your injuries him/herself, or refer you to specialists with whom he/she is in turn affiliated. Or perhaps you already have a personal physician who looks after your health needs; young dancers living at home, for instance, are often under the care, through families, of an internist, a generalist, or a family practitioner. This is a perfectly fine arrangement; it meets your basic need of having someone who knows you and your health history and will assume responsibility for dealing with new problems as they arise or coordinating the work of specialists as required.

But suppose you are on your own, far removed from family and uncovered by institutional health plans. As with anyone in the population at large, it would be a good idea, assuming that you expect to live in the same place for some time, to seek out a personal physician even before you have any specific need of one. Let the doctor take a health history and give you a general examination so he/she can use the knowledge of what your body is like in its healthy state as a baseline against which to measure any pathogenic condition that develops.

Because you are a dancer you may well be guided in your search by a desire to find a doctor who is accustomed to dealing with dancers. Before you settle on a personal physician try to find out from his/her appointment secretary if he/she has other dancers for patients. Lacking advanced information, you might ask the doctor about this on your first visit. This would also be the time to find out what this physician knows about dance in general and feels about the dancer's imperative to keep dancing and working while a problem is being managed. Assuming he/she has a general interest in dance (otherwise your relationship may be short-lived), this would be a good time to start explaining where you fit into the dance world: what type(s) of dance you do, what specific technique(s) you use, how many hours/week you study, rehearse, perform, etc.

If you are not able to identify a personal physician, you may be in an area that is served by a new type of clinic that caters to persons in all of the performing arts. These are currently located in New York City, Boston, Braintree (MA), Morristown (NJ), Cincinnati, Cleveland, Louisville, Indianapolis, St. Louis, Austin, Houston, Denver, Chicago, and San Francisco. Such a clinic includes both primary care physicians and specialists. You might also seek help at a sports medicine clinic. Although many of these have not had much experience with dancers, the health needs of athletes (especially as regards injuries) are similar enough that their doctors will be particularly well qualified to assist you.

In the Physician's Office

When you have an appointment with a physician or clinic that you have selected, prepare yourself beforehand so that your time and that of the physician can be used effectively. Review what you are going to say, so you don't forget anything important. If your visit concerns an injury, when, exactly, did it happen and under what conditions? What treatment, if any, have you had for it before your present visit? Has the injured body part been previously injured? If so, when, what treatment did you have, and what was the result? If it is an illness that brings you to the doctor, when did it start, how is it bothering you, and what have you done for it? Have you had the same thing before, and if so, when? If you have more than one illness or injury to discuss, make a list so you will remember everything.

When you are telling the physician about your problem(s), try to determine if he/she is listening to you carefully or is being distracted by the telephone or other interruptions. The physician will probably ask questions which give you an idea of whether he/she understands you correctly. You should like this person, or at least you should feel that he/she takes you and your problems seriously to heart. Don't be afraid to ask questions of your own; history-taking should be a dialogue.

When you and the physician are satisfied about your history, the physician will want to make a physical examination that is appropriate to your problem. This may include tests of your blood and urine and perhaps some x-rays. These may be done in the physician's office or elsewhere, depending on their nature. Most clinics are equipped to do their own testing.

After all information is in, the physician will give you a diagnosis of your condition. Make sure you understand exactly what it means; if you don't, ask for further explanation. You and the physician should have a good discussion of its significance for you and of what treatment may be necessary. If that will involve seeing another physician or a therapist, you should know exactly who it is you are to see, and what is to be anticipated as a result of this specific treatment. As a dancer, you should be especially careful to discuss the ramifications of the projected treatment in terms of your ability to practice your art.

Be prepared to make notes of your discussion with the physician. It may be difficult to remember everything that was said, and much may have happened during your interview and examination that was confusing. If a surgical procedure is recommended by your primary care physician and you are in any doubt about the need for it, you can always ask for a second opinion. This might also be the case if no surgery is recommended and you think it should have been.

If you are given a prescription for medicine, get it filled promptly and take it according to the physician's directions. If it is prescribed for a week, don't stop taking it after three days just because you feel better. If you think you should not continue for any reason, call the physician. Above all, don't take medicine that was prescribed for someone else. You may think it is the same as what was prescribed for you, but it may not be. It might be something that is outdated or otherwise harmful to you.

Other Professional Therapists

You may be referred by your physician to a physical therapist or an athletic trainer who is also qualified in physical therapy. With such a referral you can pretty well assume that the therapist is professionally qualified, but it does not hurt to ask about his/her qualifications.

Again, some large dance companies have begun to employ therapists as regular consultants or even as staff members. Performing arts and sports medicine clinics also employ such people. You may be referred to a strength coach. This is a distinctive field today which has its own qualifications.

We know that historically there has been a long-standing reliance of dancers on chiropractors, which continues unabated today. Although, to the best of my knowledge, the reasons for this connection have never been systematically explored, its general outlines seem clear enough; chiropractics offer an appealingly inclusive, quick-fix treatment modality, and it tends to be relatively inexpensive. Also, one assumes, enough dancers have had good results from chiropractors to continue recommending their services from one generation to another. Be that as it may, like other therapies chiropractics is primarily concerned with treatment, so to take an injury to a chiropractor before it has been clinically diagnosed is to put cart before horse.

Another mainstay of dancers continues to be the podiatrist. These people, many of whom have worked extensively with dancers, are well qualified not only to help in practical ways, but also to advise regarding preventive measures. They can provide special pads, shoe corrections and foot supports, and give local treatment for corns, bruises, nail disorders, and some more seriously disabling foot problems which are common in dancers.

Masseurs may be helpful to dancers if they are professionally trained (those who are not must be avoided). It should be noted, however, that massage is *not* the cure-all many dancers seem to think it is; indeed, if applied improperly it can be downright dangerous. A vigorous massage immediately after some injuries have occurred can be damaging to the injured tissues. As with the work of all practitioners, massage can be helpful for some injuries when applied in the right way at the right time.

Continuing Relationship

Although many physicians are not as knowledgeable about special problems of dancers as they are about those of athletes, interest and involvement are growing as more information is published and more conferences are held to discuss these matters. If the physician you select for other good reasons has much to learn about dance, he/she can learn from you as you work together to solve your problems. This learning should be mutually beneficial.

16

Dance Injuries, Health Insurance, and Workers' Compensation

Robin Chmelar, MS

Dance medicine has made tremendous strides in recent years, and dancers today have available to them better care for their injuries than ever before. However, it is important to remember that this care can be very expensive, and in order for the dancer to benefit from these services someone has to *pay* for them. Medical insurance is something that we are used to taking for granted; most people don't think about it until they need it, and by then it is often too late. Dancers in particular cannot afford to be uninformed about their insurance policies and how medical treatment for their injuries will be covered, as illustrated by the following stories:

A dancer for a nationally known company sustained an injury to her back when she fell from a set piece during a performance on tour. Like many dancers in their mid-twenties she had learned to work through previous minor injuries, and she figured this too would take care of itself in due time, although she did inform the company director of the fall. When pain from the injury continued into its third week despite rest and restricted activity she made an appointment with an orthopaedic physician.

An older dancer in the company told her that if her injury occurred "on-the-job" her medical bills should be submitted to workers' compensation (WC). The dancer obtained the appropriate forms from the company management, asked that the manager file a WC claim, and took the forms to the physician. Unfortunately, the problem with the dancer's back turned out to be serious and she eventually underwent two spinal surgeries, both of which failed. She was unable to continue working as a dancer and had considerable pain and functional impairment due to the effects of the failed surgeries.

Although she received some pay from her contract with the company, that ran out in a few months time. Because the injury happened during a performance, her company's workers' compensation carrier should have provided for wage-replacement benefits as well as benefits for any permanent disability, but as sometimes happens the insurance carrier denied responsibility for the claim on the grounds that they did not think her injury was due to a work-related accident. She then had to file her medical bills with the company's private health insurance carrier, which paid them but provided for no wage-replacement benefits.

The dancer first consulted her dance company's management about the denial of the WC claim, but no one seemed to know much about the whole process, so she went to an attorney. He told her that he felt her WC claim had been unfairly denied, and filed for a hearing with the state's industrial commission to reinstate her medical and lost-wage benefits. The court proceedings took nearly two years, but the dancer eventually received lost-wage and permanent partial disability benefits for her injury. The attorney's fees were provided for as a percent of the final settlement.

This story is in contrast to that of another dancer for a regional company who injured her knee when she fell off her bicycle. Since the injury occurred outside of her dance-related work the medical bills were filed with her company's private insurance carrier. The insurance company paid the medical bills, but the dancer was unable to tour with the company for nearly eight weeks. The dancer checked her contract with the company and found she was entitled to only two weeks of disability pay in the event she was physically unable to perform. For the remaining six weeks of her recuperation the dancer was without income except for what she was able to make teaching free-lance.

These two stories underscore just two possible scenarios involving dance injuries and insurance. They emphasize the need for dancers to have a fundamental understanding of their legal rights and contractual agreements so that in the event of an injury the financial and career losses can be minimized. The following information is intended to give a basic overview of two main types of insurance coverage for dance injuries—private health insurance and workers' compensation coverage.

Private Health Insurance

Private health insurance is usually obtained through employer group plans or directly through a carrier on an individual basis. Group rates are substantially lower than individual rates. Persons who are unemployed, self-employed, or who do not qualify for a group plan through their employer either go without private health insurance or pay for the full cost of the policy, the premium, themselves.

Health insurance premiums have risen rapidly over the last few years. In 1988 the average yearly premium for family coverage was $2,700, up 11.9 percent from 1987. Individual coverage averaged $1,056 in 1988, up 14.3 percent. Premiums vary from state to state and also according to how much coverage one wishes to buy.

Private health insurance is designed to cover costs of all necessary medical treatment, including physician's fees, lab work, testing, and medication. Hospital expenses are often covered under a separate policy and include all costs directly related to hospital stays, such as room, nursing, and emergency room care. Most policies are thus divided into major medical and hospitalization components.

Most policies also include a yearly deductible (bills which must be picked up by you) of anywhere from $100 to $1,000 before regular coverage takes effect. After the deductible is met, policies usually cover 80 to 100 percent of approved medical costs. Policies also usually include a pre-existing condition clause, which precludes coverage for illnesses or injuries diagnosed prior to coverage by the current policy. Most pre-existing condition clauses are in effect for one year. Many policies also put a limit on how much they will pay for medical costs in a given year or for a given illness or injury.

If you work full-time for a dance company you probably are covered by a group health plan, with a portion of the monthly premium taken out of your paycheck. The rest of the premium is picked up by your employer (the dance company) or the corporation managing the company. Take note, however, that an insurance carrier can cancel your group's coverage at any time and you may not always be notified of the cancellation by your employer. Be sure to keep tabs on the insurance deductions from your paycheck and, if you go on a period of unemployment and then return to your company, be sure to find out if your health insurance has been maintained.

Private health insurance should cover any injury that (a) occurs outside the confines of your employment, (b) does not arise out of an accident related to dancing while employed, or (c) is due to illness rather than accidental injury. (I will distinguish work-related vs. non-work-related injuries in more detail in the section on workers' compensation.) For example, if a dancer is injured while he/she is a student, his or her student health insurance will cover most of the costs of treatment once the deductible has been met, unless the student is still covered under his or her parents' family policy. Similarly, if an injury to a professional dancer occurs outside of a regularly paid performance or rehearsal, or if the injury is due to illness (such as bone disease), private insurance is responsible.

Trends in private insurance coverage such as Health Maintenance Organizations (HMOs) and Preferred Provider Organizations (PPOs) limit their participants to treatment by certain doctors on a pre-approved list. There are usually strict regulations as to the type of care administered by these physicians as well. HMOs have come under close scrutiny by government agencies because of some of these treatment restrictions, with many HMOs going out of business in recent years. Be sure you know if your private insurance is through an HMO or PPO and who the doctors are on the approved list.

Workers' Compensation Insurance

When we think of workers' compensation we usually think of coverage for blue collar workers and other laborers. However, in the eyes of the law, a dancer who is employed by a dance company is as much a laborer as a construction worker and is entitled to coverage by WC insurance. WC is designed to cover both the medical costs and salary losses resulting from work-related injuries and is governed by a state agency. The premiums are paid by your employer, and both medical bills and lost wages due to disability are covered. In most states all companies that employ more than two or three people *must* buy a WC policy to cover their employees.

WC insurance includes the following:
1. *Medical benefits*. Medical expenses related to your injury are fully covered *if* they are performed by a licensed health care provider. Medical expenses may include prescription drugs, orthotics, and transportation expenses, depending on the state. You are also financially compensated for any permanent disability you suffer.
2. *Wage benefits*. You receive a portion of your regular paycheck in the form of disability pay for the time you are unable to work.
3. *Rehabilitation*. Depending on the state, you are entitled to both physical and vocational rehabilitation if your injury prevents you from returning to dance.

WC laws are complex and diverse; therefore, the following is intended only to highlight some of the key issues relevant to dancers:
1. *What is the purpose of workers' compensation?* WC was designed to protect both employees and employers from the effects of work-related injuries. Founded in the early 1900s, the intent of the WC laws was to protect employees from suffering financial loss due to on-the-job accidents and to protect employers from lawsuits

involving large sums for negligence. Lost-wage benefits are usually 66 percent of your working salary (up to a maximum) for
periods during which you are medically disabled. Students are
not covered by WC.

2. *Why should a dancer be informed about WC?* Dancers who perform
for a company, in a stage production, or who teach for a living
in a university are all at some risk for becoming injured and
unable to work as a result of their employment. Because of the
WC system, you are entitled by law to receive medical and lost-
wage benefits for any periods of disability due to a work-related
injury. Financially, this can be critical in the case of a severe or
prolonged injury. As dancers depend completely on their bodies
to make a living, it is important that they be informed as to what
their disability benefits entail should they suffer serious injury.

3. *Is WC a federal law?* No. WC laws emerged by state. Although all
states use similar principles, considerable variation exists in
terms of benefits, coverage, eligibility, and administrative
arrangements.

4. *What is a WC carrier?* Just as there are many different private
health insurance companies (or carriers), there are different WC
insurance companies. Some common WC carriers are Liberty
Mutual, Travelers, Wausau, and the State Insurance Fund. All
these companies must operate under the guidelines of the WC
laws for each state, which are legislated like any other state law.

5. *Are WC medical bills covered the same as they are by a health carrier?*
No. There is no deductible for WC medical bills and there is no
copayment required on the part of the patient. Depending on
the state, there may be certain restrictions as to what types of
services are covered. For example, although chiropractic visits
are covered in most states, there are certain limitations regarding
length and type of treatment. Most alternative therapies, such
as acupuncture and body therapy techniques, are not covered.
However, most services provided by a licensed physician or
physical therapist are covered.

As for the amount of fees covered, although some states require
that WC bills be paid according to what is "reasonable and customary," many states now employ what is known as a "fee schedule" to
determine the reimbursement rates for WC. A medical fee schedule
determines the amount a physician can be reimbursed by WC carriers.
These rates are specified by your state's industrial commission and,
although they are supposed to reflect "customary rates," they are
usually much lower than the reimbursement from private carriers.
That is, if a surgeon charges $5,000 for a particular surgical procedure

and the WC fee schedule stipulates a fee of only $1,800, that's all the surgeon will get reimbursed. If the procedure were being covered by a private carrier, the physician would usually expect to get close to full reimbursement. For this reason not all surgeons will do WC-related surgery.

Even if you have health insurance, your carrier is not obliged to cover any expenses related to your WC injury. In fact, most private carriers have a WC exclusionary clause; that is, if an injury is determined to be work-related the private carrier will not pick up any unreimbursed costs. However, any health service provider who is certified by the state industrial commission is obligated to accept the fee schedule of that state for his or her procedures. When you consult a doctor for a work-related injury be sure to ask if he or she is a WC physician; however, not all states require certification and therefore it is up to the physician whether or not they will accept WC cases.

6. *How do I know if my injury should be covered under private or WC insurance?* In order to be covered by WC, the injury must be work-related according to the definition determined by the state's legislature and industrial commission. Although this varies from state to state, there are common stipulations. The basic requirements are that (1) there must be a personal injury that (2) results from an accident that (3) arises out of the employment and (4) occurs in the course of employment. It is the second requirement that usually separates compensable from noncompensable dance injuries. An "accident" has generally been interpreted to mean that (a) there had to be an unexpected aspect to the injury, and (b) the injury had to be traceable, within reasonable limits, to a definite time, place, and cause.

The first thing to be done after *any* mishap in rehearsal, teaching, or performance is to notify your company or rehearsal director that the incident occurred. This should be documented in writing and filed with the company management. Then your doctor submits a medical report to the insurance carrier, who either accepts or denies responsibility for the claim. If the claim is accepted as a WC injury, your medical bills for that injury will be paid for by your WC carrier according to the policies of your state. If you are restricted in the amount of performing or teaching you can do because of your injury, or if you are completely disabled from dancing for a period of time, your doctor should note this in his or her report as partial or total temporary disability. This is important because this information is used to determine your lost-wage benefits.

In most cases a dance injury will involve a period of time off, followed by a gradual re-entry into full-time performing. The time off from an injury must be longer than seven days to qualify for lost-wage benefits in most states. In the event that a surgical procedure must be performed as treatment for the injury, extended periods of total disability from dancing as well as some permanent partial disability usually result. It is very important that these periods be carefully documented by you and your physician.

It is also important that you and your physician agree on the anticipated recuperation period for your injury. Most dancers are anxious to get back to their performing schedules; on the other hand, no injured dancer wants to be put on the spot and expected to perform at the risk of further injury. For this reason communication between dancer and physician must encompass all work-related issues.

In one of the stories related earlier the dancer's back injury was deemed compensable because she was injured as the result of a fall during a performance. The injury would still have been compensable if this had happened during rehearsal, but since many dancers are only officially on salary (and therefore officially employed) during performances, you may be dancing in a legal loophole if you are injured during rehearsal and are not "employed" at the time. If you find yourself in such a situation consult an attorney who specializes in WC.

If you are injured during rehearsal or performance, report it to your company director or manager immediately. Even if you think you are "okay" and not really injured be sure to let someone know anyway. Sometimes the extent of an injury is not apparent until hours later when swelling sets in. It is important in filing a WC or any insurance claim that your injury be reported to a company director immediately *and that this be documented.*

If you are injured in an activity outside of your dance work, that injury is not compensable under WC, but the medical bills should be covered by your private insurance. If you are not sure if the injury is WC, you can still file a claim, although the carrier may not accept it. As might be expected, there are many gray areas regarding whether or not an injury is work-related. For example, what if you are on tour and slip on some ice in a parking lot on the way to dinner? Whether the resulting injury is covered depends on the WC laws for the state in which your company is based, or sometimes the state in which you are injured. If you are injured while traveling, be sure to consult a WC attorney regarding which state should cover your claim. Also, dance injuries such as tendinitis, stress fractures, muscle strains, or other "chronic overuse" injuries may or may not be compensable under WC, depending on the wording of your state's laws.

If you are involved in a "gray area" situation check with a WC attorney (you can get a referral from your state or county bar association). In most states a WC attorney works on a contingency basis; that is, he or she cannot charge you directly for services but must rely on receiving a set percent (determined by law) of whatever lost-wage settlement you receive. If you receive nothing, the attorney receives nothing. Check with your state's bar association regarding payment policies.

7. *What if my injury is so severe that I can no longer perform or teach for a living?* Check with your state's Department of Industrial Relations, Division of Vocational Rehabilitation, since many states have programs that will pay for re-schooling if you become injured or ill and can no longer perform your job (the disabling circumstance does not have to be work-related in many states). In California and Florida it is *mandatory* to offer vocational rehabilitation to those involved in a career-ending industrial accident.

8. *Are there any alternatives to WC for getting disability benefits?* Possibly. Private disability insurance policies are available, but in any case be extremely careful with the terms of such a policy. Be sure the terms under which you will receive benefits (i.e., wage replacement) reflect your work realities. A dance company may wish to consider including a disability policy with its group health plan. If you belong to a union you may be entitled to disability benefits through your membership. Also, if you perform for a major company check your contract to determine the company's responsibilities for disability should you become physically unable to perform. Some states have what are known as statutory benefits, which cover *all* workers for any disability (including maternity) at 50 percent of salary (with limits) for up to six months.

Words to the Wise

Knowledge of health insurance and workers' compensation issues, while hardly of interest to the healthy dancer, can become critical for the injured dancer. If nothing else, dancers should become aware of the following points:

1. For private insurance, be sure to find out *if* you are covered. A company is not required to offer group health insurance, and if it has a group plan that is subsequently dropped the company may not be obligated to tell its employees (sad, but in some states, true). Be sure you know what your company's health plan entails *before* you need it. If you are a university student, know

what your student health insurance covers. Remember, many policies have limits on how much they will cover.

2. For WC, find out if your company or theatre group is covered, and if not find out if they *should* be covered. Discuss this with your company management, but if you are in doubt contact the state's industrial commission or a WC attorney. If you teach for a university, be sure you are familiar with your institution's private health and work-related injury plans.

3. Know your rights before you need them. Discuss health insurance, disability benefits, and WC with your company management. Your management may have limited information, so you may wish to invite a WC attorney or someone from your local WC office to address your company, school, or theatre group, or provide literature. You may be able to find someone who will provide a session free of charge or in exchange for performance tickets.

4. Don't expect the insurance carriers to tell you your rights. The WC and private health insurance systems are in a state of tremendous flux. Costs are skyrocketing and insurance companies are scrutinizing claims more closely than ever. In this atmosphere the situation between the injured party and the insurance carrier can easily become adversarial. Know your rights and be prepared for some difficulties. It is unfortunate, but many in the WC system see claimants as out to get a "free ride" and avoid working. Such an attitude is so far away from the dancer's intention that it can be especially frustrating when a dancer comes face to face with a difficult insurance representative. Be prepared and don't let it get to you.

5. Whether you are involved in a WC or private insurance claim remember to *document in writing* what transpires and keep an organized record of all bills, payments, correspondence, and reimbursements. Get fee and treatment approvals in writing and document all phone calls made to the insurance carrier and your physician. If your claim is challenged you will need this documentation.

6. *Dancers are not indestructible.* It is easy to say "But I've never been injured" or "It couldn't happen to me"; unfortunately, accidents happen, unknown weaknesses in the body emerge, or poor judgments are made even in the best situations. Severe injury is certainly the exception rather than the rule in dance, but it is the exception for which you must be best prepared. It is bad enough to suffer a debilitating injury without having to go through the

trauma of financial loss as well. The fact is no one is going to look out for you but you.

Sources

Burton, J.F., ed. (1985). Disability benefits for back disorders in workers' compensation. In *New York State School of Industrial Labor and Relations*. ILR reprints. Ithaca, New York: Cornell University.

Johnson, F. (1988, May). Workers' compensation: a worker's experience. In: *Proceedings of Worker's Compensation Conference*. Syracuse, New York.

Lewis, J.H. (1989, April). Historical development and current pressures in the workers' compensation system. In: *Proceedings of Workers' Compensation College*. Tucson, Arizona: International Association of Industrial Accident Boards and Commissions.

Millikan, S.D. (1989). Intense pressures grip workers' compensation system. *Worker's Compensation Report*, 1(1),2. (Available from Alliance of American Insurers, 1501 Woodfield Road, Suite 400 West, Schaumburg, IL, 60173-4980.)

Minter, S.G. (1988). Workers' compensation in need of fine-tuning or an overhaul? *Occupational Hazards*, 50(2), 51-57.

[Staff]. (1988). Legal briefs: workers not told of group policy cancellation. *Business Insurance*, 22(12), 28.

[Staff]. (1989). New England journal calls for national health insurance. *Health Lawyers News Report*, 17(2), 5.

Workers' Compensation Research Institute. (1989). Comparing attorney fee arrangements. *WCRI Research Brief*, 5(4), 1-4.

Workers' Compensation Research Institute. (1989). Improving physician fee schedules. *WCRI Research Brief*, 5(2), 1-3.

Workers' Compensation Research Institute. (1985). Income replacement for short-term disability. *WCRI Research Brief*, 1(12), 1-3.

Workers' Compensation Research Institute. (1987). Innovative approaches to medical cost containment. *WCRI Research Brief*, 3(9), 1-3.

Workers' Compensation Research Institute. (1987). More on containing medical costs. *WCRI Research Brief*, 3(11), 1-2.

Workers' Compensation Research Institute. (1987). Workplace injuries: economic and noneconomic consequences for workers. *WCRI Research Brief*, 3(7), 1-3.

(Research Briefs available from Workers' Compensation Research Institute, 245 First Street, Cambridge, MA 02141.)

Acknowledgements

I wish to thank Donald G. Vass of the New York State Insurance Fund and Estelle Baum, RN, CIRS, for their help in preparing this manuscript.

Dance Glossary

Alexander principle: A body therapy system designed to make the participant aware of use and misuse of the body, particularly with reference to posture, mechanical efficiency, and emotion.

arabesque: A movement in which the body weight is supported by one leg. The supporting leg may be straight or half bent, while the gesturing leg is straight and extended to the rear. The arms are normally placed to provide the longest possible line from fingertips to toes. There are a number of *arabesque* positions.

assemblé: A ballet step in which one foot slides along the floor and into the air. The supporting foot then pushes off from the floor, joins the other in the air, and both feet land together in fifth position.

attitude: A position in which the body weight is supported on one leg. The supporting leg may be straight or bent, with the arm on the same side opened front, side, or back. The other leg is extended to the back and bent 90 degrees at the knee, while the corresponding arm is raised above the head.

barre: Generally a cylindrical piece of wood which is fastened horizontally to the walls of the dance studio at a height of approximately three feet six inches from the floor. Warm-up exercises are done at the *barre* at the beginning of every ballet class.

contraction: A concave curving of the lumbar and thoracic spine through use of the psoas and abdominal muscles. Throughout this action the knees bend and the shoulders remain over the hips, with the body as elongated as possible.

développé à la seconde: A movement in which the gesturing leg is raised until the thigh is at a right angle to the body, with the toe at the knee of the supporting leg. From this point, the gesturing leg gradually extends (straightens) to the side of the body.

développé: The unfolding movement described above can be performed in other directions—to the front, the back, and in parallel position—without being turned out at the hip.

demi-plié: A bending or flexing of the knees only to the point where the heels are still on the floor. *Demi-plié* can be performed in all five ballet positions, and in parallel.

demi-pointe: In this position the weight of the body is supported on the balls of the feet and plantar aspect of the toes; also known as half *pointe*.

en dedans: An inward movement in which the gesturing leg or the body turns toward the supporting leg.

en dehors: An outward movement in which the gesturing leg or the body turns away from the supporting leg.

entrechat: A springing movement into the air, beginning and ending in fifth position, in which the legs are straight and criss-cross while in the air. The feet are pointed downward. The legs criss-cross a varying number of times, depending on the type of *entrechat* being performed. In an *entrechat quatre*, for example, the legs and feet go through four positions: the beginning and finish in fifth and one criss-cross in the air.

extension: A movement in which the gesturing leg is extended out from the body. This term has also come to mean the height to which a dancer can raise the leg above waist level.

fouetté: This term applies to a variety of ballet steps which are characterized by a whipping action of the foot or leg out to an open position, and quickly back in again. This whipping action can also propel the dancer into a series of turns known as *fouetté rond de jambe en tournant*.

grand battement: A movement in which the gesturing leg is raised from the hip into the air and brought down again. *Grand battement* is performed with both knees straight. It can be done front, side, or to the back, and usually starts and finishes in fifth position.

grand plié: A bending at the knees, in which the dancer begins in an erect position and slowly flexes the knees until the heels come away from the floor. The back remains straight, with the shoulders over the hips. The *grand plié* passes through *demi-plié* and can be performed in all five ballet positions and parallel. In *grand plié* in second position, the heels remain on the floor, although the movement is larger than *demi-plié à la seconde*.

jeté: A jump from one leg to the other. The change of weight is preceded by a brushing or throwing action of the gesturing leg.

parallel position: In modern and jazz dance, a position in which the feet are placed side by side, in line with the hip sockets, with the toes of both feet pointing straight ahead.

passé: A transitional movement in which the foot of the gesturing leg passes the knee of the supporting leg as it goes from one position to another.

pilates exercises: A series of exercises developed by Joseph Pilates, designed to strengthen specific muscle groups. Many of these exercises are performed on specially designed apparatus which utilize springs to provide resistance.

pirouette: A ballet turn in which the body is whirled or spun around on one foot, either on *pointe* or *demi-pointe*. *Pirouettes* can be performed *en dedans* or *en dehors*. Momentum for the turn comes from a *plié* and arm movement. The head is whipped around so that it is last to turn, and first to arrive at front facing. There are many types of *pirouettes*.

plié: A bending movement of the knee or knees; perhaps the most basic ballet movement (see *demi-plié* and *grand plié*).

pointe: In this position the dancer moves or balances on the tips of the toes, with the aid of the toe (*pointe*) shoe.

port de bras: A movement or series of movements made by passing the arm or arms through various positions. This term also refers to a group of exercises designed to develop grace and harmony of arm movement.

relevé: The action of raising the body onto *pointe* or *demi-pointe*. *Relevé* can be performed smoothly and continuously, or with a springing movement.

rond de jambe à terre: A circular action of the gesturing leg. It moves from first position through fourth front, second, fourth back and then passes through first position again. The toe of the gesturing leg remains on the ground. This exercise can be performed *en dedans* or *en dehors*.

rond de jambe: A circular movement of the gesturing leg (see above). It can be performed in the air as well as on the ground.

saut de basque: A jumping and traveling step in ballet, in which the dancer turns in the air with one foot drawn up to the knee of the other leg.

tendue: An action in which the foot and leg are stretched away from the body. In *battement tendue* the gesturing leg is opened to the front, side, or back, while the toe rests lightly on the floor. Then it is returned to a closed position.

tour jeté: The technical name for this ballet step is *grand jeté dessus en tournant*. In this step the dancer is propelled into the air as in a leap, but in midair the body is turned quickly to face the direction from which the step originated. While the dancer is airborne both legs pass closely with the knees straight. Then the step is landed in *demi-plié* in *arabesque* position.

turnout: This is the ability of the dancer to stand and move with the legs externally rotated at the hip so that the toes are directed diagonally away from the midline of the body.

Medical Glossary*

Alpha motor neuron: The final common pathway for transmission of motor impulses from the central nervous system to the skeletal muscles. These motor neurons innervate extrafusal muscle fibers.

abductors: Muscles that draw a body part away from the median line.

acetabulum: A cup-shaped socket on the external surface of the pelvis, in which the head of the femur sits.

achilles tendon: Heel tendon; the tendon of insertion of the triceps surae (gastrocnemius and soleus) into the tuberosity of the calcaneus.

acromioclavicular: Denoting the articulation between the clavicle and the scapula and its ligaments.

adductors: Muscles that draw a body part toward the median line; in dance, often synonymous with "groin muscles."

afferent neuron: A structure which passes messages or impulses from one part of the body to another by way of an electrochemical process. In particular, afferents carry nerve impulses from sensory receptors into the spinal cord or brain.

amenorrhea: Absence or abnormal cessation of the menses.

anterior cruciate ligament: Internal ligament of the knee, which originates on the lateral femoral condyle and inserts on the anterior aspect of the tibia; a primary control of back-to-front motion and rotation of the knee.

anterior tibialis: Muscle originates on the lateral condyle, surface of the tibia, and interosseous membrane; inserts at the bases of 2nd to 4th metatarsal bones and tarsal bones, except talus; dorsiflexes and inverts the foot.

anteversion (femoral): Position of the femoral neck relative to the femoral shaft in the horizontal plane; a forward turning; in dance, refers primarily to inward rotation of the femur in the hip socket.

arthrography: X-ray of a joint, using contrast solution ("dye") to define soft tissue.

---

*These definitions draw most heavily on *Dorland's Medical Dictionary*, 26th edition; Miller and Keane, *Encyclopedia and Dictionary of Medicine, Nursing and Allied Health*, 4th edition; G.B. Sage, *Introduction to Motor-Behavior: a Neuropsychological Approach*, 2nd edition, and *Motor Learning and Control: A Neuropsychological Approach*; and *Stedman's Medical Dictionary*, 24th edition.

arthroscopic surgery: A technique for diagnosis or surgical treatment within a joint, done by passing surgical instruments through a rigid metal tube containing a light and fiberoptics (an endoscope).

arthrosis: Disease of a joint.

autogenic reflex: The reflex, the simplest functioning unit of the nervous system, operates automatically. This particular reflex serves the role of triggering muscular relaxation to protect a muscle from excessive tension.

basal ganglia: A group of nuclei or cluster of cell bodies within the brain which are located in the inner layers of the cerebrum surrounding the lateral portions of the thalamus. These structures project a rich supply of nerve fibers to the spinal cord, and also up to the motor cortex. Collectively, the basal ganglia are part of the system which organizes motor activity.

biceps brachii: A muscle of the arm; inserts on the tuberosity of the radius and flexes and supinates the forearm.

calcaneus: The heel bone; the largest of the tarsal bones.

capsule: A membranous structure that envelops an organ, a joint, or any other part.

cerebellum: A structure lying behind and below the cerebrum which has two hemispheres and a very convoluted appearance. Knowledge about the precise functioning of various parts of the cerebellum is incomplete; generally, it seems to be important in the coordination and monitoring of complex patterns of skilled motor activity.

cerebral cortex: The outermost layer of the cerebrum, or large umbrella-like dome of the brain. The cerebrum is divided into two hemispheres by the longitudinal fissure or groove. The cortex is about one-fourth inch thick, and composed mostly of tightly packed neuron cell bodies. The cerebral cortex receives and interprets sensory information; organizes complex motor behaviors; and stores and utilizes learned experiences.

chondromalacia: Degeneration or softening of cartilage, most commonly on the undersurface of the patella.

coccyx: The small bone at the end of the vertebral column, formed by the union of 4 (sometimes 5 or 3) rudimentary vertebrae; articulates with the sacrum.

collagen: The main protein of connective tissue, cartilage, and bone.

corticospinal tracts: The neurons which have axons and nerve fibers which originate in the cerebral cortex and descend to the spinal cord, making up a motor transmission network. The axons of this system are some of the longest in the body. This structure is also known as the pyramidal system.

cuboid, cuboidal: Pyramidal bone, on the lateral side of the foot, in front of the calcaneus; articulates with the calcaneus, lateral cuneiform, 4th and 5th metatarsal bones, and occasionally the navicular.

cuneiform: Three bones of the foot—intermediate, lateral, and medial—on the distal row of the tarsus.

disc: A structure between the bodies of adjacent vertebrae, composed of an outer fibrous part that surrounds a central gelatinous mass.

efferent neuron: A neural structure which transmits impulses from the central nervous system out to effector organs such as muscles or glands.

elastin: A yellow elastic fibrous mucoprotein; a major connective tissue protein of elastic structures.

endomysium: The sheath of delicate reticular fibrils which surrounds each muscle fiber.

enzyme: A protein secreted by cells that acts as a catalyst to induce chemical changes in other substances.

evert: To turn outward.

external rotators: Muscles by which a part can be turned externally; of special concern to dancers are the hip rotators (see Clippinger).

extensor digitorum longus: A muscle which originates on the lateral condyle of the tibia and anterior margin of the fibula; inserts by tendons to the dorsal surfaces of the bases of the 2nd to 5th toes; serves to extend the four lateral toes.

extensor hallucis longus: Long extensor muscle of the great toe; originates on the lateral surface of the tibia and interosseous membrane; inserts at the base of the distal phalanx of the great toe.

extrafusal: Muscle fibers which make up the main skeletal muscles (in comparison to intrafusal fibers, which are located in muscle spindles).

extrapyramidal: The part of the motor system which comprises a second motor pathway, including all of the motor axons not found in the pyramidal tract. It is believed that the extrapyramidal neurons modify some of the operations of the pyramidal system by refining and smoothing out movements, and carrying a large part of the impulses for postural adjustment and reflex movements.

facet: A small smooth surface on a bone or other firm structure.

femoral anteversion: (see anteversion).

femoral condyle(s): A rounded projection at the distal end of the femur; articulates with the tibia; affords attachment to the cruciate ligaments.

femur: The thigh bone; the longest and largest bone in the body. The head of the femur fits into the acetabulum of the pelvis.

fibula: The lateral and smaller of the two bones of the leg.

fibroblast: A stellate or spindle-shaped cell. It is present in connective tissue, and is capable of forming collagen fibers, fibrous tissues in the body, tendons, aponeuroses, and supporting and bending tissues of all sorts. Such cells also proliferate at the site of chronic inflammation.

flexor digitorum longus: A muscle which originates on the posterior surface of the tibia and inserts by tendons into the bases of the 4 lateral toes; flexes the 2nd to 5th toes.

flexor hallucis longus: A muscle which originates on the posterior surface of the fibula; inserts at the base of the great toe; flexes the great toe (see Norris).

fusiform muscle: A spindle-shaped muscle; one that has a fleshy belly, tapering at either extremity.

gamma efferent pathway: Motoneurons which begin in the gray matter of the spinal cord, and which have axons passing through spinal nerves to the specialized fibers of the muscle spindles.

gamma (stretch) reflex: The reflex that results when the extrafusal fibers are suddenly stretched. The muscle spindle will be stretched, and spindle afferents will be activated which will then reflexively produce extrafusal contraction to reduce the stretch.

gastrocnemius: A two-headed muscle which originates from the popliteal surface of the femur, upper part of the medial condyle, and capsule of the knee; combines with the soleus to form the tendocalcaneus (achilles tendon), which inserts into the lower half of the posterior surface of the calcaneus; plantar flexes the foot and flexes the knee joint.

gemellus inferior: A muscle which originates on the tuberosity of the ischium; blends with the tendon of the obturator internus and inserts into the inner surface of the greater trochanter; rotates the thigh laterally.

genu recurvatum: A condition of hyperextension of the knee.

genu valgum: "Knock knees"; a deformity in which the knees are abnormally close together and the space between the ankles is increased.

genu varum: Bowleg; an outward bowing of the lower extremity at the knee.

glucose: Dextrose, or starch sugar; it is the product of complete hydrolysis of cellulose, starch, and glycogen.

gluteals: The muscle group which includes the gluteus maximus, medius, and minimus.

gluteus maximus: A muscle which originates on the dorsal aspect of the ilium, the posterior surface of the sacrum and coccyx, and the sacrotuberous ligament; inserts on the iliotibial band of the fascia lata and the gluteal ridge of the femur; extends, abducts, and rotates the thigh laterally.

gluteus medius: A muscle which originates on the lateral surface of the ilium; inserts at the greater trochanter of the femur; abducts and rotates the thigh.

glycogen: Animal or liver starch; found in most tissues of the body, especially those of the liver and muscles; the principal carbohydrate reserve, it is readily converted into glucose.

Golgi tendon organs: A muscle receptor which detects and signals tension on a tendon. It is usually found at the origin or insertion of a muscle, rather than in the tendon itself.

greater trochanter: A broad, flat process on the femur, at the upper end of its lateral surface, to which the following muscles are attached: gluteus medius and minimus, piriformis, obturator internus and externus, and gemelli.

groin muscles: The muscles attached at the junctional region between the abdomen and the thigh.

hamstrings: Inner hamstring comprises the tendons of the gracilis, sartorius, semimembranosus and semitendinosus muscles; outer hamstring is the tendon of the biceps femoris muscle.

hip flexors: Generally considered to include the psoas, rectus femoris, sartorius, and iliacus muscles.

hyperextension: Extension of a limb or part beyond the normal limit.

hypertonia: The condition of having an abnormally high degree of muscular tension.

hypotonia: The condition of having an abnormally low degree of muscular tension.

idiopathic: Denoting a disease of unknown cause.

iliac crest: The lateral, flaring portion of the pelvis.

iliacus: A muscle which originates on the iliac fossa; inserts into the psoas tendon on the lesser trochanter of the femur and capsule of the hip joint; flexes the thigh and trunk.

iliocostalis: The lateral division of the erector muscle of the spine, having three subdivisions: lumborum, which extends, abducts and rotates lumbar vertebrae; thoracis, which does the same for the thoracic vertebrae; and the cervicis, which similarly services the cervical vertebrae.

iliofemoral ligament: A Y-shaped ligament that covers the anterior and superior portions of the hip joint. It is attached above to the lower part of the anterior-inferior spine of the ilium, and diverges to form two bands; inserts on the intertrochanteric line.

iliopsoas: A compound muscle, consisting of the iliacus and the psoas major.

ilium: The broad flaring portion of the pelvis; joins the pubis and ischium to form the acetabulum.

induction: The appearance of an electrical impulse as a result of the presence of another electric current or field nearby.

internal rotators: Muscles by which a part can be turned internally; e.g., semitendinosus and popliteus at the leg, and pectineus at the thigh.

interneuron: A neural structure which originates and ends totally within the central nervous system; interneurons make up 95 percent of all neurons in the nervous system.

intrafusal: Muscle fibers which are not part of the main skeletal muscle, but which are located in muscle spindles, and which have specialized sensory and motor functions.

irradiation: The dispersion of a nervous impulse beyond the normal path of conduction.

ischial apophysitis: Inflammation of the bony outgrowth (process, or tuberosity) on the lower posterior portion of the hip bone.

ischial tuberosity: Bony projection at the junction of the lower end of the body of the ischium and its ramus.

isometric: A form of muscular contraction in which the muscle is engaged in a static contraction against resistance. This condition can be contrasted to isotonic muscular contraction, in which movement occurs through range of motion against resistance.

kyphosis: Posterior convexity in the curvature of the thoracic spine.

lamina(e) (vertebral): The flattened posterior portion of the vertebral arch from which the spinous process extends.

lateral collateral ligament: The cordlike band of fibrous tissue that passes from the lateral epicondyle of the femur to the head of the fibula; serves to stabilize the knee laterally.

lateral meniscus: A crescent shaped fibrocartilage in the knee joint attached to the lateral border of the upper articular surface of the tibia. With the medial meniscus it helps to absorb shock.

lesser trochanter: A short conical process on the posteromedial part of the femur below its neck. It receives the insertion of the psoas major and iliacus (iliopsoas) muscles.

limbic system: A network of subcortical structures located in the forebrain which are connected to other structures in the brain and are also interconnected. Recent studies indicate that parts of the limbic system are involved in arousal.

Lisfranc joint: A junction between the medial cuneiform bone and the proximal head of the 2nd metatarsal in the foot.

longissimus (thoracis): A muscle which originates from the transverse and articular processes of the lower thoracic vertebrae; inserts by lateral slips between transverse processes of all thoracic vertebrae and 9 or 10 lower ribs; extends thoracic vertebrae.

lordosis: A concave posterior curvature of the lumbar spine (hollow back, swayback).

lumbar: The part of the back between the thorax and the pelvis.

malleolus: A rounded process on either side of the ankle joint.

medial collateral ligament: The broad fibrous band that passes from the medial epicondyle of the femur to the medial margin and medial surface of the tibia; serves with the lateral collateral ligament to stabilize the knee for side-to-side motion.

medial meniscus: A crescent shaped fibrocartilage in the knee joint attached to the medial upper articular surface of the tibia.

medulla: One of the parts of the brainstem. It is the superior extension of the spinal cord, and contains: sensory nerve tracts ascending to the brain; descending motor tracts which extend toward muscles and glands; and another collection of neurons and nerve tracts that regulate vital processes like respiration and blood pressure.

menarche: Beginning of the menstrual function.

metatarsal: Distal portion of the foot between the instep and the toes; consists of the 5 long bones articulating proximally with the cuboid and cuneiform bones and distally with the phalanges.

multifidus: The state of being cleft into many parts.

myotatic reflex: The automatic response of muscular contraction when a muscle is stretched. A common example of this type of reflex is the knee jerk which occurs when the patellar tendon is hit, causing the quadriceps muscle to be stretched and thus to contract in response.

navicular: A bone at the medial side of the foot, it articulates with the head of the talus, the cuneiform bone, and occasionally the cuboid.

neuromuscular spindle: A structure located in skeletal muscles which contains both sensory receptors and muscle fibers. It consists of a fluid-filled capsule tapering at both ends.

obturator externus and obturator internus: Two of the muscles that insert on the greater trochanter near the upper extremity of the femur, and serve to rotate the thigh laterally.

osseous: Bony.

osteoid osteoma: A small, benign but painful tumor of bone occurring especially in the bones of the extremities and vertebrae, most often in young persons.

osteophyte formation: A bony outgrowth secondary to degenerative processes; "bone spur."

paraspinal muscles (erector spinae): A name applied to the fibers of the more superficial of the muscles of the back, originating from the sacrum, spines of the lumbar and the 11th and 12th thoracic vertebrae, and the iliac crest, which split and insert as the iliocostal, longissimus and spinalis muscles; extend the vertebral column.

paresthesias: The state of having an abnormal sensation.

pars interarticularis: A supporting bar of bone between the superior and inferior facet on each side of the vertebral arch (see Trepman).

pectoralis major: A muscle which originates at the clavicle, sternum, the six upper ribs, and the aponeuroses of the external oblique and rectus abdominis; inserts at the head of the humerus; adducts, flexes, and medially rotates the arm.

pedicle(s): One of the paired parts of the vertebral arch that connect a lamina to the vertebral body.

pennate muscle: A feather shaped muscle (see Teitz).

peroneus brevis: The shorter of the peroneal muscles. It originates on the lateral surface of the fibula and inserts at the base of the 5th metatarsal. With the peroneus longus it helps to evert, abduct, and plantar flex the foot.

peroneus longus: The longest peroneal muscle; originates at the lateral condyle of the tibia and the lateral surface of the fibula; it inserts by a tendon passing behind the lateral malleolus and across the sole of the foot to the medial cuneiform and base of the first metatarsal; plantar flexes, everts, and abducts the foot.

peroneus tertius: Originates at the anterior surface of the fibula and the interosseous membrane; inserts at the base of the 5th metatarsal; assists in dorsal flexion of the foot.

phalanges: The long bones between joints of the fingers or toes.

piriformis: A muscle of the hip; originates at the greater sciatic notch of the ilium and 2nd to 4th lumbar vertebrae; inserts on the upper border of the great trochanter; rotates the thigh laterally.

plantar fasciitis: A painful condition of the foot, secondary to tightness or inflammation of the plantar fascia, the thick central portion of the fascia investing the plantar muscles.

plantaris (the aponeurosis plantaris): Radiates toward the toes from the medial process of the calcaneal tuberosity and gives attachment to the short flexor muscle of the toes.

plica: A general term for a ridge or fold, commonly found on the inside of the knee joint capsule.

popliteus: A muscle which originates at the lateral condyle of the femur and inserts on the posterior surface of the tibia; flexes the knee and rotates the leg medially.

posterior cruciate ligament: Is stronger but shorter and less oblique than the anterior. It attaches behind the spine of the tibia, to the popliteal notch, and inserts into the inner condyle of the femur, stabilizing the knee.

pronation: Eversion and abduction of the foot, causing a lowering of the medial edge; "rolling in" (see Kravitz).

proprioception: The collection of sensations coming from the body, including those from the skin, joints, muscles, and vestibular apparatus.

prostaglandins: Physiologically active substances present in many tissues that stimulate contractility of smooth muscle, lower blood pressure, regulate acid secretions, body temperature, and platelet aggregation; also control inflammation.

proteoglycan: A group of glycoproteins found primarily in connective tissue.

psoas (major): A muscle which originates at the bodies of the vertebrae and intervertebral discs from the 12th thoracic to the 5th lumbar; inserts on the lesser trochanter of the femur; flexes the thigh. Psoas minor originates at the bodies of the 12th thoracic and 1st lumbar vertebrae and discs; assists with flexion of the spine (see Solomon).

pyramidal: The motor transmission network made up of neurons beginning in the cerebral cortex with axons descending to the spinal cord. The name comes from the wedge-shaped bulges the fibers of this system form on the surface of the medulla. This system is also known as the corticospinal tract.

quadratus femoris: A muscle of the thigh which originates at the tuberosity of the ischium; inserts on the intertrochanteric crest and quadrate tubercle of the femur; adducts and rotates the thigh laterally.

quadratus lumborum: Quadrate muscle of the loins; originates at the iliac crest, iliolumbar ligament and transverse process of the lower lumbar vertebrae; inserts at the 12th rib and transverse process of the upper lumbar vertebrae; flexes the lumbar vertebrae laterally.

quadriceps femoris: Quadriceps muscle of the thigh; originates by four heads: rectus femoris, vastus lateralis, vastus intermedius, vastus medialis; inserts by a common tendon that surrounds the patella and ends on the tuberosity of the tibia; extends the leg and flexes the thigh by the action of the rectus femoris.

reciprocal reflex: An automatic response which acts as a protective reflex to prevent muscle injury. When a given muscle contracts maximally the antagonist muscle or muscles are reciprocally inhibited from contracting. Also known as reciprocal inhibition.

rectus abdominis: Straight muscle of the abdomen; originates on the crest and symphysis of the pubis; inserts on the xiphoid process and 5th to 7th costal cartilages; flexes the vertebral column, and draws the thorax downward.

rectus femoris: A muscle of the thigh; originates on the ilium and upper margin of the acetabulum; inserts to a common tendon of the quadriceps femoris at the base of the patella, on the tuberosity of the tibia; extends the leg and flexes the thigh.

reticular formation: A formation consisting of a net-like mass of inter-woven neurons extending from the brainstem up to the thalamus. This formation has both ascending and descending axons with neu-rons extending throughout the central nervous system. Evidence has shown that the reticular formation is important in arousal or attention, sensory integration, and motor aspects of neural function.

reticulospinal tracts: The nerve fibers of the reticular formation, extending between that formation and the spinal cord.

retinaculum: A strong fibrous band. The patella has both a lateral and medial retinaculum, which attach to the tibia.

retroversion: Position of the femoral head relative to the femoral shaft in the horizontal plane; a backward turning; in dance, refers primar-ily to outward rotation of the femur in the hip socket.

rhomboid: The greater rhomboid muscle originates from the spinous processes and supra-spinalis ligaments of the 2nd, 3rd, 4th and 5th thoracic vertebrae; inserts on the medial border of the scapula; draws the scapula toward the vertebral column.

rubrospinal tract: The nerve tract extending from the red nucleus to the spinal cord.

sacrum: The wedge-shaped segment of the vertebral column forming part of the pelvis; formed by the fusion of five originally separate sacral vertebrae; articulates with the last lumbar vertebra, the coc-cyx, and the hip bone on either side.

sartorius: A muscle which originates on the anterior superior spine of the ilium; inserts at the medial surface of the tibial tuberosity; flexes the thigh and leg.

scapular humeral joint: The joint at which the shoulder blade articu-lates laterally with the bone of the upper arm (humerus).

sciatica: Pain in the lower back and hip radiating down the back of the thigh into the leg (see Trepman).

scoliosis: A lateral deviation (curvature) in the vertical line of the spine. It includes rotation (see Trepman).

semispinalis: The superficial part of the transversospinalis muscles; comprised of the capitis, cervicis and thoracis; serves to extend and rotate the head and vertebral column.

serratus anterior: A muscle which originates on the first eight or nine ribs; inserts at the medial border of the scapula; draws the scapula forward and rotates it to raise the shoulder in abduction of the arm.

soleus: The deeper of the two major muscles of the leg (with the gastrocnemius). It originates from the shaft of the fibula and middle third of the tibia and is joined by the achilles tendon to the calcaneus; plantar flexes the foot.

spinalis muscles: Spinal muscles of the head, neck and thorax, originating on the spinous process of the respective vertebrae; serve to extend the vertebral column.

spinous process: A prominence or projection of bone; part of the vertebrae projecting backward from the arch, giving attachment to muscles of the back.

spondylolisthesis: A forward displacement of a vertebra over a lower segment, usually due to a defect in the pars interarticularis (see Trepman).

spondylolysis: A degenerative lesion or stress fracture of the pars interarticularis.

static stretches: A form of stretching achieved by holding the body in a position that elongates the target muscle or muscles, usually for a period of 30-60 seconds.

sternoclavicular joint: One of the joints at which the medial aspect of the clavicle articulates with the sternum.

sternum: The breast bone, forming the middle of the anterior wall of the thorax and articulating with the clavicles and cartilages of the first seven ribs.

subluxation: Incomplete or partial dislocation.

subtalar: Below the talus (ankle bone); second largest of the tarsal bones; as in subtalar joint (see Fitt).

supination: Inversion and abduction of the foot, causing elevation of the medial edge.

synapse: A submicroscopic gap between the end of one nerve cell and the cell membrane of another; the point at which one neuron affects the firing rate of another cell by the release of a transmitter substance.

synovial fluid: A transparent alkaline viscid fluid (joint "oil"), secreted by the synovial membrane; contained in joint cavities, bursae, and tendon sheaths.

synovial joints: A specialized form of articulation permitting more or less free movement; bony elements covered by articular cartilage, and surrounded by a capsule lined with synovial membranes and containing synovial fluid.

talus: The "ankle bone"; second largest of the tarsal bones; articulates with the tibia and fibula to form the ankle joint.

tarsus: The "instep"; the seven bones of the foot: talus, calcaneus, navicular, three cuneiform bones, and the cuboid.

tectum: The structure which makes up the roof of the midbrain. It is composed of the superior and inferior colliculi, or rounded elevations on either side of the midbrain.

tensor fascia lata: A muscle which originates on the iliac crest and inserts at the iliotibial band of the fascia lata; serves to flex, abduct, and rotate the thigh medially.

tibia: The inner and larger bone of the leg below the knee. It articulates with the femur and head of the fibula above and with the talus below.

tibial torsion: Twisting of the larger bone of the leg.

tibialis posterior: A muscle which originates on the tibia, fibula and interosseous membrane; inserts at the bases of the 2nd to 4th metatarsal bones and tarsal bones, except the talus; plantarflexes and inverts the foot.

transcutaneous electrical muscle stimulation: A therapeutic procedure in which mild electrical stimulation is applied by electrodes in contact with the skin over a painful or weak area.

transverse process: A prominence on either side of the vertebrae, projecting laterally from the junction between the lamina and the pedicle.

transversus abdominis: A muscle of the abdomen which originates at the cartilages of the six lower ribs, the thoracolumbar fascia, and the iliac crest; forms the conjoint tendon which inserts with the rectus sheath into the pubic crest; compresses abdominal viscera.

trapezius: The "cowl muscle"; originates on the occipital bone, the nuchal ligament, and the spinous processes of the 7th cervical and all thoracic vertebrae. It inserts at the clavicle, acromion, and spine of the scapula; draws the head to one side or backward and rotates the scapula.

triceps surae: Muscles of the calf; gastrocnemius and soleus considered as one muscle.

vascular: Relating to or containing blood vessels, or indicative of a copious blood supply.

vastus medialis: A thigh muscle which originates on the medial aspect of the femur; inserts at the tibial tuberosity by a common tendon of the quadriceps femoris and patella ligament; extends the leg.

vestibular apparatus: A structure which contributes to the collection of proprioceptive sensations. It is located adjacent to the inner ear and is sensitive to positions of the head in space and to sudden changes in direction of movement of the body.

Index

X

X-rays, 134, 140
  (*see also* Radiographs

Z

Zen, 191